LOWER YOUR BLOOD PRESSURE IN 8 WEEKS

A Revolutionary Programme
for a Longer, Healthier Life

Dr Stephen T. Sinatra
and Jan Sinatra

PIATKUS

ஃ Visit the Piatkus website!

Piatkus publishes a wide range of best-selling fiction and non-fiction, including books on health, mind, body & spirit, sex, self-help, cookery, biography and the paranormal.

If you want to:
• read descriptions of our popular titles
• buy our books over the Internet
• take advantage of our special offers
• enter our monthly competition
• learn more about your favourite Piatkus authors

VISIT OUR WEBSITE AT: www.piatkus.co.uk

First published in the USA in 2003 by
The Ballantine Publishing Group,
a division of Random House, Inc.

First published in the UK in 2003 by
Judy Piatkus (Publishers) Limited
5 Windmill Street
London W1T 2JA
e-mail: info@piatkus.co.uk

The moral right of the author has been asserted

Consultants for UK edition: Dr Naomi Craft and Kathy Cowbrough

*A catalogue record for this book is available
from the British Library*

ISBN 0 7499 2428 4

This book has been printed on paper manufactured
with respect for the environment using wood from
managed sustainable resources

Data manipulation by Phoenix Photosetting, Chatham
Printed and bound in Great Britain by
MPG Books, Bodmin, Cornwall

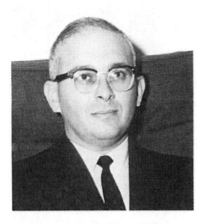

To Dr Gerald S. Kanter, who interviewed me for the Albany Medical College class of 1972. I will always remember our conversation in the early autumn of 1967. Your faith in me as a human being opened the door for my acceptance into medical school. Thank you for giving me a chance.

Contents

Acknowledgments

To Norman Goldfind, president of Basic Health Publishing, Inc., who published some of my previous books and suggested this one. To Deborah Chase, for writing an excellent outline. To Donna Chaput, Anne Lodge, and Ni Bushnell, for endless hours of typing and retyping the manuscript.

To Mark Tavani, editor at Ballantine, for your patience in making this project happen.

To Rhonda Brownbill, M.S.R.D., for her tedious and meticulous assessments in the recipe portion of this book, including taste-testing, nutritional analysis, and meal planning.

To my colleagues and friends at Phillips Publishing, including Thomas L. Phillips, Kevin Donoghue, John Missner, Glynnis Mileikowsky, Meg deGuzman, Bill Todd, Robert Austen, Erica Bullard, Gail Diggs, Eva Cover, Sue Petersen, Lynn Nopper, Elisa Novak, Michele Raynor, Anne Marie Bethel, Robert Kroening, Lauren Bach, Damien Thompson, Lisa Fleige, Roger DiFato, and Peggy Sullivan.

To my copy editors, Steve Kupritz, Richard Stanton Jones, and James Punkre.

To my partners, Sun King Wan, M.D., F.A.C.C., and Saqib Naseer, M.D., F.A.C.C.; thanks for your support.

To Jo-Anne Piazza, my dedicated executive assistant and faithful "right arm."

To my entire staff at the New England Heart and Longevity Center, for your utmost patience, support, and loyalty during this project, including Susan Graham, Rosemary Pontillo, Janet Hill, Kathleen Hunt, Caron Maker, Alethea Parsons, Rebecca Rossick, and Janet Rulon.

To my health food restaurant chefs, including Lois Chapman, Leanne Fortin-McCue, Lindsey Rashaw-Tsokalas, Tracy Shepley, and Sandra Tsokalas, for supplying fantastic recipes.

To my Optimum Health International staff, including Jo-Anne Renna, Marcelle Ringbloom, Karen Leppo, Laurie Oliva, Sharon Dumouchel, Alice Urban, Jennifer Dionne, Alison Lodge, and Craig Kelly.

To Stan Jankowitz and Raj Chopra, for supporting my nutriceutical endeavours in the pursuit of preventive and anti-ageing medicine.

To Dr. Robert Lang and Dr. Nicholas Perricone, two Connecticut conventional/alternative practitioners who have experienced the loneliness of going out on a limb.

To Susy Sinatra, who supported me with friendship, humour, and grace in my earlier years.

To our children, MarchAnn, Step, Drew and Donna, Kristin and Greg.

To my wife and co-author, Jan Sinatra, M.S.N., A.P.R.N., for working incessantly on this book. Your love, affection, and loyalty are cherished deeply.

And finally, to all my patients, past and present, for helping me stay humble, asking me to seek out the truth, and keeping me in touch with the true nature of healing.

Introduction

by Jan Sinatra, MSN, APRN

There's no magic bullet or quick fix that will get your blood pressure down to a healthy level. Instead, Steve's progressive eight-week programme has at its foundation his concept of the four pillars of good health: diet, supplements, stress reduction, and exercise. Each component of his approach includes a number of lifestyle changes. Steve has learned that if he gives patients the complete list of instructions in a single visit, they get overwhelmed, find them harder to follow, and are more likely to be unsuccessful.

But by the end of Steve's eight-week plan, most patients find that their blood pressure has dropped so significantly that they can start cutting down on the number and dosage of the medications they've been taking. Not infrequently, over time they are even able to eliminate medication entirely. That could happen for you if you follow this plan.

Steve has found that gradually building the programme concepts provides the support patients need to succeed. And there's another reality that's promoted the writing of this book: Most people cannot come to the New England Heart and Longevity Center. Even for those who can, Steve hasn't the kind of schedule that would allow him to see many people on a weekly basis for two months.

So Steve has written this book to bring his unique blood-pressure-lowering programme to you, right in your own home.

The step-by-step, week-by-week guidelines in this book will put you on the road to lowering your blood pressure safely and effectively. Chapters are organized to build your knowledge base and gradually introduce information and selections to enhance your success.

Chapter 1 provides you with an overview of high blood pressure as a health problem, along with a thumbnail sketch of traditional medical interventions currently in use. Your primary focus in this first week is to get some background on the topic, so you are motivated to move forward into action.

Chapter 2 is Week 1 of your actual lifestyle change. You'll read about Steve's Pan-Asian Modified Mediterranean eating plan, or PAMM diet for short, and why it's the best dietary approach to bring those blood pressure numbers down, down, down. You'll then be stepping into your own kitchen to pitch and toss foods that will thwart your blood pressure lowering efforts. Your primary activity this week is to restock your refrigerator and pantry with items you'll be needing to stay with the programme. You'll be getting weekly updates on foods in the remaining chapters

Chapter 3 focuses on the various nutritional supplements that you'll be adding to your program weekly, in addition to your first "Diet Update." Chapters 4 and 5 follow the same format, introducing first exercises, then mind-body techniques. After these topics are explained, then each subsequent chapter will provide you with weekly updates on these special areas of focus. By Week 6, each chapter will contain update sections on diet, supplements, exercise, and mind-body approaches so that you can add variety to your programme, creating a lifelong plan you can live with.

I hope you find that *Lower Your Blood Pressure in 8 Weeks* has come to you at just the right time in your life to make that all-important difference. Just by buying this book, you've taken that critical first step on an incredible health journey.

I wish you the very best of health.

Part One

Part One

1 Hypertension 101

Maybe you're picking up this book because you've just been told you have high blood pressure and you're looking for some answers. Or maybe you were diagnosed a long time ago and you're just tired of taking all that medication. Or perhaps traditional medicine has failed to keep your blood pressure under control, and you're searching for a new approach.

Well, my friend, whatever your reason for opening this book, I'm just glad you're here. High blood pressure is something you need to know about, and something you need to take seriously. I hope this book informs you and provides you with some new options. I've learned a lot about treating hypertension these last thirty years, and I've found some really novel approaches that have turned my patients' lives around, so I think I can help.

It's hard to overstate the impact of high blood pressure on our health, but let's just start with the cold, hard facts:

- About 10 million people in the UK have high blood pressure.
- Hypertension is more common in men and in people over sixty-five years of age.
- About half of people over sixty-five are hypertensive in the UK.
- High blood pressure is more common in black and South Asian people than in Caucasians.
- Hypertension is serious because it places you at increased risk for blindness, kidney damage, heart disease, an enlarged heart, heart attack, and stroke.

- Americans spend more than $3 billion on antihypertensive prescription drugs, more than for medications for any other diagnosis.
- According to the British Heart Foundation, of those who are treated over two thirds remain hypertensive.
- Despite new drugs and diagnostic techniques, the death rate from hypertension has risen by 36 percent in the past decade in the US.

Clearly, traditional drug and diet therapies for hypertension are falling far short of their intended goals. I believe that part of the problem is that, as doctors, we're taught to refer to the step-by-step process of a one-size-fits-all algorithm in designing a programme of care for our hypertensive patients. What's an algorithm? Basically, it's a step-by-step protocol to be followed. In treating hypertension, the algorithm goes something like this: Step one is that we are to prescribe drug A. After a month or so, if treatment A doesn't work, then we are to prescribe drug B. If B worked somewhat but we didn't get the results we were seeking, then we add in drug C, possibly juggling the dose of A or B. A typical algorithm doctors follow for treating blood pressure includes the following: a diuretic first, followed by a beta blocker or calcium channel antagonist, then an ACE inhibitor or angiotensin receptor blocker (ARB). This is a very structured, precise system . . . but that's just not how the human body functions.

Now don't get me wrong. There is an appropriate place for algorithms. They work best in an emergency situation such as a hypertensive crisis or a heart attack, when time is critical and the doctor may have just met the patient and knows little about him or her. Algorithms establish the standard of care that you receive, and that's a good thing. But once the crisis is over, you want to receive a more personalized treatment plan that takes into consideration your personal needs and your own physiology.

Each of us is an individual, with a unique body chemistry and physiology. An algorithm can only work so far, for I have found that blood pressure control is really more of an art than a science. As a cardiologist, I need to tune in to each individual to design a hypertension reduction programme that gets at the root of his or her problem. To understand how this approach works, I need to explain some of the basic concepts behind the problems. Let me fill you in on what I consider as I sit across from a new hypertensive patient who's seeing me in my clinic.

Simply stated, blood pressure is a measurement of how hard your heart has to work to circulate blood through your body. Chronically elevated blood pressure can hurt your body in a number of ways, primarily by adding to the workload of your heart and arteries. And when your heart must work harder than normal for a long period of time, like any other muscle in your body, it gets bigger and bigger. Slightly bigger may be okay, but if your heart gets extremely enlarged and sluggish, it will begin to fail. Then it will have a hard time meeting your body's oxygen demands.

When your blood pressure is too high, the excessive shear force of blood coursing over your arterial walls causes the cells there to become weakened and porous. Put simply, when the pressure in your heart and arteries is high, the blood goes through the twists and turns of your arteries much like racing cars hugging the walls on the tight turns in the Grand Prix.

Over time, the blood's high shear force under pressure wears down the healthy, glistening surface of your arterial walls, carving out little vulnerable patches. These worn, inflamed areas are open invitations to toxic substances such as heavy metals, the chemicals in cigarette smoke, high insulin levels, or excessive amounts of low-density lipoprotein (LDL) or "bad" cholesterol that are just looking around to take up residence somewhere, preferably the smooth muscle lining of your coronary arteries and arteries in other locations such as the brain and neck.

Add to this the fact that as you age, your arteries become stiffer and less elastic, decreasing their ability to stretch with the pulsation of each heartbeat. Picture this scenario as it builds momentum with time, and you have an image of what's going on in your own body, right now, if your blood pressure is still elevated. There's no time to waste. You must take action.

I hope that now you have a better understanding of how high blood pressure tends to speed the process we called atherosclerosis or arteriosclerosis. Hardened or narrowed arteries may not be able to supply the amount of blood your body's organs need; the end result is that they can't work properly. Another risk is that a blood clot may get stuck in an artery roughened and narrowed by atherosclerosis, depriving part of the body of its normal blood supply and potentially resulting in a stroke or a heart attack.

If a blood vessel gets clogged in the brain, you can have what we call a thrombotic stroke (*thrombus* = clot). Or you can have what we call a haemorrhagic (bleeding) stroke if a cerebral artery wall weakens to the point of rupture. A heart attack used to be called a coronary thrombosis, referring to a blot clot lodging in a coronary artery, cutting off blood flow to a region of the heart muscle. Now we use the term "myocardial infarc- tion" (MI), which indicates the damage it causes (*myo* = muscle, *cardio* = heart, *infarct* = area of tissue death).

THE STATISTICS ARE STAGGERING

Now you can better understand the statistics. Compared to people with controlled high blood pressure, people with uncontrolled high blood pres- sure are:

- seven times more likely to have a stroke
- three times more likely to develop coronary heart disease
- six times more likely to develop congestive heart failure (CHF)

Untreated, high blood pressure is the number one cause of strokes. And hypertension didn't get the nickname "the silent killer" for nothing. Often a person with hypertension has no symptoms warning of the condi- tion, so high blood pressure can go undiagnosed for years. That's where regular check-ups and blood pressure screening programmes come in, and I advise everyone to take advantage of them.

We've just looked at how hypertension can cause heart disease, but note that it actually triples your risk for it, and that's independent of other traditional risk factors you may have, including family history, obesity, smoking, elevated lipid levels, sedentary lifestyle, being over fifty, being male and stress. I even check for newer risk factors such as Lp(a) or lipoprotein, C-reactive proteins (CRP), oxidized LDL, homocysteine, and others that are screened with blood testing. Lp(a), for example, is a highly inflammatory cholesterol particle that accelerates artherosclerosis.

In fact, recent research has shown that a person with hypertension and high levels of homocysteine is more likely to have a stroke. Increasing folic acid intake could substantially reduce the risk of a heart attack and stroke.

Congestive heart failure happens when the heart is unable to pump enough blood to meet the needs of the body's tissues. Your heart muscle can become weak due to a variety of causes, such as scarring from heart attack(s), stretching and enlargement from hypertension, or other diseases. The bottom line is that a weak heart can't keep the blood moving in a forward fashion; some of it backs up to the lungs, then the tissues. People with CHF may notice swollen ankles and fingers. A doctor or nurse can even hear fluid crackling in the lungs with a stethoscope. When the fluid backs up abruptly, making it nearly impossible to breathe, then CHF has progressed to pulmonary oedema, a medical emergency.

The long and short of it is that high blood pressure puts you at high risk for the medical problems I've described and others, including damage to your kidneys, your eyes, and more.

WHO GETS HIGH BLOOD PRESSURE?

Hypertension is an equal-opportunity disease. Rich or poor, black or white, male or female, high blood pressure can strike anyone, often without warning. Unlike other diseases and ailments, you can't feel high blood pressure and it isn't heralded by chest pain, dizziness, or any other signs of an imminent problem.

And, as you can imagine, because there are no symptoms or warning signs, nearly one-third of the 10 million British people walking around with hypertension don't even know that they have it. All too often, the first sign of trouble is a stroke or heart attack.

Practically every day in my consulting room, a patient is shocked and frightened to be told that his or her blood pressure is too high. While no one wants to hear bad news, I assure the patient that the discovery of hypertension is the best thing that could have happened! Now that we know there's a problem, we can at least do something about it. It didn't take a crippling stoke or fatal heart attack to reveal the threatening situation.

While we don't fully understand the causes of hypertension, some people seem to be more likely to develop the problem. Black and South Asian people develop high blood pressure more often than Caucasians, and for them it also tends to occur earlier and be more severe. In fact, hypertension affects about one out of every three Black and South Asian persons. And in my experience African American women are actually my toughest population to treat for blood pressure. In fact, after twenty-five years, I can honestly say that for black women, medicines alone are almost never successful. They are one group who more often needs to add lifestyle modifications, such as diet and exercise, to help reduce body mass index (if overweight status is the problem causing the hypertension).

Additionally, Mexican Americans and other Hispanics are more likely to suffer from high blood pressure than white Americans.

Heredity also seems to play a role. Hypertension runs in families, so if your parents or other close relatives have high blood pressure, then you're more likely to develop the problem. In general, advancing age is a risk factor for developing high blood pressure; it occurs most often in people over age thirty-five. Men seem to develop it most often between thirty-five and fifty, while women are more likely to see their blood pressure start climbing after the menopause. Men have a greater risk of becoming hypertensive than women until age fifty-five, when their respective risks are similar. But by the time they've reached age seventy-five and beyond, women are more likely to develop high blood pressure than men are.

WHITE-COAT HYPERTENSION

Anxiety, stress, fear, and worry can influence blood pressure levels. Some people experience high blood pressure only when they visit the doctor. This condition is called "white-coat hypertension". The name reflects the fact that blood pressure rises when the doctor walks into the consulting room in his or her white coat. Although the effect also occurs without the white coat the name has stuck. If your doctor suspects this, you may be asked to monitor your blood pressure at home or wear a device called an ambulatory blood pressure monitor. This device is usually worn for twenty-four hours and can take your blood pressure every thirty minutes.

If you suffer from white-coat hypertension, here are some tips for taking more accurate readings at home or at the doctor's surgery:
- Do something relaxing beforehand.
- Avoid caffeine, smoking, or exercising before taking a reading.
- Take your reading in a serene place.
- Do it at the same time each day.
- Remove your arm from your sleeve instead of simply rolling up your sleeve.
- Breathe deeply.
- Don't talk during the reading.
- Wait a few minutes between readings to allow blood vessels to return to normal.

WHAT IS BLOOD PRESSURE?

Your blood pressure reading consists of two numbers: The top number represents the force of contraction of the heart's main section, the left ventricle, and the lower number corresponds with resistance to blood flow in the arteries. Everybody has and needs blood pressure. Without pressure gradients, the blood can't circulate through the body. Without circulating blood, vital organs can't get the oxygen and food that they need to work. Every cell in the body requires constant blood flow to transport oxygen and other nutrients to it as well as to remove waste products.

Here's what happens: When the heart beats, it pumps blood to the arteries and creates pressure in them. This pressure—blood pressure— results from two forces. The first force is created as blood pumps into the arteries and through the circulatory system, while the second is created as the arteries resist the blood flow. It is recorded as two numbers—the systolic pressure (as the heart beats) over the diastolic pressure (as the heart relaxes between beats). The measurement is written one above or before the other, with the systolic number on top or first and the diastolic number on the bottom or last. Blood pressure is measured in millimetres of mercury, which is expressed as mm Hg.

Another thing about blood pressure is that it changes constantly. With each beat, the heart exerts a surge of pressure that sends blood through the body's arteries. Influencing it is the time of day (for example, blood pressure is lowest in the morning), your psychological state, and even how much physical exertion you do. Anxiety and anger are two emotions that are particularly good at raising your blood pressure.

Later, we'll get into the details of how blood pressure is generated.

In the UK blood pressure of less than 140 over 85 is considered normal for non-diabetic adults. A systolic pressure of 140 to 159 or a diastolic pressure of 90 to 99 needs to be watched carefully and may need treatment in patients who are at high risk of a stroke or heart attack. A blood pressure reading equal to or greater than 140 (systolic) over 90 (diastolic) is considered high.

Blood pressure (mm Hg)	Optimal	Normal	Mild hypertension	Hypertension
Systolic (top number)	Less than 120	Less than 140	140–159	160 or higher
Diastolic (bottom number)	Less than 80	Less than 85	90–99	100 or higher

WHAT IS "NORMAL"?

In the UK systolic blood pressure (the upper or first number in a blood pressure reading) below 140 and diastolic pressure (the lower or second number in a blood pressure reading) below 85 are considered normal. National recommendations advise doctors to treat blood pressure in patients who are not diabetic and have no other medical problems when it goes over 160/100. Such treatment can include weight loss, stress management, improved diet, and/or blood-pressure-lowering drugs.

About 70 percent of people with high blood pressure have mild to moderate hypertension, which refers to systolic pressure between 140 and 159 and diastolic pressure between 90 and 99. While it's tempting to think that heart attacks occur only in people with extremely high blood pressure, it's not exactly accurate. About two-thirds of all heart attacks occur in people whose blood pressure is only mildly elevated.

HOW CAN YOUR DOCTOR TELL IF YOUR BLOOD PRESSURE IS ELEVATED?

You can find out if you have high blood pressure by having your pressure checked regularly. Most doctors will diagnose a person with high blood pressure on the basis of at least two readings per visit taken on four different occasions. They will probably use a device called a sphygmomanometer (pronounced "sfig-mo-ma-no-me-ter"). This common test involves wrapping an inflatable cuff around your upper arm. Air is pumped in, and you feel the cuff get tighter and tighter until your circulation is cut off. Then a health care professional will place a stethoscope on the artery just under the cuff and listen to the sound that your blood makes as air is released from the cuff. At first there is silence. Then as the air is slowly let out of the cuff, blood flow resumes at the point where the pressure in the cuff is equal to the pressure in the left ventricle of the heart, and that can be heard through the stethoscope.

Named after the phase in the cardiac cycle that we call *systole*, when the left ventricle contracts to eject blood out into the aorta, the largest artery in your body, the systolic reading reflects how high the pressure forces a column of mercury to rise in a tube. That's why blood pressure readings are reflected in millimetres of mercury (abbreviated mm Hg). Now we have gauges that use air, or are even computerized, but the first gold standard was a column of mercury, so everything that's come after is corrected to equilibrate with mm Hg.

As more and more air is let out, the pressure exerted by the cuff lessens until the sound of the blood pulsing against the artery walls becomes less and less audible. The point at which silence is again heard through the stethoscope is the point of lowest pressure, called diastolic pressure. Diastole is the resting phase of a cardiac cycle, when the heart is filling with blood and awaiting the next heartbeat, or contraction. Diastolic blood pressure actually reflects the amount of resistance, or tone, against which the heart is pushing to move blood through the arteries.

You see, if there's too much resistance to blood flow (reflected in a high diastolic number), then the pressure inside the left ventricle (systolic pressure) will need to kick up in order to keep the blood moving forward. That's why you may have heard your doctor caution you, saying something like "Your top number is okay, but that bottom number is creeping up, and that concerns me." A good number for diastolic pressure is 80mm Hg, plus or minus about 5mm Hg. Most doctors will start to be more concerned when your diastolic pressure starts to hover around 90mm Hg.

I'll bet I can guess what you're thinking: Why isn't a diastolic pressure of zero the best thing? Diastolic pressure also reflects tone in your arteries, right? Well, this muscle tone creates gentle pulsations that help the blood flow through the arteries in between heartbeats, delivering it where it's needed. Isn't the human body amazing?

TREATING BOTH "NUMBERS"

A factor contributing to the vast undertreatment of hypertension is that many doctors still pay more attention to the diastolic reading than they do to the systolic reading, despite widely recognized recommendations that patients be treated for high blood pressure based on both numbers. Why?

Some doctors disregard systolic pressure because, starting thirty years ago, most of the studies in the medical literature that looked at treating high blood pressure focused on diastolic, not systolic, pressure. But at least three large studies now show that treating systolic pressure is, in fact, beneficial even when diastolic pressure is in the normal range. This condition is referred to as isolated systolic hypertension, or ISH. It is the most common form of high blood pressure in elderly patients.

About 5% of people aged 60–69, 10% aged 70–79, and 20% aged 80+ have systolic readings greater than 160, the threshold point of ISH. In two landmark studies, the treatment of high systolic pressure lowered rates of heart attack and stroke by more than one-third!

Reducing systolic pressure by 12 points—a goal that can easily be achieved without drugs—can lower your risk for heart attack by 30 percent.

THE CAUSES ARE AS ENIGMATIC AS THE SILENCE

In 90 to 95 percent of cases, the cause of hypertension is unknown. This type of high blood pressure is called essential hypertension. In the remaining cases, high blood pressure is a symptom of a recognizable underlying problem, such as a kidney abnormality, a tumour of the adrenal gland, an overactive thyroid gland, or a congenital defect of the aorta. In these 5 to 10 percent of cases, after the root cause is corrected, blood pressure usually returns to normal. This latter type of high blood pressure is called secondary hypertension.

Although medical science doesn't understand why most cases of high blood pressure occur, we have identified a number of risk factors that are closely linked to the development of hypertension:

- *Weight gain.* Studies have shown that increased body weight or increased body mass index are related to higher blood pressure levels. Losing just 10 percent of your body weight can have a significant effect on blood pressure levels. This can be done simply by incorporating lifestyle modifications such as following a healthy diet and by walking one to two miles a day.
- *Inactivity.* People who don't exercise are up to 52 percent more likely to develop high blood pressure than their more active counterparts, according to the American Heart Association. Exactly why exercise has such a potent effect on hypertension is not completely understood, but several theories exist. Some doctors believe that the effect may be due to reductions in body weight and body fat, while others suggest that exercise may also

affect certain chemicals in the body known to influence blood pressure, such as nitric oxide.

- *Diet.* High sodium (salt) levels are also known to be part of the problem. The average American consumes twenty to thirty times more sodium than is needed. Did you know that in the United States the number one source of sodium is processed foods, not table salt? Salt locks fluid in the blood vessels, giving the heart more work to do.

Fatty cold-water fish such as salmon and mackerel are the best source of heart-protective omega-3 essential fatty acids (EFAs). Omega-3s have multiple health benefits including lowering blood pressure. Fresh fruits and vegetables are rich in blood-pressure-lowering minerals and antioxidants. Hearty whole grains are the best sources for minerals and B vitamins. In general, we use far less olive oil than people living in the Mediterranean, and less soya foods than the Japanese, two dietary elements that provide so many health benefits for people in these regions.

Four servings a month of fatty cold-water fish, which contain high levels of omega-3 EFAs, were associated with a 50 percent reduction in cardiac arrest. Just think about it—you can significantly reduce your risk of cardiac death by eating fish once a week!

- *Stress.* Chronic anxiety or stress is not only irritating and upsetting emotionally, but it can be extremely harmful to your health. Negative emotions, including anger, depression, frustration, and fear, provoke the release of adrenaline and cortisol in the body, all of which can raise your blood pressure. Research shows that people who experience more depression or anxiety are more likely to become hypertensive.
- *Alcohol.* There is a strange dichotomy to alcoholic beverages. Epidemiological studies have shown that one or two drinks a day can be cardioprotective, primarily by raising HDL ("good") cholesterol. But ingest larger amounts and the picture changes radically. More than three to five drinks a day significantly increase your risk of serious heart disease.

- *Tobacco.* Cigarettes have both a long- and short-term impact on blood pressure. From your first puff of a cigarette, you're pulling nicotine into the lungs. Nicotine constricts blood vessels, making it harder for the heart to do its job and therefore elevating blood pressure. Over time, the nicotine and carbon monoxide in the smoke decrease oxygen levels in the blood, increasing the risk of clotting events and promoting artery-blocking plaque development. Yuck! Smokers with hypertension have three times the risk of stroke and twice the risk of heart attacks.

The X Files

Sometimes hypertension is part of a syndrome that is finally getting the attention it deserves. Syndrome X, also referred to as insulin resistance syndrome, includes the four situations described below. I'll be discussing insulin resistance in greater detail later, but realize for now that it's part of a cluster of problems that must be considered if you want to get to the bottom of treatment-resistant hypertension.

You need to know if you have any of the following:

- impaired carbohydrate tolerance
- abnormal blood fats (low HDL and high triglycerides)
- weight gain in the abdominal area
- high blood pressure

When hypertension is not an isolated problem but is combined with these other three considerations, it becomes a prescription for disaster. This deadly quartet tends to be especially resistant to conventional medical treatment, yet places you at great risk for heart disease and stroke. I believe that most people who fail to respond to standard hypertension medication actually have syndrome X.

When it comes to syndrome X, it's been my experience that some doctors tend to swing to extremes, depending on whether or not they recognize it as an issue. Many doctors either under-diagnose or overtreat this medical condition. In the former situation, the doctor who's been tracking blood pressure readings makes the diagnosis of hypertension but fails to look deeper for the other three components. Then when a patient fails to respond to the prescribed drugs, wham! The doctor just increases the number and dosage of medications. But this still misses the point. On the other hand, some doctors go into medical intervention overload right off the bat. Not only do they prescribe the usual medications for hypertension, they write prescriptions for more: drugs to lower your triglyceride levels and help raise HDL, and insulin-sensitizing agents normally reserved for diabetics.

I have to confess right here and now that I have my own personal pet peeve about drugs to alter blood lipids (fats). I'm troubled that they are handed out so readily to treat a lone elevated cholesterol level. The problem is, statin drugs have been linked to many undesirable reactions—in fact, one widely used pharmaceutical agent from this class was removed from the market after it was associated with thirty-one deaths! And they lower your levels of coenzyme Q10, an important nutrient that, among other attributes, acts as a membrane stabilizer to keep your blood pressure stable. (I will say more about coenzyme Q10 later.)

But insulin-sensitizing drugs are not harmless medicines, either. One was banned because of the unacceptable number of liver failure cases found in people who were taking it. Another diabetes-type medication used to treat syndrome X was found to cause significant digestive problems for about 30 percent of people swallowing it, and has been known in rare cases to cause fatal lactic acidosis.

If an overly zealous doctor starts right off with this three-drug regimen, and treats other conditions, a patient can wind up taking as many as five or six different medications, each with its own set of side effects and each with its own risks of potentially fatal reactions.

If I'm treating high blood pressure that's the result of insulin resistance, I know I can't make an impact if I fail to treat the core problem; otherwise those blood pressure numbers just won't be going anywhere on conventional drugs alone. That's the bad news. The good news is that hypertension, whether it occurs as a lone wolf, or as part of syndrome X, responds beautifully to my natural blood pressure lowering programme. My patients are able to control their blood pressure without a drawerful of medications. Many come to a point where together we can gradually, but dramatically, reduce the number and type of medications they need. At least 85 percent of them can discontinue at least one or two of their antihypertensive medications. And a number of really successful people are eventually able to eliminate their drugs entirely.

In the next section, I'm going to discuss how these drugs work and the adverse reactions they may cause. Then we'll start to look at safer and more effective alternatives.

PHARMACOLOGICAL DRUGS

Now that we've nailed down some of the blood pressure basics, it's time to get a little more specific about the physiological havoc some of the treatments for this condition can wreak on your body.

There are over sixty-five different drugs used to lower high blood pressure. Many people are on a cocktail of different medications that bring with them a host of unpleasant and often unbearable side effects. In my opinion, too many people take potent drugs such as ACE inhibitors, diuretics, and calcium channel blockers to control their hypertension, even when their blood pressure is only mildly elevated. All these drugs have potential side effects, including impotence, loss of libido, fatigue, drowsiness, dry cough, light-headedness, and even depression.

These adverse effects are particularly intolerable for patients whose high blood pressure caused them no real physical symptoms—and remember, that's most people! They're left frustrated and often don't comply with medication schedules because the cure is so much worse than the disease. All too often, people start to skip pills or stop taking them entirely. They actually feel better without their prescribed drugs, even though the hypertension is silently continuing to weaken their heart and blood vessels.

Choices, Choices, Choices

In this section, I want to discuss the different therapeutic options for hypertension, exploring the way they work and the problems that they can cause. In the following table you will find thirty-one of the top two hundred drugs by number of prescriptions dispensed in 2000 in the US. The primary purpose of most of these drugs is blood pressure lowering.

Top Antihypertensive Medications

Drug Class, Examples	Method of Action	Typical Side Effects
ACE Inhibitors Tritace (ramipril); Capoten (captopril); Gopten/Odrik (trandolapril); Staril (fosinopril); Carace/Zestril (lisinopril); Accupro (quinapril); Innovace (enalapril); Coversyl (perindopril)	Blocks the conversion of of angiotensin I to angiotensin II (A-II). A-II is one of the main hormones that causes blood vessel constriction, which contributes to hypertension.	Cough; dizziness; kidney dysfunction; excessive potassium retention; taste alteration.

A-II Receptor Antagonists Cozaar (losartan); Diovan (valsartan)	Blocks action of angiotensin II (see ACE inhibitors).	Well tolerated.
Calcium Channel **Blockers** * *Rate-limiting*: Cordilox/ Securon (verapamil); Tildiem/ Adizem SR/Angitil SR (diltiazem) * *Non-rate-limiting*: Adalat LA/Adalat Retard (nifedipine); Istin (amlodipine); Plendil (felodipine)	Both classes of calcium channel blockers dilate blood vessels, reducing blood pressure.	* *Rate-limiting*: fluid accum- ulation; slow heart rate; con- gestive heart failure; GI disturbance. * *Non-rate-limiting*: oedema; heart palpitations; faster heart rate; headache; GI disturbance. * Both can weaken the heart muscle.
Beta Blockers Corgard (nadolol); Inderal (propranolol); Lopresor/Betaloc (metoprolol); Tenormin (atenolol); Monozide 10 (bisoprolol + hydrochloro- thiazide)	Decrease heart rate and heart output; interfere with the produc- tion of renin, a hormone that increases blood pressure.	Bronchial spasm in asthma patients and COPD patients; increase in triglycerides; nervous system disturbances (confusion, nightmares, depression, excitement); slow heart rate; left ventricular dysfunction; impotence.
Diuretics * Thiazide: bendrofluazide * Loop: Burinex (bumetanide); Lasix (furosemide/frusemide) * Potassium-sparing: Aldactone (spironolactone); Aldactide (hydroflumethiazide +spironolactone); TriamaxCo/Triam-Co/Dyazide (hydrochlorothiazide + triamterene) Dytac (triamterene); Amiloride (amiloride HCL)	These decrease the volume of blood, which decreases heart output, so less blood is being pumped through the blood vessels. With continued therapy they relax peripheral blood vessels.	Mineral depletion, including sodium, potassium, and magnesium; increased blood glucose, LDL, and triglyce- rides; impotence. Loop diuretics have a shorter duration of action and generally cause more nutrient depletion.
Alpha-Adrenoceptor **Blockers** Cardura (doxazosin); Hypovase (prazosin); Hytrin (terazosin)	These drugs relax smooth muscles in blood vessel walls.	Heart palpitations; inconti- nence; sexual dysfunction; dizziness; excessive lowering of blood pressure on standing; dry mouth and eyes.

Diuretics

Diuretics are my first line of treatment for blood pressure lowering in most people and especially African Americans. Diuretics, sometimes known as "water pills", are drugs that draw excess fluids and salt (sodium) from the tissues of the body and convert them into urine. They do this by disrupting the normal action of the kidneys. The kidneys usually remove water, minerals, and waste products from the bloodstream. Most of the water and minerals are subsequently returned to the bloodstream after the waste products have been filtered out via the urine. Diuretics reduce the amounts of sodium and water that are reabsorbed into the bloodstream. They draw excess fluid from tissues, reduce the water content of the blood, and increase urine output (thus increasing the number of trips you make to the bathroom each day—note that urine output usually peaks one to two hours after you take a diuretic, so you may want to plan accordingly).

As the diuretics facilitate enhanced urine output, your tissues become less waterlogged and the workload on the heart is lessened, as it has less blood volume to move around. Diuretics cause you to lose potassium in your urine, so if you have a prescription for a diuretic, then another one for a potassium supplement probably accompanies it. Or potassium-retaining drugs can also be taken along with diuretics.

The primary side effects of diuretics are low potassium levels, which can cause muscle cramping, fatigue, weakness, and impotence.

There are several types of diuretics your doctor may prescribe for hypertension:

Thiazide Diuretics

Bendrofluazide	Nephril (polythiazide)	Natrilix (indapamide)
(bendrofluazide)	Diurexan (xipamide)	Metenix 6 (metolozone)
Navridrex (cylopenthiazide)	Hygroton (chlortalidone)	

Thiazides work by blocking the reabsorption of sodium in the kidney. Thiazide diuretics are used in a low dose which reduces blood pressure but has minimal effect on potassium, glucose, and uric acid levels.

Loop Diuretics

Torem (torsemide)	Burinex (bumetanide)	Lasix (furosemide/frusemide)

The loop diuretics get their name because they work in the loop of the distal tubule in your kidney. This class of "water pills" can deplete your body's stores of vitamins B1 and B6, calcium, magnesium, potassium, and zinc while they block the reabsorption of sodium, potassium, and water. They have an extremely rapid action and for this reason are sometimes used in emergencies (for example, to relieve rapidly accumulating fluid in the lungs in situations known as pulmonary oedema).

People with impaired kidney function who do not react well to thiazide diuretics may use loop diuretics, but the potassium-depleting action of loop diuretics can be more powerful than that of the thiazides. Those of you taking a loop diuretic must also avoid licorice products, as well as any foods and herbs that have diuretic properties, such as asparagus, blessed thistle, burdock, butcher's broom, buchu, chaparral, chickweed, corn silk, dandelion, dog grass, grape vine, hawthorn, horse-tail, ho shou wu, hydrangea, juniper berries and nettle.

Potassium-Sparing Diuretics

Aldactone	Dytac (triamterene)	Amiloride (amiloride HCL)
(spironolactone)	TriamaxCo/Triam-Co/Dyazide	
Aldactide	(triamterene +	
(spironolactone +	hydrochlorothiazide)	
hydroflumethiazide)		

Another group of diuretics is the potassium-sparers. These block the reabsorption of sodium and water without affecting the body's potassium balance. They're relatively mild and may be prescribed together with a thiazide or loop diuretic to prevent the body from losing excess potassium. These diuretics, however, deplete the body of folic acid and calcium.

ACE Inhibitors

Tritace (ramipril)	Staril (fosinopril)	Vasotec (enalapril)
Capoten (captopril)	Carace/Zestril	
Gopten/Odrik (trandolapril)	Accupro (quinapril)	
Coversyl (perindopril)		

ACE inhibitors lower blood pressure by dilating or widening arteries, which interferes with the body's production of angiotensin, a chemical that causes the arteries to constrict. They deplete the body of zinc, tend to increase potassium levels in the body, and may interact negatively with arginine. Side effects can include dry cough, skin rash, and high potassium levels. ACE inhibitors are not recommended for people with moderate to severe kidney disease or pregnant women.

A newer generation of ACE inhibitors includes the ARAs, or **Angiotensin II Receptor Antagonists**, such as Cozaar (losartan) or Diovan (valsartan). These drugs are usually well tolerated with minimal side effects. In fact, they could be the better choice of drug for treating high blood pressure.

In March 2002, an audience of cardiologists at the American College of Cardiology's annual meeting gave Swedish researcher Dr. Bjorn Dahlof an extended ovation—a rare occurrence among cardiologists. The reason? In his study of 9,193 hypertensive men and women, all of whom had heart wall thickening (a sign of heart deterioration) from high blood pressure, Dr. Dahlof found that Cozaar, a well-known A-II receptor antagonist, was more effective at reducing blood pressure than Tenormin (atenolol), a widely used beta blocker. Cozaar didn't stop there: It also reduced the new onset of diabetes by 25 percent, cut stroke risk by 25 percent, and decreased the risk of death from all causes by 13 percent.

Beta Blockers

Corgard (nadolol)	Betaloc/Lopresor	Monozide 10 (bisoprolol +
Inderal (propranolol)	(metoprolol)	hydrochlorothiazide)
Cardicor/Emcor/Monocor	Tenormin (atenolol)	Celectol (celiprolol)
(bisoprolol)	Eucardic (carvedilol)	Trandate (labetalol)

Beta blockers are an invaluable heart medicine, and I believe that they're among the best drugs we have in cardiology to date. They work by doing just what the name suggests—they block the beta limb of the autonomic nervous system, the part that's responsible for gearing up your body for action. When fully activated, your beta-adrenergic system raises alertness, heart rate, and blood pressure.

Beta blockers also blunt exaggerated physiological responses to stress, so they're great when it comes to treating things such as performance anxiety. I often prescribe them for actors who get stage fright on opening night, as well as my professional golfers, whose steady putting hand is crucial to their success in an important tournament. In this type of high-stress, peak-performance situation, beta blockers can be used in a single-dose format, not on a regular basis as in blood pressure lowering. But I just want to paint you a picture of how they can be used to help kick down that high adrenaline level, assuaging the fight-or-flight response for people who tend to live their lives in overdrive, for whatever reason.

Make no mistake about it: beta blockers offer important cardioprotection and have been cited definitively for lowering the risk of sudden death due to lethal arrhythmia—a sudden change in the heartbeat. Their antiarrhythmic effect is the result of their ability to keep cell membranes stable, especially for the cells that conduct electricity in the heart. Beta blockers assist your conduction system to resist blood level surges in catecholamines, such as adrenaline, that can provoke life-threatening arrhythmias, especially in vulnerable populations whose heart muscle is less stable, such as survivors of a previous heart attack. Clinical research from several studies has documented that beta blocker treatment resulted in a 20–50 percent reduction in mortality for people who had previously had a heart attack. Research published in the *Journal of the American Medical Association* reported mortality for elderly patients given beta blockers to be 43 percent lower than for those who were not.

Like all drugs, beta blockers are no panacea, and are not without their own set of problems. Patients report side effects that range from fatigue and nightmares to wheezing, impotence, and depression. And because they can block the symptoms of low blood sugar and can even promote bronchospasm, I can't use them for my patients who are diabetic or asthmatic.

Despite these drawbacks, though, beta blockers have a strong therapeutic record and remain my first choice of medicines whenever they're medically appropriate. In my opinion, the best drug combination for the treatment of high blood pressure is a low-dose beta blocker, plus an ARB. If you can't lower your blood pressure naturally, at least bring in the drugs that will reduce your overall risk of cardiovascular events, providing much more benefit than you'd expect from lowering blood pressure alone.

Calcium Channel Blockers

Adalat LA/Adalat Retard (nifedipine)	Tildiem/Adizem SR/ Angitil SR (diltiazem)	Istin (amlodipine)
Cordilox/Securon (verapamil)		Plendil (felodipine)
		Cardene (nicardipene)

Another class of antihypertensive medications, called calcium channel blockers (also known as calcium antagonists), improves blood flow and vascular tone through narrowed blood vessels. Some of these drugs relax smooth muscles in the inner lining of blood vessels, preventing spasm and helping them stay open. Although the antihypertensive effect of calcium channel blockers are equal to other classes of blood-pressure-lowering medications, their long-term record is troubling. In a metanalysis of nine large-scale clinical trials, calcium channel blockers were associated with 25 percent higher rates of both acute heart attacks and heart failure compared to other types of medication.

Calcium channel blockers have their own side effects, including swollen ankles, constipation, fatigue, headache, and dizziness. However, despite the side effects and increased rate of myocardial infarction, some research shows a reduction in stroke for patients taking calcium blockers. I prescribe this class of drugs only to patients with high blood pressure and a family history of stroke.

Alpha-Adrenoreceptor Blockers

Cardura (doxazosin)   Hytrin (terazosin)   Hypovase (prazosin)

Slowly but surely we are learning which drugs provide the most benefit for the majority of patients. To illustrate, a class of antihypertensive drugs called alpha-adrenoceptor blockers can lower your blood pressure, but they also activate the central nervous system, an undesirable effect. These drugs are also prescribed to relieve tension in the prostate gland and are used by many urologists for improving urine flow as well. However, alpha-adrenoreceptor blockers do come with a long list of side effects, including dizziness, light-headedness, heart palpitations, and even loss of consciousness when abruptly rising from a sitting position.

And to make matters worse, a large clinical trial found that patients taking doxazosin had 25 percent more serious complications than a controlled group taking diuretics. The risk of developing congestive heart failure was 1 percent per year in the diuretic group and doubled to 2 percent for those taking the alpha-adrenoreceptor blockers. The study involved more than forty-two thousand high-risk patients at 623 clinical sites in the United States, Puerto Rico, Canada, and the Virgin Islands. A total of about nine hundred patients developed congestive heart failure during the study. These findings were so disturbing that a clinical alert about alpha-adrenoreceptor blockers was raised at the American College of Cardiology sessions in Anaheim, California.

On the more positive side, the diuretic drugs as well as the alpha-adrenoreceptor blockers were similarly effective in preventing heart attacks and reducing the risk of death from all other causes. The heart failure outcome was the major concern. Indeed, drugs can have a dark side.

DANGERS IN YOUR MEDICINE CABINET

Most over-the-counter cold and flu products contain decongestants that can raise your blood pressure. Decongestants (and also appetite suppressants) containing phenylpropanolamine (PPA) have been taken off the market because they increase the risk of haemorrhagic stroke in people who take them. But the American Heart Association recognizes that other decongestants have been reported to increase blood pressure and even to interfere with blood pressure medications. Additionally, chronic use of OTC and prescription anti-inflammatory drugs including ibuprofen (Nurofen, Advil) and naproxen sodium (Arthosin/Timprou) may also drive up your blood pressure.

WHEN GOOD DRUGS GO BAD

Any cardiologist who's treating critically ill patients will tell you that many of the medicines now available to us are truly indispensable. Untold numbers of people would have died if they did not have the opportunity to take these lifesaving drugs. Perhaps many of you have experienced improved physical and mental health because of prescription drugs. But any pharmacological agent that impacts cardiodynamics is very powerful and has the potential to cause harm as well as improve heart function.

Several years ago, the *Journal of the American Medical Association* (JAMA) reported that improperly prescribed medications in a hospital environment were the fourth leading cause of death in the United States. In the year of this survey (1994) over a hundred thousand deaths were attributed to drugs given to hospital patients because of administration errors, adverse reactions, and drug interactions. The article noted that the elderly were particularly at risk because their kidneys and livers don't always metabolize medications at the rate seen in younger people.

The American Medical Association (AMA), which estimates that reactions to prescription and over-the-counter drugs kill more people annually than all illegal drug use combined, has confirmed these hazards. Obviously, this is one of the major reasons why natural blood pressure lowering is the most preferred treatment.

If you are currently on medication, then don't stop without your doctor's knowledge and approval. To avoid adverse reactions, here a few of the guidelines that I give my patients:

- Do keep your medications in a place that's dry, cool, and away from the light (in other words, not a windowsill).
- Never take medication with grapefruit juice, a combination that may cause severe blood pressure drops.
- Read labels and package inserts carefully, and ask your pharmacist for information if you start a new drug.
- Never take medications in the dark, or in poor lighting, or without your glasses. You could take the wrong one.
- Never take someone else's prescription, thinking it's the "same drug".
- Never take your first dose of medication and then drive a car.
- Never take your first dose of a new medication if there isn't someone at home with you.
- Never take alcohol within two hours of taking medication.
- Work with your doctor to introduce medication in smaller doses, moving to higher doses as needed.
- If you ever feel that you are having an adverse reaction to a drug, then don't take the next dose until you've consulted with your doctor.

WOMEN AND HIGH BLOOD PRESSURE

Many women and some doctors don't believe that heart disease is a widespread health problem for women of all ages. They couldn't be more wrong. And even modest increases in blood pressure put women more at risk than their male counterparts.

High blood pressure is a major risk factor for heart disease—and this has special implications for women. Whether they like it or not, heart disease is every woman's concern. One in ten American women aged forty-five to sixty-four has some form of heart disease, and this increases to one in five women over age sixty-five. Another 1.6 million women have had a stroke.

So how does high blood pressure factor in? Hypertension greatly increases a woman's chances of developing cardiovascular disease, and it's the most important risk factor for stroke. Even slightly elevated blood pressure doubles a woman's risk, and more than half of American women will develop high blood pressure at some point in their lives.

One out of every two American women will die of some form of heart disease. That's over half a million women every year, making heart disease the number one killer of women in the United States. Largely due to the hard work of breast cancer advocates, most women are more afraid of breast cancer than heart disease. But the latest statistics have been convincing enough to shift health concerns to include heart disease as well.

By comparison, breast cancer kills approximately forty thousand American women yearly. Heart disease is the leading killer of women aged fifty-five and older, and women are six times more likely to die of heart disease than breast cancer. So heart disease prevention and awareness of heart disease risk factors such as hypertension are vital to every woman's health. For more on heart disease and women, see my earlier book *HeartSense for Women* (Plume, 2001).

SUCCESSFUL BLOOD PRESSURE CONTROL

Most people who are diagnosed with hypertension leave their doctor's surgery with a fistful of prescriptions and vague advice to cut back on salt and fat and try to lose some weight. Now that you've seen the current health statistics on hypertension, I think you understand why this approach alone is clearly not working. I have spent the past twenty years developing a more effective approach to hypertension.

Instead of relying on powerful medicines that alter body physiology, I searched relentlessly for ways to directly address the four major risk factors: dietary problems, lack of targeted nutritional supplements, inactivity, and stress. The result is a four-part programme that includes nutrition, supplementation, exercise, and stress reduction strategies. I've learned that tweaking the traditional approach to hypertension not only leads to effective blood pressure lowering but can eventually reduce, and in some cases even eliminate entirely, the need for medicines.

THE FOUR PILLARS OF MY BLOOD-PRESSURE-LOWERING PROGRAMME
- Nutrition (Pan-Asian/Modified Mediterranean Diet)
- Supplementation (antioxidants, vitamins, and minerals)
- Exercise
- Stress reduction

I often see patients who have tried everything else and are willing to do whatever it takes to lower their blood pressure. Traditional medications and diets have failed, leaving them weakened and frightened for their future. They're amazed that my programme works so well, and grateful for the success. Others are like Dr. K., who was sceptical that a natural approach could work better than traditional medicine. Here's his story.

A fifty-year-old doctor, Dr. K. was astonished when an annual examination revealed a blood pressure of 160/100. This blood pressure elevation is considered moderately severe and carries with it a significantly increased risk for stroke or heart attack. A non-smoker and non-drinker, Dr. K. had always followed a reasonably healthy diet. Just five to ten pounds over his ideal weight, he'd watched his sodium intake, avoided junk food, and made a point to eat fresh fruit and vegetables every day.

After one month on a calcium channel blocker his pressure was 140/95 . . . better, but still too high. Rather than increasing his medication dosage or adding another drug, Dr. K. decided to follow my dietary recommendations. He added several fish meals a week, changed his breakfast from bagels to oatmeal, and practically eliminated white flour, pasta made with white flour, white rice, all sugars, and high-fat cheese, replacing them with four to five servings of fruits and vegetables a day. He made a point of having an apple in the afternoon and a big salad at dinner.

Within ten days his blood pressure had dropped to 130/85. By the end of the month it was down to 120/80—a healthy, normal level. Dr. K. was equally delighted to find that his cholesterol had dropped from 7.2 to 4.8 mmol/l. Feeling better than he had in years, Dr. K. agreed to overcome his long-held scepticism toward supplements, and even incorporated coenzyme Q_{10} and vitamin E for further cardioprotection.

Getting a handle on your blood pressure requires a number of lifestyle changes.

In the next eight weeks I am going to provide you with complete plans for this journey. Each chapter will provide step-by-step advice, including daily menus, a supplement schedule, exercise programmes, and stress reduction techniques. Each week you will build new knowledge and new skills. In the first week we are going to focus on a diet programme that I call the Pan-Asian/Modified Mediterranean Diet. My patients just call it a lifesaver.

2 The Pan-Asian/Modified Mediterranean (PAMM) Diet: A Lifesaver Week 1

The foundation of my approach to controlling high blood pressure is a nutritional plan that I call the Pan-Asian/Modified Mediterranean Diet, or PAMM for short. Like most cardiologists, I used to recommend that my patients follow the American Heart Association (AHA) guidelines—similar to the British Heart Foundation guidelines—a diet that was low in fat and high in energy-releasing carbohydrates. Sounds great, right? Trouble is, it wasn't, but it took us years to figure that out.

These AHA guidelines made perfect sense when they first came out, and it made sense to those of us in the medical establishment who felt that less fat in the diet would mean less fat in the bloodstream. So we adhered to that plan to prevent our own heart disease. We figured that carbohydrates, such as bread, pasta, and rice, would be very beneficial or at the very least harmless. Unfortunately, it didn't work out quite the way we had hoped.

We later found that by encouraging people to replace fat calories with carbohydrates, we had unknowingly promoted a diet that contributed to the development of insulin resistance and hypertension, problems that increase and accelerate the development of heart disease. Now, after years of study, I've gone 180° on the subject of carbohydrates.

Let me explain. Insulin is a hormone—that's right, a hormone—just like testosterone, oestrogen, thyroid, or growth hormone. It is secreted by the pancreas and helps your body break down and absorb sugar and other carbohydrates. But when you're eating excessive amounts of carbohydrates—as we were on the high-carb, low-fat plan—your body requires more and more insulin to metabolize those carbohydrates, over and over and over again. Excessive amounts of this hormone in turn send out a signal to your body: "Store those carbs, because we don't have enough effective metabolism or calorie burning going on!" And you know what happens next—weight goes up . . . and up . . . and up.

Carbohydrate cravings → carbohydrate overload → high blood sugar → high insulin levels → fat storage → more carbohydrate cravings

---

Extra body weight translates all too easily into blood pressure numbers that climb and climb. In addition, chronically high levels of circulating insulin provoke the release of inflammatory chemicals that encourage the development of atherosclerotic plaque, which in turn constricts your blood vessels—yet another reason for your blood pressure to climb. This is a very, very vicious circle! No wonder these high-carb, low-fat diets produced more problems than they ever solved!

After recommending the AHA diet, I noticed something very unnerving in my patients: They were developing insulin resistance, and so was I. (Even my dog Charlie, who was on the same "healthy plan" for his heart, packed on the pounds.) Despite our best motivation and effort, my patients—and I—were gaining weight and watching our cholesterol and triglyceride levels rise. I couldn't figure it out! Concerned about both the long- and short-term effects of the AHA diet, I began to explore other ways of eating that might offer better cardiopreventive benefits.

As I did the research, I became particularly impressed by the health patterns of people living in the Mediterranean regions of Italy, Greece, and Spain, as well as the heart disease trends in Asian cultures. Natives of these cultures experienced a rate of heart disease that's a fraction of what is seen in northern Europe and the United States. Of course, the statistics come from the years before these countries became Westernized and were invaded with fast-food restaurants. Thanks to "modernization", their younger generations, and those who have moved to the West and don't follow their traditional diets, see an incidence of hypertension and heart disease that is catching up to that of people in the West.

In a nutshell, too much insulin causes excessive wear and tear on cellular membranes (oxidative stress), which ages your blood vessels, resulting in higher blood pressure.

We now know that the typical Mediterranean diet, which includes helping after helping of fresh fruits and vegetables, local fish, home-produced olive oil, fresh garlic, and nuts, is a key source of the southern Europeans' enviable health statistics. And the Asian diet—bountiful in fish, fresh veggies and fruits, locally harvested seaweeds, and soya products—offers many of the same protective properties, and then some. For instance, there isn't even a word for "hot flush" in Japanese because most of the women in Japan follow their traditional diet and pass through the menopause with no troublesome symptoms.

THE LYON ROARS . . . WITH THE EVIDENCE

My observations were supported by the 1996 medical journal publication of the results of the Lyon Heart Study. In this French trial, more than six hundred patients who had suffered a heart attack were assigned to one of two diets: a Mediterranean-style diet or the diet recommended by the American Heart Association. Four years later, research showed that those on the Mediterranean diet were up to 70 percent less likely to have experienced cardiac problems, such as a second heart attack, unstable angina, heart failure, or cardiac-related death. Even better, separate analysis showed the death rate for all causes to be almost 50 percent less for the Mediterranean diet group.

When I reviewed the initial findings of the Lyon study, I was determined to explore why the Mediterranean diet offered so many health benefits. I found that this diet not only provided optimal levels of nutrients to promote better health, but was and still is very low in those foods known to cause health problems. Over the years I've found in my practice that when patients truly understand the role that each food choice plays in their overall health, they're more likely to be able to follow the plan and enjoy it. So before I start giving you menus and recipes, I'd like you to try to understand the principles behind the food choices of the PAMM diet.

NO WONDER ZORBA DANCED!

The Mediterranean portion of the PAMM diet is based on the eating tradition of the people of Crete and other olive-growing regions up until the 1960s. For decades, epidemiologists studying the dietary habits in these areas wondered how it was that the inhabitants maintained such excellent health, even though almost 40 percent of their daily caloric intake came from *fat*. Adult life expectancy in these areas was among the highest in the world, and rates of coronary disease, certain cancers, and other diseases were among the lowest.

This finding led researchers to look more closely into what role certain fats play in making us healthy, because Mediterraneans were eating a lot of olive oil and fatty fish. Other no-table aspects of their diet were seasonal fresh fruits and vegetables, whole grains, legumes, nuts, and seeds. Dairy products—primarily yogurt and cheese—and fish and poultry were consumed in low to moderate amounts; red meats were used primarily to flavour sauces. People drank a glass or two of red wine with meals, and ate sweets containing sugar or honey only a few times a week. Another essential aspect of the Mediterranean lifestyle was that it included regular physical work in the field or kitchen. The culture was associated with little obesity.

Fortunately, you don't have to live in Greece or farm for a living to improve your diet and reap significant health benefits. It may take some changes, but it's easy to incorporate the Mediterranean diet and moderate activity into your life.

THE GREENING OF THE WESTERN MEALTIME

The Mediterranean diet, like the Asian diet, includes fruits and vegetables at every meal. This wonderful fresh produce is packed with disease-fighting antioxidants, bioflavonoids, and phytonutrients. Just about every fruit and vegetable offers something special. For example, strong-tasting veggies such as cabbage, broccoli, and cauliflower contain anticancer agents such as indole-3-carbinol and isothiocyanates. Spinach is rich in the antioxidant lutein as well as vitamins C and E. Tomatoes offer the carotenoid lycopene, which helps to prevent and fight cancer, especially prostate cancer.

Lycopene, a powerful antioxidant, is the bright red colour of a luscious, ripe tomato. A member of the carotenoid family, this free-radical fighter has been shown to be a powerful ally in the war against cancer and heart disease. Lycopene made front-page news several years ago when scientists reported that men who ate tomatoes ten or more times a week cut their risk of prostate cancer by 35 to 40 percent, when compared to those who had consumed less than one and a half servings of tomatoes weekly.

The health benefits of this free-radical scavenger are equally impressive. Because lycopene has antioxidant properties more potent than beta-carotene, scientists believe it can have a positive impact on cholesterol metabolism. The best source of lycopene is deep red, ripe tomatoes and watermelon. And interestingly enough, the lycopene in cooked tomatoes and tomato products is more bioavailabile than that in raw fresh tomatoes. So tomatoes are one veggie that confers more health benefits when cooked.

In fact, your best health results are reported with five to seven servings of tomato sauce per week. Because this many servings may be more of a good thing than most people want, this week you will notice that a lycopene supplement is already a part of your nutritional programme. Taking a couple of milligrams a day, in addition to eating tomatoes, is the best way to maximize your lycopene intake on the programme.

For instance, did you know that a single serving of kale has as much calcium as a glass of milk? And that dates, figs, and raisins are outstanding sources of minerals such as calcium, iron, and magnesium? And that practically all fruits and vegetables are excellent sources of different types of fibre that can help lower your cholesterol? Even the onions and garlic we use as seasonings in the Mediterranean diet provide allicin, a cholesterol-lowering nutrient. These foods are all rich in a type of nutrient called flavonoids. Black tea, apples, and onions are the most studied because they contain amounts of quercetin, a flavonoid, similar to those found in the red grapes used in making red wines. We've come a long way toward understanding the old adage "an apple a day keeps the doctor away". Fresh fruits and vegetables containing precious quercetin help block the oxidation of LDL cholesterol. Onions are your best dietary source of this magical flavonoid.

VALIDATING THE VIDALIA'S VASODILATING EFFECTS

You may be amazed, as I was, to hear how onions combined with small amounts of other nutrients can help lower your blood pressure. In a German study of twenty-four relatively young subjects with hypertension (average age was 45.1 years), researchers were curious about the effects of a product with the essential ingredients of the Mediterranean diet. They compared the results of a daily 270mg capsule of onions macerated in olive oil against an olive oil placebo after just one week. Each onion–olive oil capsule also contained 50mg grapeseed extract, 30mg L-carnitine, 3 mg vitamin E, 2mg ascorbyl palmitate, 1mg lycopene, and 44mcg folic acid. Four of these onion–olive oil capsules are equivalent to a mean daily dose of 2.5g of fresh onions.

Just five hours after dosing, the onion–olive oil capsules led to a significant reduction in systolic (7mm Hg) and diastolic (3.1mm Hg) blood pressures. After seven days, the treatment group had an average systolic blood pressure of 138.1mm Hg, compared to the placebo group mean of 142.6mm Hg systolic pressure. In addition to a lower blood pressure, there was a significant reduction in plasma viscosity (thickness), suggesting to investigators a vasodilative effect from the onion–olive oil product. In fact, those with the greatest increase in blood fluidity had the strongest effects in terms of blood pressure lowering. So adding more onions, including spring onions, to your dishes may be one way to lower your blood pressure and to prevent strokes and heart attacks.

I'll be addressing the benefits of some of the other ingredients in these capsules, such as grapeseed extract, L-carnitine, and vitamin E, in upcoming chapters. But for now, I just want to impress upon you the importance of the polyphenols found in onions.

I've also been impressed by a study of Japanese women whose LDL levels were inversely correlated with their dietary intakes of flavonols, flavones, and isoflavones. These substances of plant origin belong to a class of flavonoids totalling approximately four thousand compounds in nature with varying biological activities. The woman surveyed received 45.9 percent of these health-promoting flavonoids from onions and 37 percent from tofu. The researchers commented that their high consumption of both flavonoids and isoflavones might be the reason that Japanese women have such a low incidence of coronary heart disease when compared to women in other countries.

If you still have your doubts, consider a Finnish study where researchers looked at a cohort of 5,133 Finns, age thirty-nine to sixty-nine, from thirty Finnish communities. They explored the relationship between the dietary intake of flavonoids, coronary disease, and total mortality. Finns have one of the highest rates of coronary disease in the world, and the researchers were looking to find out why. Their results suggested that those with the lowest flavonoid intake had the highest risk for coronary disease, even when investigators controlled for variables such as blood pressure, smoking, serum cholesterol, and body mass index. Another European study in Holland reported that Dutch men, aged sixty-five to eighty-four, reduced their risk of heart attack and sudden death when they ate more onions.

By now, I hope that you can appreciate my excitement about the Pan-Asian/Modified Mediterranean Diet, because you reap the benefits of two cultures that eat quite similarly in many ways. The Mediterraneans and Asians are so compatible, in fact, that my Japanese friend Chizuko teased me—a Sinatra—about how her son-in-law taught her to cook Italian, like his own family. "It is easy for me!" she joked proudly. Now I know why!

THE SKINNY ON FATS IS A LITTLE FISHY

Another important aspect of the Mediterranean and Asian diets is the type and quantity of the fats that are included in—as well as the fats that are excluded from—the plans. Both diets are generous in fish that are high in protein but low in saturated fat. Fish also contains important chemicals that provide critical health benefits. Fish and seafood, particularly fatty cold-water fish such as salmon, halibut, and mackerel, are abundant sources of powerful cardioprotective compounds called omega-3 fatty acids. Studies have shown that even one serving of fish each week will help protect you from stroke and heart attack and can lower your risk of colon, breast, and prostate cancer. Doctors also report that omega-3s help relieve the pain and inflammation of rheumatoid arthritis.

A landmark Italian study evaluated a group of about eleven thousand people who had survived a heart attack within the preceding three months. The patients were divided into four equal groups. Participants in one group were given 850mg of omega-3 fatty acids daily, while a second group took 300mg of vitamin E. A third was given both nutrients, while a fourth group was given a placebo. The results were astonishing! People taking the omega-3 supplements had a 20 percent reduction in total mortality and a 45 percent reduction in sudden cardiac death, regardless of their vitamin E intake. How can that be?

Omega-3 fats contain two types of essential fatty acids—eicosapentaenoic acid (EPA) and docosahexaenoic acid (DHA). Essential fatty acids are just that: essential. EFAs are chemicals that your body needs in order to make hormones and other compounds necessary for life itself. EFAs, which cannot be manufactured by your body, penetrate tenacious layers of cholesterol-laden plaque, soothe inflamed blood vessels, and prevent blood clots from attaching to the lining of coronary arteries. We'll look at my EFA recommendations in more detail in the "Diet Update" section of Chapter 4. But for now just know that EFAs have two very important cardioprotective properties: They've been noted to prevent spasm of the coronary artery vessels and to prevent the rupture of unstable arterial plaques.

OMEGA-3 FATTY ACIDS IN FISH AND SHELLFISH
Not all fish are created equal. Fish are an important part of the PAMM diet because they are so rich in coenzyme Q_{10} and precious omega-3 fats that help reduce blood pressure, inflammation, and clotting. One fish meal a week can cut your risk of sudden death in half! But one word of caution: Not everything that swims is healthy. With all the pollution in today's waters, I'd steer you to the fish below.

These statistics reflect the amount of good fat in 100g of some of the most popular fish.

Salmon, Atlantic*	2.50g	Flounder or sole*	0.56g
Anchovy, canned* in		Crab, canned, drained*	0.36g
olive oil, drained	2.11g	Shrimp*	0.35g
Salmon, pink, canned*	1.76g	Tuna, yellow fin*	0.31g
Salmon, sockeye*	1.42g	Tuna, light, canned	
Mackerel, Atlantic*	1.42g	in water**	0.28g
Swordfish**	1.06g	Mackerel, Pacific*	0.27g
Tuna, white, canned		Haddock*	0.27g
in water**	0.95g	Cod, Atlantic*	0.17g
Halibut*	0.67g	Lobster, northern**	0.09g
Trout, sea*	0.58g		

*Indicates these fish/shellfish are safe to eat two or three times a week.

**Indicates these fish/shellfish are safe to eat once every two months being higher in pollutants.

However, omega-3 fatty acids are not the only health-promoting nutrients that you'll find in fish. Fish is also a great source of coenzyme Q10, a vitamin-like nutrient that has been shown to lower blood pressure by reducing oxidative stress in blood vessels that have been damaged by free radicals. I'll be giving you more information on coenzyme Q10 in Chapter 3.

The Mediterranean diet is also rich in another essential fatty acid: alpha-linolenic acid (ALA). Found in high amounts in nuts and a leafy green vegetable called purslane (which grows wild in Greece), alpha-linolenic acid can be transformed in small amounts of the omega-3 fatty acids DHA and EPA. Walnuts and flaxseed are naturally good sources of alpha-linolenic acid, and I use them frequently in the menus of this eight-week programme.

Many doctors also credit the enhanced longevity and health patterns of the Mediterranean people to the large quantity of olive oil in their daily meals. Epidemiological studies have demonstrated that those consuming a significant amount of olive oil have much lower rates of heart disease and breast cancer, while other research points to benefits for arthritis and diabetes. Great stuff, huh? And it's all there on your plate—if you follow the PAMM Diet!

And there's more. Research conducted in Spain indicates that olive oil may help prevent colon cancer, while studies from the Harvard School of Public Health suggest that women who use olive oil more than once a day are at 25 percent less risk of developing breast cancer. On a molecular level, scientists have discovered that the cardioprotective effect of olive oil may be due to its impact on LDL cholesterol.

HEALTH FACTS ABOUT OLIVE OIL
- Olive oil contains flavonoids and polyphenols, potent antioxidants that help prevent free radicals. Polyphenols support immune function and healthy blood pressure. Ten grams of extra virgin olive oil contain 5 mg of polyphenols.
- Olive oil is high in squalene, an important immune protective factor. The average American consumes 30mg of squalene daily, whereas people in Mediterranean countries typically take in 200–400mg/day. Studies show that olive oil may help reduce the incidence of colon and skin cancers. Also, Greek and Spanish women have a far lower incidence of breast cancer than American women.

- Just one tablespoon of olive oil provides you with 8 percent of the RDA for vitamin E. Olive oil also contains a high percentage of monounsaturated oleic acid, a fatty acid that reduces LDL ("bad") cholesterol and increases HDL ("good") cholesterol.

Here's a little background on what's happening, so you'll understand why the PAMM Diet is so key to heart health. Everyone probably knows by now that there are basically two forms of cholesterol—the "good" HDL cholesterol and the "bad" LDL cholesterol. The higher your LDL ("bad") cholesterol, the greater the risk of coronary artery disease.

Actually, there's a bit of *somewhat* good news. We now realize that LDL cholesterol isn't dangerous in its own right. It's only when LDL cholesterol becomes oxidized that it becomes a danger to your circulatory system. Once allowed to oxidize in reactions with free radicals, LDL molecules will irritate the walls of your arteries, making them puffy and inflamed, thereby promoting the development of fatty streaks that cling to their surface. You then have artery-blocking plaque that impedes coronary blood flow. Left untreated, this plaque will eventually close off the affected artery entirely, leading to angina, and possibly heart attacks or strokes. But even if your LDL is high, you can help block this negative effect with antioxidants.

GOOD FATS, BAD FATS, AND KILLER FATS

The very low levels of unhealthy fats consumed in the Mediterranean diet boost the health benefits of olive oil. Chemically, fats and oils are made up of chains of carbon atoms edged with hydrogen and oxygen atoms. When the carbon chain is completely filled with hydrogen, it is a saturated fat, such as butter. When the chain is missing two hydrogen atoms, it's a monounsaturated fat, such as olive oil. If the carbon chain is missing four or more hydrogen atoms, then the fat is said to be polyunsaturated, as in the case of corn oil. Each type of fat has different properties and therefore different effects on your body. Saturated fats, which are solid at room temperature, are found primarily in animal products like marbled meats. High saturated fat intake has been linked to heart disease, hypertension, stroke, and diabetes, as well as breast and ovarian cancer.

On a cellular level, scientists have determined that unsaturated fats, such as peanut oil, contain arachidonic acid, which sets into motion a cascade of biochemical events that raise your blood pressure and block your body's arteries. Arachidonic acid is highly inflammatory and is also produced by the body in response to free radicals generated by the oxidation of saturated fats found in meats. Several fatty acids convert to arachidonic acid in the body.

The Mediterranean and Asian diets are very low in saturated fats. Red meat and full-fat dairy products (such as cheese and cream) are eaten infrequently and in very small portions. In the PAMM programme, I follow this very healthy pattern. Lean beef, pork, and lamb should be on the menu only once or twice a week and only in small portions. Substitute fat-free milk for whole milk and cream, and avoid butter, sour cream, and most types of cheese.

Polyunsaturated fats from vegetable sources such as corn oil, safflower oil, and canola oil were once the darlings of nutritionists because of their ability to lower LDL cholesterol. Unfortunately, they also lower HDL, the "good" cholesterol. Even more troubling, polyunsaturated fats become oxidized faster than you can say "Rumplestiltskin", making your body's cells more vulnerable to degenerative diseases such as cataracts, cancer, Alzheimer's disease, and heart disease.

To make matters even worse, the hydrogenated polyunsaturated fats that you'll find in processed foods such as margarine and commercial baked goods turn themselves into trans fatty acids almost in the blink of an eye. Hydrogenation is adding extra hydrogen atoms to make the fat more solid at room temperature and also to extend shelf life. Trouble is the trans fats can increase Lp(a) in the blood. This kind of fat actually rockets your risk of heart disease and certain types of cancers. Trans fats are entirely absent in the fresh, natural diets of Greece, Italy, and Asian countries such as Japan, so I urge you to follow their example by substituting healthier fats such as olive oil and sesame oil.

As part of my PAMM programme, I include 1 to 2 Tbsp. of olive oil each day, to be used in salad dressings or as a condiment for vegetables and grain dishes. Small amounts of olive oil can be used in cooking, but remember that heat damages the health-enhancing compounds in the oil, so uncooked olive oil is best.

OLIVE OIL NUTRITION FACTS (ALL VARIETIES)
Serving size: 1 Tbsp. (15ml)

Calories: 120	Fat Calories 120
	% Daily Value*
Total Fat 14g	22%
Saturated fat 2g	10%
Polyunsaturated fat 1.5g	
Monounsaturated fat 10g	
Cholesterol 0mg	0%
Sodium 0mg	0%
Protein 0g	0%

CULINARY TIPS

- Light or extra-light olive oil has the highest smoke point, meaning that you can heat it gently. It's good for stir-frying, frying, or even baking. Olive oil seals in the flavour while producing a thin, greaseless crust.
- Extra-virgin olive oil has the *lowest* smoke point and is best used in light sautéing, drizzled on cooked foods, and for salad dressings.
- Brush extra-virgin olive oil over fish, meats, or vegetables to seal in flavour and juices when grilling. The antioxidants in olive oil protect against the adverse effects of grilling, but remember to limit your grilling in general. Charcoal-grilled meats, especially chicken, have higher amounts of carcinogens in their flesh.
- In baking, the tocopherols (vitamin E) are antioxidants. They also help keep baked goods fresher for a longer period of time. Light olive oil contains fewer tocopherols than extra-virgin oil, but it has less olive oil taste and allows the flavour of other ingredients to come through.
- Drizzle light olive oil over air-popped popcorn for a more satisfying flavour.
- Fill a kitchen spray bottle with light or extra-light olive oil and use instead of nonstick baking sprays.

USING OLIVE OIL IN PLACE OF BUTTER OR MARGARINE

If the recipe calls for this much butter/margarine:	Use this much olive oil:
240g	180ml (6fl oz)
180g	160ml (4–5fl oz)
120g	70ml (2.5fl oz)
80g	60ml (2 fl oz)
60g	45ml (1½fl oz)
15g	11ml (⅜fl oz)
10g	6.5ml (¼fl oz)
5g	3.75ml (⅛fl oz)

COMPLEX VERSUS SIMPLE CARBOHYDRATES: IT'S NOT THAT SIMPLE

For many years, carbohydrates were divided into two groups: simple carbohydrates (such as sugar and honey) and complex carbohydrates (such as wheat and corn). Simple carbs were considered inherently bad because they packed on the pounds, caused dental cavities, and failed to offer any real benefits.

Complex carbohydrates were considered the good guys, because they were believed to be absorbed more slowly. Most doctors, including myself, recommended generous servings of complex carbohydrates at every meal. We were well intentioned, but we were only half right.

Now, rather than looking at sugars as either simple or complex, we've learned to rate carbohydrates based on the way they affect your blood sugar levels, using a chart known as the glycemic index. A food's glycemic index (GI) is a numerical value that reflects the rate at which its sugars enter your bloodstream. Every food is given a value from 1 to 100. Pure glucose, which has the quickest rate of absorption, has a glycemic index of 100. I like to think of it as pure jet fuel—100 percent combustible.

Foods such as pretzels, potatoes, and biscuits have a GI of over 80 and are considered high-glycemic-index items. Foods such as wholemeal and brown rice fall into the 55–70 range, placing them in the moderate-glycemic-index category. Fresh fruits and vegetables, such as cherries, broccoli, apples, and lentils, are considered low-glycemic-index sources, with a GI between 18 and 55.

THE GLYCEMIC INDEX
The higher your blood sugar, the faster you age. Reducing daily sugar intake lowers cholesterol and triglycerides, promotes weight loss, increases energy, and reduces the risk of degenerative diseases such as diabetes and heart disease.

The best way to keep insulin and blood sugar levels low is to eat carbohydrates that rank low on the glycemic index, which indicates the rate at which carbohydrates break down into sugars that enter the bloodstream. Foods with a high glycemic index (greater than 70) release glucose into the bloodstream quickly, causing a rapid rise in blood sugar and subsequent rise in insulin. Low-glycemic-index foods (less than 55) usually contain more fibre and release glucose into the blood stream at a slower rate.

If you are vulnerable to insulin resistance, you must be especially careful of carbohydrates that can cause blood sugar to soar. Among the worst offenders are beer (which contains maltose), bread, rice, bagels, crackers, pasta, potatoes, corn and processed cereals, especially Corn Flakes and Rice Krispies. When you do eat high-glycemic-index foods, be sure to mix them with healthy fats, protein and lower-glycemic-index carbs so you can prevent insulin spikes. You'll preserve your insulin response, increase your HDL ("good") cholesterol, and protect your blood vessels.

High-Glycemic-Index Foods (GI>70)

Glucose	100	Waffles	76
Baked potato*	93	Chips	75
Red-skinned potato*	88	Digestive biscuits	75
Corn Flakes	84	Raisin Bran Flakes	73
Pretzels	83	Short-grain white rice	72
Rice Krispies	82	Bagel	72
Jelly beans	80	Watermelon*	72
Vanilla wafers	77	Corn chips	72
Rye bread	76		

Moderate-Glycemic-Index Foods (GI 55–70)

White bread	70	Shortbread	64
Wholemeal bread	69	Beetroot*	64
Shredded Wheat	67	New potatoes*	62
Melon*	65	Ice cream	61
Sucrose	65	Long-grain white rice	56
Raisins*	64	Brown rice	55
Oatmeal biscuits	55	Bananas	55
Sweet corn	55	Popcorn	55

Low-Glycemic-Index Foods (GI<55)

Stone-ground wholemeal bread	53	Plums	39
Sourdough bread	52	Meat ravioli	39
Kiwi fruit	52	Pears	38
All-Bran with extra fibre	51	Apples	38
Pumpernickel bread	51	Flavoured low-fat yogurt	33
Chocolate	49	Chickpeas	33
Oatmeal	49	Skimmed milk	32
Green peas	48	Egg fettuccine	32
Baked beans	48	Dried apricots	31
Orange juice (fresh)	46	Lentils	30
Grapes	46	Whole milk	27
Bran Buds with psyllium (see p 282)	45	Kidney beans	27
Oranges	44	Cherries	22
Apple juice (fresh in season)	40	Peanuts	14

* These foods have other benefits, such as a high antioxidant level. Don't avoid them just because of the glycemic index value.

High-glycemic-index foods surge quickly into your blood stream, rapidly shooting up your blood sugar. And your body reacts with equal speed, signaling your pancreas to crank out insulin to lock that free-floating glucose into its appropriate receptor sites on the outsides of the cells. As your blood sugar levels soar, your metabolism tries to keep up with the pace, pouring out more and more insulin.

In the short term, these high insulin levels encourage your body to store excess carbohydrates as fat. As the needle on your scale goes up, your body becomes less and less responsive to insulin (which is called insulin resistance), and your weight creeps even higher. This vicious circle leads to carbohydrate cravings, crashing your efficiency for burning carbs and leading to more insulin resistance, more weight gain . . . and eventually higher blood pressure.

The long-term effects of this scenario are even more troubling. Consistently high levels of circulating insulin damage your insulin receptor sites, making it increasingly difficult for your body to utilize glucose. The extra insulin tends to increase adrenaline levels, promote atherosclerotic plaques, increase blood clotting, and constrict blood vessels—all of which increase blood pressure. Increased adrenaline levels can impair the metabolism of the cells lining your blood vessels, and that can raise your blood pressure.

Thirty years ago, when I was in medical school, we were taught that 80 percent of hypertension was of unknown origin, or what doctors call "idiopathic". I now believe that in many cases where we can't find the root cause of high blood pressure, the underlying physiology has to do with insulin resistance.

The PAMM programme is rich in low-glycemic-index foods such as green vegetables, tomatoes, fish, and legumes, as well as monounsaturated fats that don't elicit an insulin response. Not surprisingly, high-glycemic-index foods are used only infrequently on the PAMM diet. I believe that the insulin-protective aspects of the PAMM programme make it the most effective blood-pressure-lowering and weight-loss programme I have ever encountered. The low-glycemic-index foods found on this programme help your body avoid overshooting your insulin production and developing insulin resistance.

TIP OF THE DAY
Perhaps the most important finding in treating hypertension in the last three decades is understanding the phenomenon of insulin resistance, a condition that can be reversed only with diet and exercise.

DON'T DRINK YOUR MILK

We all grow up being told to drink lots and lots of calcium-rich fresh milk to build strong bones and teeth, right? Doctors believed that two to four servings of milk daily were essential for healthy development. However, the increased fat and sodium content of most dairy products was something we didn't need to sink our teeth into. This way of eating raised our cholesterol levels and increased our risk of heart disease.

There's relatively little fresh cow's milk in Mediterranean areas such as Greece, or in Asian countries like Japan where the intake of saturated fat from cheese and cream is very low. Greeks are simply stingy with their use of dairy products, using only small amounts of feta and kasseri cheeses or fresh unflavoured yogurt as dairy choices. The Japanese consume very little dairy—80 percent of Japanese, in fact, are lactose-intolerant, meaning they cannot easily digest lactose, the sugar found in milk products.

To get yourself a healthy milk alternative, try drinking soya milk. If you like your tea or coffee light, then use small amounts of fat-free milk or give your body an additional health boost with soya milk. Avoid all types of full-fat dairy foods, including cream cheese, sour cream, and whipped cream. I'm not a fan of the so-called low-fat cheeses because they're high in chemicals and sodium. Some even contain those dreaded trans fatty acids. Read those food labels, and, to satisfy your cheese cravings, look for soya cheese, especially kinds made with limited amounts of salt.

THE XO FACTOR

It's actually the homogenization of milk that makes it unhealthy. This process creates very small compounds that get inside blood vessels, causing injury. One of these, xanthine oxidase or XO, causes inflammation and injury to your blood vessels. Even though xanthine oxidase is an enzyme involved in the conversion of uric acid, the consumption of bovine xanthine oxidase has been associated with atherosclerosis in humans. My advice is to limit your homogenized milk products (whole milk, skimmed and semi-skimmed milk).

I recommend that you do as I do: Limit or eliminate your intake of cow's milk, and substitute soya milk instead. If you must have the taste of milk in your coffee and tea, then try a mixture of one-third pasteurized heavy cream and two-thirds skimmed milk. Even with the fat content of heavy cream, it's a safer choice than risking the havoc that XO can wreak with your blood vessels.

A WELCOME WEIGHT LOSS

If you're like most of my patients with high blood pressure, you're probably carrying around at least ten to fifteen more pounds than you should. It's estimated that every extra pound of fat requires over 5,000 miles of blood vessels to support it. And pumping blood to reach all that excess body fat requires extra work from your heart, an effort that's reflected in elevated blood pressure. The extra stress and strain that obesity places on your heart is what prompts doctors to urge their overweight hypertensive patients to lose weight.

While the PAMM programme is touted for its anticancer and cardio-protective benefits, it's also one of the most sensible, metabolically correct, and easy-to-follow weight loss programmes that I've ever seen. Even my patients who have tried and failed on every other diet plan have been thrilled to discover how easily they can drop those unwanted pounds on my healthy PAMM programme.

WHY CHANGE A GOOD THING?

The traditional Mediterranean-style diet is based on the eating habits of people living in the Mediterranean countries of Greece, Italy, and Spain. The problem with exporting this diet to the United States and northern Europe is that we tend to embrace only the parts of the plan that we like, such as the olive oil, bread, tomato sauce, and cheese, while ignoring the legumes, fruits, vegetables, and fresh fish. If you simply add olive oil and bread to your usual diet, all you're likely to get is an increase in cholesterol and a wider waistline. Remember olive oil does contain small amounts of saturated fat that can translate into higher cholesterol levels so less is more!

Dining more regularly at your favourite Italian or Greek place doesn't necessarily mean that you're eating like a southern European. As I studied the nutritional components of this diet, I recognized important opportunities for new health benefits. On the downside, the traditional Mediterranean diet contains generous servings of white bread, pasta, and rice. This level of carbohydrates concerned me, so I've sharply limited the ingestion of these items in my menus. In addition, I recommend that people with high blood pressure limit the amount of sodium in their diet. Let me tell you why.

AN OVERVIEW OF THE RESEARCH FINDINGS ON THE MEDITERRANEAN DIET
Helps prevent heart disease
- As compared with a typical Western diet, the traditional Mediterranean style of eating has been shown to predispose you to lower blood pressure.
- A number of large European and U.S. studies have shown beyond a doubt that a diet high in saturated fats—as is common in the United States and northern European countries—raises LDL cholesterol and is linked to a high incidence of coronary artery disease.

Supports healthy blood sugar
- Cross-cultural comparisons and studies on vegetarians show that a high intake of complex carbohydrates and dietary fibre—such as is found in the Mediterranean diet—and the low intake of saturated fats could lower the risk of insulin resistance and diabetes.
- The traditional Mediterranean diet meets all the demands of an adequate diabetes diet. That's because it's based on fibre-rich whole grains, legumes, and vegetables and is low in saturated fats. The absolute sugar content can be varied to individual needs. If you're diabetic or managing your sugar balance, then choose lower-glycemic-index grains, vegetables, and fruits.

Supports healthy inflammatory response
- Studies conducted on olive oil have shown that it can be beneficial in inflammatory and autoimmune diseases, such as rheumatoid arthritis.

Helps in weight management
- Low in saturated fat, but high in essential fatty acids, complex carbohydrates, and fibre, the Mediterranean diet gives you varied and delicious food options for optimum energy intake, and can protect against obesity.

A PINCH OF SALT MAKES THE MEDICINE GO DOWN

My PAMM programme limits the amount of salt used to season your daily meals. As you well know, a diet high in sodium will increase your water retention. This increased volume of fluid forces the heart to work harder to move blood through your body. In past decades, some doctors believed that, except for a small group of salt-sensitive people, sodium restriction wasn't important for hypertension control. I disagree. It's been my experience that my patients do better when I limit their intake of this mineral.

Taking the salt shaker off the table is the first step. But it's just that: a first step. It's estimated that the bulk of our sodium intake—a whopping 80 percent—is actually ingested from hidden sources. Virtually all packaged and prepared foods, such as frozen meals (even heart-healthy or dietetic ones), soups, ice cream, bread, canned vegetables, and pickles, carry a heavy salt payload.

In order to gauge their salt intake, I encourage my patients to keep a food diary for several days, and then go back and look up the sodium content of each item on their list. They're usually shocked to find that they've been consuming between 5 and 10g every day, without sprinkling a single grain of salt on their food! To bring hypertension under control, I advise them to limit their sodium intake to 2–3g a day.

TOP TEN FEATURES AND BENEFITS OF MY PAMM DIET

1. A cornucopia of fresh fruits and vegetables are loaded with antioxidants and other phytonutrients that are associated with a lower incidence of free-radical-induced diseases, including cancer, cardiovascular disease, premature ageing, and cataracts.
2. Cold-water fish such as mackerel, sardines, and salmon are packed with beneficial omega-3 essential fatty acids that reduce arterial clotting and inflammation. They're also excellent sources of coenzyme Q_{10}, an energy-boosting nutrient.
3. Low-glycemic-index legumes such as lentils, chickpeas, and soya beans provide vegetable protein without the insulin spike that can lead to hyperinsulinemia and its deadly offspring, heart disease, obesity, high blood pressure, and high LDL ("bad") cholesterol.
4. Nuts and seeds, including almonds, walnuts, and flaxseed, are rich in essential fatty acids and provide another healthy source of fats, protein, and fibre. Phytosterols are nutrients present in nuts and seeds that inhibit the body's ability to absorb dietary cholesterol.
5. Small quantities of dairy products and meat equate with less methionine, an amino acid precursor to homocysteine, which is associated with a higher risk of coronary heart disease, stroke, and peripheral vascular disease.
6. Low intake of saturated fats creates less arterial plaque—a major precursor to heart disease—and helps support a healthy weight.
7. High fibre intake from vegetables, fruits, whole grains, nuts, and seeds supports a healthy lower bowel and helps stabilize blood sugar by slowing the absorption of carbohydrates.
8. Liberal amounts of garlic and onions give you two terrific heart supporters noted for their antioxidant benefits.
9. The monounsaturated fat in olive oil supports a healthy cholesterol level and can help lower the risk of cardiovascular disease. It may also protect against certain cancers such as those of the colon and breast. Olive oil is a far healthier fat choice than margarine, which contains trans fatty acids.
10. Small amounts of red wine and/or green tea provide rich sources of health-promoting polyphenols, beneficial compounds that help protect against coronary heart disease.

THE PAN-ASIAN CONNECTION

The PAMM programme goes even further to add what I like to think of as the best of both worlds: an East-meets-West approach to eating that allows you to add some new foods with critical nutritional advantages to your diet. Many of these foods are popular in Japan, China, and Thailand. That's why these days I've come to describe my approach as a Pan-Asian Modified Mediterranean programme.

Along with appetizing fish, olive oil, fresh fruit, and vegetable selections from the Mediterranean plan, I've incorporated tasty soya and other healing foods such as flaxseed, Japanese mushrooms, and great moderate/low-glycemic-index grains such as spelt and brown rice. Each of these foods offers you powerful disease-fighting activity. For example, soya beans alone can lower your cholesterol and protect you against different types of cancer, especially cancers of the breast and prostate.

These foods are unusual in taste and texture, and scintillating to the palate. I strongly urge you to learn to use them for variety and additional health perks. Over the coming weeks, I'll be integrating them into your meal plans and explaining how to use them simply and deliciously. For example, in Week 3 I'll be introducing you to soya products in the form of tofu and easy-to-make, tasty soya shakes. Later on, I'll be introducing you to Japanese mushrooms—not just for their great flavour, but for their disease-protective benefits as well.

At times on your eight-week programme you may be dining out, so I encourage you to stay on the plan by dining at a Japanese eatery, an experience that may be new to some of you. Sometimes people associate Japanese food with raw fish dishes and so elect to dine elsewhere. But Japanese foods include all the healthy features of fresh fruits and vegetables, plus the exciting tastes of unique seasonings and soya products. For some tasty ideas on great Japanese selections that will help with blood pressure lowering, check out my favourite choices in the sidebar. If you get to feeling really adventurous, try the maki rolls, fish, crab, or shrimp. Cooked fish choices (if that's more to your liking) are also available.

DR. SINATRA'S TOP PICKS, JAPANESE STYLE

Green salad with ginger	Shiitake mushrooms
Tofu	Steamed broccoli with sesame seed oil
Okinawa pork	Seaweed and cucumber maki rolls
Omelette with spring onions	Green tea

PUTTING THEORY INTO PRACTICE

On my PAMM programme, I recommend that only 20 to 25 percent of your calories come from protein, 30 to 35 percent from healthy fat, and 45 to 50 percent from slow-burning, low-glycemic-index carbohydrates that include whole grains and fresh fruits and vegetables. For the average person, this breaks down to two to three servings of protein per day, 2 Tbsp. of olive oil, and five to seven servings of fruits, vegetables, nuts, and grains. And I must urge you to incorporate organic foods as much as possible into your diet, because there's absolutely *no* doubt that the pesticides, antibiotics, and hormones used to produce many foods are contributing to the wide range of diseases and disorders that plague us.

Whenever I raise the topic of changing to the PAMM programme with my patients, I can see a wave of concern come over their faces. I know that they're imagining the end of their favourite foods, such as chocolate, wine, and ice cream. But you know, I believe that there's a big difference between an ideal diet and a *real* one. In an ideal world, our diet would look like plateful after plateful of disease-fighting nutrients. The fact is that very few of us can stay on such an ideal diet. But this doesn't mean that you can't have small amounts of chocolate or wine to add a little taste and pleasure to your foods. Completely denying yourself these foods can doom any diet to failure, but allowing a small portion may actually help you stay on the programme.

For example, if you're a chocoholic, then having a bite of bittersweet chocolate at the end of your meal twice or maybe three times a week will allow you a moment of satisfaction and pleasure, and it will allow you to believe you've had a real treat without sacrificing the strides you've made on your healthy meal plan. Remember, small and infrequent portions of your favourite but less healthy food choices can be a great way to reward yourself at planned intervals. But do remember that I said "small"; portion size is key if you want to be successful, so savour a few delicious morsels of your favourite taste sensations! Similarly, a glass of wine one or two times a week will provide the same kind of emotional and psychological pleasures that will keep you on a healthy dietary routine.

I know this diet can work for you as well as it has for me and my patients, because it's one you can *live* with! Each week I'm going to be easing you into more and more aspects of the PAMM programme. In the first week I will give you the foods that you are most used to eating and that are easily available in American and northern European coffee shops, restaurants, and supermarkets. Over the following seven weeks, as you build on your nutritional knowledge and your dietary expertise, you will be adding new foods and changing food habits. But this first week, I just want you to feel comfortable and familiar with this new approach. There are a lot of new pieces of information to absorb, as well as new ways of preparing and eating foods. You can't make all these changes at once and be successful. I've laid it out for you, step by step, so you'll be able to change the way you eat.

For example, in this first week, you'll find meal plans advising that you select whole-grain toast for breakfast, and sandwiches on whole-grain bread or pitta for lunch. This number of bread selections will gradually be tapered down each week as we move you to other low-glycemic-index carbohydrate choices. The first week, your primary goal is to focus on eliminating the biggest problem foods in the Western diet: saturated fats, sodium, heavily processed foods, and sugary snacks and desserts.

KITCHEN CLEAN-UP: THE FIRST STEP

To help you stay on the programme, take the time this first week to set up your PAMM kitchen. To do this, you're going to need to throw out the foods that will sabotage your diet, and replace them with healthy foods that will naturally lower your blood pressure. So take the phone off the hook, put on your favourite music to clean by, grab a few rubbish bags, a bucket of soapy water, and a sponge, and let's get serious!

Open that refrigerator door, grab sugary condiments such as jams, jellies, and cranberry sauce, and toss them! These are high-glycemic-index foods, and they're going to provoke those high insulin levels that will drive up your blood pressure. Pour out the last of the full-fat milk and throw away any opened containers of fruit juice and regular soft drinks. You won't be needing any of them.

Now start tossing out those bad fats. This means hard cheeses (Parmesan is okay), margarine, mayonnaise, flavoured sweetened yogurt, sour cream, and bacon. Out they all go . . . even those low fat cheeses! Ditch that leftover packet of fried chicken, the prawn-fried rice, and anything that looks even remotely like luncheon meat.

Now get ready to raid the freezer. Be bold! That French-bread pizza? Low-calorie chicken dinner? Out! If you check the sodium content on the product labels, each small serving probably contains more than about half of the recommended daily allowance for sodium. They're also loaded with high-glycemic-index carbohydrates that you can't afford if you're serious about controlling your blood pressure without medication. Make a clean sweep! Now's the time to toss out that frozen pasta that you've stored away "for emergencies". With the freezer nice and empty, you'll be able to fill it with fresh poultry and unseasoned frozen vegetables.

After you've finished going through the refrigerator and freezer, it's time to restock your kitchen with a bounty of healthy foods. And you're going to need plenty of space to store these delicious, fresh blood-pressure-lowering choices, so let's move on to the pantry.

ATTACKING THE KITCHEN CABINETS

As a start, you can head straight for those boxes and boxes of cereals. For the first meal of the day, the last thing you want is a so-called healthy cereal loaded with everything that you don't want to eat, including trans fatty acids, sugars, and preservatives. Pick up each box and read the label carefully. If the first or second ingredient is sugar, toss it! Keep your shredded wheat and old-fashioned oatmeal for healthy, blood-pressure-lowering breakfasts.

Now sort through those containers of "white" stuff: white rice, white flour, white sugar, pasta made with white flour, instant mashed potatoes, crackers, bread crumbs from white bread, cake mixes with white flour, jelly powder, and pudding mixes—even those sugar-free and fat-free foods. Turn to the canned goods and boxes, chucking cans of soup, pizza mix, and any canned fruits, vegetables, pastas, and salsas. The same fate awaits your jars and cans of juice, except for tomato and low-sodium V8. Give away those fancy gourmet sun-dried tomatoes—even if they are packed in olive oil, they are probably saturated with sodium and preservatives. Eliminate all bottles of oil except flaxseed and extra-virgin olive oil.

Save the sweetest job for last. Don't even think about keeping sugar for company! They don't need the insulin blast from simple sweeteners any more than you do. Don't stop with the white sugar. Be equally ruthless with brown sugar and artificial sweeteners. Keep only pure honey and maple syrup in your PAMM kitchen. They are the healthiest ways to sweeten, and certainly far healthier than the artificial sweeteners, which actually tend to raise your blood pressure.

Take one last look for foods to get rid of. Look for boxes of drink mix, squashes, hot chocolate, flavoured coffees, and jars of chocolate syrup, as well as the "salties": crisps, pretzels, and salted nuts.

RESTOCKING THE PAMM KITCHEN

Now for the real fun! Let me accompany you to the supermarket to fill your kitchen with great-tasting, fresh foods that will keep your weight and your blood pressure in check. Grab a big shopping trolley and head down the dairy aisle. If you must have milk, look for organic skimmed milk. Then pick up some plain low-fat organic yogurt, soya milk, organic fresh eggs, and fat-free cottage cheese, as well as chunks of imported Parmesan cheese. In a few weeks you'll want to add a small block of feta or a package of soya cheese, but for now we're just going to cover the basics.

Next, wheel your trolley over to the produce aisle. Look for fresh lemons, dark green lettuce, broccoli, spinach, blueberries, melons, tomatoes, cucumbers, onions, garlic, and celery. When they're in season, stock up on shiny purple aubergine and brilliant red and green peppers. Try to buy as much organic produce as possible. Still staying on the periphery of the supermarket, park yourself at the butcher's section. Ask for skinless and boneless chicken breasts, and toss in a boneless turkey breast. Make sure you're buying poultry that hasn't received any antibiotics or hormones, such as free-range chicken and turkey. When you get home you can divide the poultry into individual portions and store them in the freezer. With these low-fat proteins tucked away, you'll never be at a loss for a healthy main course.

Stop at the fishmonger for tonight's dinner. Fish needs to be eaten when it's very fresh, and it's always best to purchase it the day you plan to eat it. Freezing damages the flavour and texture of fish, so avoid freezing fish at all costs. I'll bet it's frozen fish that has given fish its bad reputation with some people.

Until now, you've stayed safely on the perimeter of the supermarket. The interior aisles hold many of those tempting foods you want to avoid, including processed foods, breads, white breads, biscuits, snacks, and diet drinks. Walking quickly, let's pick up some old-fashioned oatmeal, some packages of green tea, and a bottle of extra-virgin olive oil. In the canned vegetable section, stock up on no-salt-added beans, including black beans, kidney beans, chickpeas, and soya beans.

Add to your shopping trolley cans of whole tomatoes, unseasoned tomato sauce, and crushed tomatoes, preferably processed without additional sodium. Look for cans of salmon and sardines packed in olive oil or water. Avoid canned fish packed in vegetable oil or sunflower oil. Be sure to include cans of no-salt-added chicken stock, which can be used to add healthy flavour to soups and sauces. Mustards, both grainy and smooth, are another wonderful source of flavour, provided they do not contain sugars. Choose a selection of vinegars, including red wine, tarragon and balsamic, to add variety to your salads.

The natural seasonings of the Mediterranean are bursting with incredible flavour and fragrance and won't add a grain of salt and/or a pinch of sugar to your diet. Stock up on fresh basil, oregano, bay leaf, marjoram, thyme, rosemary, and fennel. My motto is: Fresh is always better, for taste and nutrition. Yum! You can use these herbs and seasonings in dried form as well, but they are *much* tastier when they're fresh. And what aromatherapy for your kitchen! But all of you may not have a shop near you that has such a wide selection of fresh herbs, so buy the dried form if that's all that's available. And remember to avoid prepared combinations such as "Italian seasoning" or "lemon pepper marinade", which are often sky high in sodium. Check the labels.

Asian seasonings are equally important. Look for dried herbs and spices including coriander seeds, cardamom pods, cumin, ground ginger, sesame seeds, cloves, and Szechuan peppercorns. Steer clear of condiments such as hoisin sauce, mango chutney, and fish sauce, all of which contain large amounts of salt and/or sugar.

When you get home, put everything away. Stand back and check through your supplies. Put the dairy items in one part of your refrigerator, the vegetables in the bottom part, and the fruits on the middle shelves. To preserve freshness, don't wash fruits or vegetables until you're ready to eat. Okay, relax. Now you're ready to begin.

3 Magical Nutritionals and Phytonutrients Week 2

This week, we're going to look at the role that antioxidants, vitamins, and minerals play in lowering your blood pressure. One commonly asked question that I address every day in my practice is "What supplements are best for reducing hypertension and lowering my risk for heart disease?" Let me share with you what I tell the people who travel to my surgery for a consultation.

We know that smoking cigarettes and consuming trans fatty acids, alcohol and high-glycemic-index foods place us at risk for high blood pressure. What is less well known is that these health-threatening behaviours share a common denominator at the cellular level: They all provoke the development of free radicals.

Free radicals are oxygen molecules with an unpaired electron. They are not happy molecules. They crash around the cells, looking for an extra electron to provide the stability they crave. In the process, they tear into fragile cell walls, preventing waste products from getting out and blocking nutrients and oxygen from getting in. Once inside the cell, free radicals become irritants that can disrupt DNA replication and provoke a wild inflammatory response that injures blood vessel walls. Research shows that this injury causes spasm and constriction, tightening up blood vessels and causing blood pressure surges. As by-products of normal metabolism, free radicals are a kind of cellular trash. These molecules are constantly produced during everyday activities such as digesting food, walking in the sun, or even fighting off infection.

FREE RADICALS AND YOUR BLOOD PRESSURE

Scientists now believe that free radicals contribute to high blood pressure by triggering a kind of response-to-injury cascade of events that includes the release of an adrenaline-like substance that constricts blood vessels. This reaction is almost like a stealth fight-or-flight response that stimulates the heart muscle to pump more forcefully.

A typical physiological stress response includes the constriction of blood vessels to prevent excessive bleeding in case of injury, the shunting of blood away from nonessential organs such as the stomach, and the shifting of blood to critical areas such as the brain, heart, and skeletal muscles. The body also shuts down urine production, which in turn increases blood volume—another threat to blood pressure levels. All of this prepares us for survival—to ward off the enemy or to escape. These typical fight-or-flight reactions can be lifesaving in an emergency, but confronting saber-toothed tigers several times a day at the office or at home will have destructive effects. Living with chronic stress fans the fires of hypertension by causing an excessive free-radical load.

THE MYSTERY OF NITRIC OXIDE

Free radicals also do major damage by inactivating nitric oxide—a key, newly discovered pathway in the regulation of blood pressure.

Nitric oxide (NO) plays a role in a number of disorders that include congestive heart failure, arteriosclerosis, muscular dystrophy, circulatory shock, and male sexual dysfunction. For now, let's just focus on how the NO pathway in your body contributes to blood pressure lowering.

NO is produced by an enzyme called nitric oxide synthase (NOS) when the amino acid L-arginine is oxidized and converted to L-citrulline. It's quite a complicated process, but suffice it to say that the end result is that NO is believed to reduce blood pressure—and the tone in your vasomotor system, which relaxes blood vessels—by both a direct action and an indirect effect. NO works *directly* as a vasodilator, and *indirectly* by blocking the part of your sympathetic nervous system (part of your central nervous system) that sometimes constricts your blood vessels (a good move if you've just been badly cut).

Animal research on nitric oxide is encouraging. Even essentially normotensive mice engineered to overexpress the gene involved in NOS production had mean blood pressure levels 18 mm Hg lower than baseline. There are also interesting results in the rat model. In spontaneously hypertensive rats, one intravenous injection of the DNA material that encodes eNOS almost completely normalized blood pressure for five to six weeks. I predict you'll be hearing more about this in the future.

It may be that if we can find ways to help the body produce sufficient NO, we may discover a potential new form of anti-hypertensive therapy. And that makes total sense to me. I've been working the NO angle for years now. Let me tell you why.

You see, I know that one benefit of having my patients use L-arginine as part of their blood-pressure-lowering supplement plan (I'll address this in more detail later) is that it encourages NO production and subsequent vasodilation. Let's look at an example that many people can relate to. Consider the popular drug Viagra. Have you ever wondered exactly how it works?

Like L-arginine, Viagra stimulates the production of nitric oxide and is known for its ability to help the penis fill with blood, thus becoming erect. But there can be side effects, such as nasal stuffiness and headache when other local blood vessels become swollen, too. And if Viagra is taken with cardiac drugs, excessive vasodilation may occur, with possible serious consequences. I've encouraged my cardiac patients to take extra arginine instead to improve their love life. Although it is less potent, there are no dangerous side effects.

Deaths on Viagra have been reported, and some of you may have wondered which cardiac patients are at risk, and how death can occur. Because of its effect on nitric oxide production, Viagra is a potent vasodilator, helping the penis fill with blood. But if Viagra is taken with other medications that lower blood pressure, there is serious risk of blood pressure suddenly dropping too low, which can cause the collapse of the circulatory system and cardiac arrest. An especially dangerous combination is taking nitroglycerine under the tongue, as it's used for angina, when Viagra is in your system. Be aware that Viagra can affect your circulation for up to four hours after ingestion.

It would now seem that we're realizing that NO production is another effect of some of the cardiac medication that you may be taking. For instance, both HMG-CoA reductase inhibitors (statin drugs) and exercise have been noted to increase endothelial NOS (eNOS) in blood vessel walls. This may explain the blood-pressure-lowering effects of exercise. Some angiotensin-converting enzyme (ACE) inhibitors mentioned in Chapter 1 act by breaking down bradykinin, resulting in a receptor-mediated activation of eNOS that improves vasodilation. In fact, it may explain why many women have normal blood pressure until they hit the menopause.

Indeed, fully understanding the NO mystery and how it relates to hypertension may be one vital breakthrough in treating people with high blood pressure in the next few years. Later we will learn about the use of supplements in enhancing NO levels in blood vessels.

Nitrates are a class of drugs commonly used in cardiology to relax and expand coronary arteries—even the aorta. This vasodilatory effect helps lower the workload of the heart, making nitrates appropriate in the treatment of congestive heart failure (CHF) and angina. They may even be used in combination with other cardiac medications to lower blood pressure. Though nitrates aren't first-line antihypertensives, many doctors select them for hypertensive patients who also have CHF and angina. It's the two-for-the-price-of-one effect, so to speak—a drug that can treat two conditions at the same time. The benefits: fewer side effects, enhanced cost-effectiveness, improved compliance, and increased patient satisfaction. Most doctors consider all these factors, as well as others, when selecting medications.

HOW WE FIGHT THE FREE-RADICAL ONSLAUGHT

Our bodies have a natural defence against free radicals. The body produces elaborate enzyme systems—involving chemicals such as catalase and superoxide dismutase—that stop free-radical carnage by interacting with the out-of-control molecules and offering them the electron they so desperately crave. Once neutralized, the free radical ceases to be a problem. Foods containing large amounts of antioxidants (coenzyme Q10 and vitamins A, C, and E, to mention a few) can assist the body in this battle.

Under ideal conditions your body's level of free radicals is neutralized by the antioxidants you consume in your diet and what your body can make. But we don't live in an ideal environment. Each year we seem to be bombarded with more and more toxins as our environment becomes more polluted. Each day we are exposed to an assault of new elements that provoke the development of billions and billions of free radicals during every twenty-four-hour period.

Excessive exposure to the ultraviolet radiation in sunlight, cigarette smoke, trans fatty acids, air pollution, strenuous exercise, and everyday pharmaceuticals all provoke the production of more free radicals than the body is prepared to handle. Even more troubling is that as we age, our bodies are less able to maintain those elaborate antioxidant enzyme systems, so the damage of free radicals builds as the years go by.

In the first week of my natural approach to blood pressure lowering, you started off with the diet. This week, we are going to start using targeted nutritional supplements, beginning with my core programme. We will start off with the holy trinity of antioxidants—vitamins A, C, and E. We are also going to add three minerals that are at least as important to antioxidant protection—calcium, magnesium, and potassium. To round off this week, I am going to add two important nutriceuticals—L-carnitine and coenzyme Q_{10}. You may not have heard of these before, but after a week you won't even be able to imagine how you ever got along without them.

VITAMINS

Vitamin A and Beta-Carotene

Vitamin A is essential for the development of healthy bones, mucous membranes, skin, and hair. You can find this nutrient primarily in fish oils and dairy products. Not only does it enhance your immune system, it's critical for the prevention of both night blindness and cataracts. Vitamin A helps protect your body from the free radicals that are produced by radiation and chemical pollutants. Because it's fat-soluble (stored in the body's fat reserves)—like vitamins D, E, and K—your body tends to store vitamin A, so be careful. You can overdose on this nutrient!

In large doses, vitamin A has been reported to cause liver damage and brain dysfunction. Very recent evidence suggests that even 5,000 international units (IU) of vitamin A per day from dietary sources for more than twenty years may increase the chance of hip fractures for women, so you don't want to overdose.

To ensure that you get the benefits of vitamin A without risking problems, I recommend provitamin A, the precursor to vitamin A that is commonly known as beta-carotene. Beta-carotene is the yellowish compound found in foods with yellow, orange, or dark green hues. A single serving of carrots, pumpkin, spinach, broccoli, or melon provides more than enough vitamin A for the entire day. It's no coincidence that the PAMM diet is rich in these antioxidant-packed foods.

Studies have shown that people eating foods high in beta-carotene have fewer heart attacks, and scientists report that this nutrient might help prevent colds and flu while offering a degree of lung protection from polluted city air. There are also a couple of other beta-carotene perks. Higher blood levels have been associated with a lower risk of prostate cancer, and boosted levels of beta-carotene in subcutaneous fat are associated with a lower incidence of heart disease for men.

But as health-promoting as it can be, beta-carotene, too, is not without a downside. Too much beta-carotene alone can be harmful to some populations, such as smokers and those individuals exposed to asbestos, greatly increasing their risk of developing lung cancer. So beta-carotene is not safe to take as a stand-alone kind of nutrient. To be on the safe side, incorporate other carotenoids, such as lycopene, lutein, and alpha-carotene, along with beta-carotene for additional protection against cancer, macular degeneration, and heart disease. Your most health-
promoting and cost-effective approach is a vitamin/mineral combination that contains vitamin A, its precursor beta-carotene, and a mix of other carotenoids, such as the ones I've just named. That's what I recommend to my patients, and that's what's included in your eight-week programme.

In the US the adult Recommended Daily Allowance (RDA) for vitamin A is 5,000 IU (1500µg retinol). And you can safely add to that the RDA dose of beta-carotene, which is also 5,000 IU (300µg carotene equivalent), for a total of 10,000 IU (2,000µg retinol equivalents).

But for complete antioxidant coverage, I like to reduce the vitamin A and increase the carotenoid combination. So I use either one of the following daily:

Vitamin A	2,500 IU (750µg retinol)
Beta-carotene with mixed carotenoids	7,500 IU (4,500µg carotene equivalents)
or	
Vitamin A from carotenoid complex containing alpha-carotene, beta-carotene, gamma-carotene, lycopene, zeaxanthin, cryptoxanthin, and lutein	10,000 IU (6,000µg carotene equivalents)

It's also important that you know several things interfere with vitamin A absorption. Those include antibiotics, antacids, excessive alcohol and caffeine intake, and some cholesterol-lowering drugs, as well as laxatives. People with low thyroid states, people who drink excessive quantities of alcohol (more than three to five drinks daily) and smokers should use beta-carotene supplements with caution. Taking beta-carotene supplements in amounts of more than 25,000 IU (15,000µg carotene equivalents) a day—which I don't recommend anyone do—may cause harm. As long as you stay within the guidelines we've discussed, then you'll get the most from your supplement programme without risking negative consequences.

Vitamin C

Vitamin C is a powerful antioxidant that's essential for tissue growth and repair. Found in citrus fruits and dark green leafy vegetables, vitamin C also plays an important role in the proper utilization and absorption of calcium and iron. When you are under emotional and psychological stress, vitamin C may become depleted. Therefore, vitamin C supplements are often administered to protect the body from the physical effects of prolonged stress. The impact of vitamin C on heart health is widespread and compelling. Studies have shown that low vitamin C intake is associated with increased risk of cardiac problems.

Vitamin C is also important in hypertension control. In a recent double-blind, placebo-controlled study of thirty-nine mildly hypertensive patients, 500mg of vitamin C were given as the only therapy for one month. Investigators reported the patients' systolic pressures to be lowered by 11mm Hg, while diastolic pressures were down 6mm Hg, significantly larger results than with placebo.

Although other small clinical studies of vitamin C's effect on blood pressure have shown mixed results, one thing is for sure: Antioxidants like vitamin C have a favourable impact in terms of knocking down levels of the treacherous superoxide radical, one of the most unguided free radicals. By increasing the production of chemical mediators such as nitric oxide, vitamin C has the potential to help lower your blood pressure while helping to protect the inner membranes of your blood vessels.

We have other data to support the notion that hypertensive people should be taking vitamin C. It's a known fact that many groups of people at risk for heart disease, especially those with high blood pressure—men, the elderly, smokers, diabetics, and some women on oral contraceptives—have lower levels of vitamin C. A British study evaluating the health of over twenty thousand people aged forty-five to seventy-five found that men and women who were consuming 109 to 113mg of vitamin C daily cut their risk of death in half compared to those who were only getting about 51 to 57mg a day.

Whether you are male or female, your blood level of vitamin C is directly related to your chance of dying from just about any natural cause. The lower your blood level, the greater your chances of death—especially from ischaemic heart disease.

There's only one caveat to taking vitamin C in amounts greater than 500mg daily: it could potentially bring about iron overload states. Vitamin C can help mobilize iron reserves, so should you have any hereditary diseases that cause this condition (such as hemochromatosis or thalassemia major), vitamin C should not be used in doses greater than 200mg per day. And because there are about thirty-five million people who carry the gene for hemochromatosis, I'm not a big believer in megadosing this nutrient.

Also, no one should be taking supplemental iron except young children, menstruating women, and those who have been prescribed iron for anaemia. Check your multivitamin/multimineral supplement for iron. Men especially can increase their risk of heart disease if their iron level is too high, and should never supplement it unless a doctor has ordered them to do so.

So, where can you find natural sources of this vitamin? Fresh produce such as citrus fruits and red peppers are naturally rich in vitamin C, but the actual vitamin payload available to you depends on the handling of the foods before they are eaten. Because it's so vulnerable to heat, cold, and exposure to the air, the real vitamin C content in the foods you eat can vary widely. Even if you eat a well-balanced diet, I recommend the safety-net range of 400 to 500mg in your vitamin C supplement each day.

To avoid upsetting your stomach, take this nutrient in divided doses. Spreading out your doses of vitamin C also helps keep your antioxidant blood levels even throughout the entire day. Just remember that vitamin C is water-soluble (it dissolves in water, so you will lose extra in the urine) and can't be stored by the body, so you need to replenish your stores of this powerful antioxidant daily.

Vitamin E

As a cardiologist, I have a hard time not admiring vitamin E. Many studies have suggested the cardioprotective effects of this fat-soluble nutritional powerhouse. However, what about its value in blood pressure lowering?

For those of you with hypertension who have pre-existing heart disease, or those of you looking to prevent it, you need to know why this nutrient is especially good for you. Vitamin E has several properties that make it a must in my blood-pressure-lowering protocol. Most notably, it serves as:

- an antioxidant, to help prevent the oxidation of HDL
- an anticoagulant, to reduce your risk of stroke and heart attack
- a plaque stabilizer
- a vasodilator

In a recent (2001) review of five major trials that looked at vitamin E supplementation, the statistical analysis of the data seems to suggest that vitamin E is appropriate for anyone with a history of heart disease. In healthy people without cardiac risk factors, supplemental vitamin E as a primary preventive intervention has yet to be substantiated by research. However, its many other health benefits make it a reasonable plan of action. But which vitamin E preparation is best for you?

Whenever considering vitamin E supplements, it's important that you realize that Mother Nature intended us to get various forms of vitamin E. There are approximately eight, so I always recommend that people take several when they supplement. There are many mixed-tocopherol supplements on the market. Be sure that *gamma*-tocopherol is included in your basic formula. And note that *alpha*-tocopherol consumed in the absence of gamma-tocopherol may be ineffective when it comes to inhibiting the oxidative damage that's caused by dangerous peroxynitrate radicals. It can also compete with and displace gamma-tocopherol. Rich dietary sources of gamma-tocopherol are almonds, sunflower seeds, wheat germ, and wheat germ oil.

Vitamin E requirements are influenced by dietary intakes of polyunsaturated fatty acids (PUFA). Average diets containing 7% energy from PUFA would require 6mg of Vitamin E for women and 8mg for men. The best natural sources are found in vegetable oils and nuts, but you'd need to eat almost a pound of peanuts just to meet the RDA. For complete antioxidant protection and vasodilation effects, I recommend daily supplements of 6–8mg of vitamin E per day in the form of mixed tocopherols, including gamma-tocopherol, and tocotrienols (related vitamin E compounds).

THE GRITTY TRUTH ABOUT MINERALS

Minerals seem to have a much less glamorous image than vitamins. I find that many people fail to appreciate the contribution that minerals make to a healthy heart. For instance, there's a direct relationship between magnesium and blood pressure.

Magnesium

Magnesium is indeed the cardiologist's mineral, because it has such profound influence on coronary vascular tone and reactivity. Episodes of angina and cardiac arrhythmia have been successfully treated with magnesium, and several studies have shown it to be effective in the first few hours after a heart attack. It can stabilize cell membranes and prevent life-threatening arrhythmias such as ventricular tachycardia.

Magnesium acts much like a calcium channel blocker by preventing blood vessel spasms. Magnesium also gives you more energy, reduces muscle cramping, and helps encourage a sense of well-being. Even better, it starts those blood pressure numbers on a downward course.

Research has shown low levels of magnesium to be associated with higher blood pressure. Moreover, insulin resistance (particularly Type 2 diabetes) is often accompanied by magnesium deficiency. Given this connection, it's not surprising that many diabetics suffer from hypertension. Magnesium is endothelial-cell-friendly, helping your arteries stay smooth and elastic. We have documentation that inadequate magnesium levels cause blood vessel spasm and constriction. Any narrowing of your blood vessels makes the heart work harder, resulting in higher blood pressure.

Given the fact that we've documented profound magnesium deficiencies in the American population, and that people with cardiovascular disorders respond so well to magnesium supplementation, it's a virtual no-brainer to add this vital mineral to a blood-pressure-lowering programme.

Nutritional tables in the UK now recommend a daily magnesium intake of 300mg a day for adult men and 270mg for women, and up to 500mg daily is fine for healthy people. When it's used in the treatment of blood pressure, I recommend using up to 800mg per day, as long as you have good kidney function. This dose is also helpful for migraines, depression, chronic fatigue syndrome, and diabetes. Magnesium chloride is the most absorbable supplement form of this mineral. Good food sources of magnesium include kelp, figs, tofu, and pumpkin seeds.

Successful blood pressure lowering with magnesium—especially when it's combined with calcium and potassium—has been reported in the medical literature. But remember that too much magnesium can cause frequent loose stools or even diarrhoea (milk of magnesia is a laxative, after all), so always use your body as a barometer and cut back your dose as needed.

Calcium

Calcium is the most abundant mineral in your body. You need calcium to help muscles contract and to promote normal blood clotting. It also plays a major role in electrical conduction and transmission of nerve impulses. Research has shown that a calcium-rich diet can help to lower your blood pressure.

Studies have suggested that calcium supplementation can lower blood pressure because of its additive relationship with magnesium, as previously mentioned. Calcium essentially keeps your muscles well toned by assuaging tension in the muscular walls of the arteries. Though there's little in the literature about the relationship between calcium and high blood pressure, we do know that folks with low blood levels of calcium are more prone to have higher blood pressure readings. Calcium supplementation is believed by some researchers to be helpful, although a recent review published in the *Annals of Internal Medicine* reported a fall in blood pressure that averaged only 1mm Hg. Even if this last observation is be true, a point here and a point there, as multiple nutrients are used and blood pressure starts to fall over time, can add up.

In the UK, 700mg is recommended for adults, with more advised for teenagers and lactating women. Postmenopausal women, however, are better off taking up to 1,500mg daily. For best results, everyone should take this in two or three divided doses daily. And always take calcium supplements with food to avoid the formulation of calcium oxalate stones—never take them on an empty stomach.

Potassium: The Mineral of Life

Potassium is one of the most important minerals in the treatment of high blood pressure. Essential for the health of nerves, cells, and membranes, altered potassium levels put you at risk for a range of heart problems. Because I believe potassium to be so important in terms of blood pressure lowering, I've included a fairly detailed discussion of the subject.

You see, potassium helps to balance the sodium/potassium ratio in blood vessels, which is critical for relaxing the smooth muscle cells that line your blood vessels. Potassium also helps promote the excretion of sodium, a very good thing, because too much sodium, as most people know, raises blood pressure. Therefore, this property is particularly helpful for blood pressure lowering, especially if you're salt-sensitive.

There are also interesting population studies on this phenomenon. Caribbean natives who cook their foods in salt water have high blood pressure. Northern Japanese farmers, who have one of the highest incidences of hypertension and stroke in the world, consume enormous quantities of sodium in their typical diet, which is high in salted smoked fish, seaweed, and soy sauce. Indeed, excessive sodium can be a killer and extra potassium a saviour. Sound research on large population groups supports these observations. So to balance sodium, it's important that you keep your potassium levels on an even keel.

A diet high in potassium has been observed to help protect against stroke-related deaths. At Harvard Medical School, researchers followed 3,738 men age forty to seventy-five for eight years and found that those with the lowest potassium intake (average 2g daily) had a significantly greater risk of stroke compared to men whose potassium consumption was higher (average 3g per day).

A second study reported in the *New England Journal of Medicine* was able to correlate potassium levels more specifically with blood pressure. In a group of 859 Southern California-based men and women aged fifty to seventy-nine, investigators compared baseline twenty-four-hour potassium intake to stroke outcomes for twelve years. In a multivariate analysis, those who had the highest intake of potassium had a 40 percent lower risk of stroke-related mortality compared to those who had the lowest intake. This was true even after researchers had painstakingly controlled for other typical cardiovascular risk variables, such as gender, cholesterol level, obesity, fasting blood sugar, and smoking.

Even product developers have jumped on the potassium bandwagon, seizing the opportunity to capitalize on the health-conscious adult market. Products such as Lucozade were created to replace potassium (and other minerals) lost through the heavy perspiration of strenuous exercise. A normal serum potassium level should be somewhere around 3.5 to 5.0meq/L (milliequivalents per litre).

Those of us in medicine know that low potassium (hypokalemia, or serum potassium less than 3.5meq/L) levels can create cardiac arrhythmias. People with congestive heart failure are vulnerable to deficiencies because potassium is often lost with diuretic therapy. Remember, if you're taking a diuretic, then you're probably taking a potassium supplement, too. However, in the presence of kidney problems, potassium supplements should be avoided; individuals with such a condition should instead look to potassium-rich foods for this nutrient.

Studies also indicate that people who consume a lot of alcohol and caffeine have particularly low levels of potassium. Most people can ensure good potassium levels from a healthy diet. Best sources include fruits (especially bananas, figs, and raisins), orange juice, vegetables (especially potatoes and garlic), yogurt, and whole grains.

There is a risk in taking too much potassium. This is probably most often seen in those taking additional potassium that's prescribed during diuretic therapy and in those who have developed problems clearing the potassium through the kidneys due to low fluid intake or kidney problems. Elevated serum potassium (hyperkalemia, or serum potassium greater than 5.0meq/L), can be dangerous. It can cause the heart to stop. Therefore, doctors are usually cautious and check the blood levels of patients they are treating with potassium.

FOODS WITH HIGH POTASSIUM CONTENT

Food	Potassium (mg)
Potato, 1 med. baked w/skin	844
Avocado, ½ med.	549
Yogurt, low-fat vanilla, 200g	498
Orange juice, 240ml	496
Melon, 175g (7oz)	494
Banana, 1 med.	467
Spinach, 10g (2½oz), boiled	419
Milk, nonfat, 240ml	406
Kidney beans, 90g (3oz), boiled	357

Source (with revision): USDA Nutrient Database for Standard Reference, available at: www.nal.usda.gov/fnic/foodcomp

For the average person with mild or severe hypertension, or even the general population looking to prevent it, we definitely have enough conclusive clinical evidence and scientific research at this point to make the recommendation that we should all be looking to get enough potassium in our diet. However, you will not find an over-the-counter potassium-only supplement at your health food store, due to the potentially lethal risk of overdosing. Because of the dangers of hyperkalemia, multivitamin and mineral supplements can only add 99mg to their daily formulations. These formulations are the safest way for you to supplement your diet if you are looking to include a very small dose of this mineral to your programme. That's the dose you will find on my eight-week plan.

NUTRIENTS: THE DYNAMIC DUO—COENZYME Q_{10} AND L-CARNITINE

Anne, aged forty-six, came to my office with a blood pressure of 180/100, inquiring about taking coenzyme Q_{10}. She'd heard I'd been using it for a long time in my practice. For the past two years she had been taking standard antihypertensive drugs, including beta blockers, calcium channel blockers, and ACE inhibitors. Her quality of life was unsatisfactory for her, as she suffered with severe fatigue and a chronic cough. She had wanted to change her medications, but her doctor had insisted that this was the best plan for her.

I started Anne on hydrosoluble coenzyme Q_{10} (CoQ_{10}) at a dose of 15mg, the equivalent of 50mg of standard CoQ_{10}, which she took three times daily. Her total CoQ10 intake for the day was the equivalent of about 150mg regular CoQ10. I advised her to discuss with her doctor the possibility of discontinuing her ACE inhibitor, the most probable cause of her chronic cough.

Six weeks later, she returned with a smile on her face, renewed energy, no cough, and lower blood pressure. Anne was delighted to report that she had been able to stop one of her drugs (the ACE inhibitor), and now she wanted to see if she could get her blood pressure enough under control with CoQ10 to start lowering her other two medications. Her ultimate goal was to be truly drug-free. Her motivation to feel even better was so high that she undertook a total lifestyle change. She modified her diet, started exercising, and asked for more supplements that might enhance the CoQ10 effect.

I boosted her CoQ10 dose to 15mg four times a day (the equivalent of 200mg regular CoQ10) and told her that I would work with her doctor to try to meet her goal of discontinuing her medication. Although Anne is still on a low dose of a beta blocker, she is working toward her final goal with much success. She's also teaching her doctor about alternative approaches to blood pressure lowering. Coenzyme Q10 is the pillar nutrient around which I build my blood-pressure-lowering support system. But what is CoQ10 all about?

The Magic of Coenzyme Q10

Coenzyme Q10 is a vitamin-like substance that's commonly found in natural food sources—particularly sardines, salmon, mackerel, and pork heart and liver—and is also made by the human body. Every cell in the human body makes CoQ10, but its endogenous production starts fading after the age of forty. By the time you've lived eighty years, your cells have more difficulty in making this compound. In fact, some researchers believe that falling CoQ10 levels can lead to accelerated ageing and diseases such as heart disease and cancer.

In essence, the vitamin-like actions of CoQ10 prevent the depletion of substances that recharge the cellular energy systems in your body. If you remember from biology classes at school, the mitochondria are the little "powerhouses of the cell" where vital ATP (adenosine triphosphate) is formed. In these mitochondria, CoQ10 helps support the formation of ATP, and ATP provides the energy that your body needs all day and night.

Because the heart muscle continuously metabolizes oxygen and consumes huge amounts of energy, heart muscle cells require substantial amounts of CoQ10 to work at peak performance. In fact, tissue levels of CoQ10 are usually ten times higher in the healthy heart than in any other organ in the body—including the brain! We now know that a CoQ10 deficiency is most likely to affect the heart more readily than any other organ, and is a major contributing factor in congestive heart failure.

Research also estimates that approximately 39 percent of patients with high blood pressure have a CoQ10 deficiency. Since the heart requires an enormous amount of energy in the body, it also contains the largest amount of mitochondria per cell. I was amazed to find out that a typical heart cell contains approximately five thousand mitochondria. Contrast that to a skeletal muscle cell, where you'll find an average of two hundred mitochondria.

As you can appreciate, the energy production for the heart is enormous when compared to the energy production required for other tissues of the body. And because your heart requires a constant supply of CoQ10 to meet its energy needs, it's extremely vulnerable to nutritional deficiencies, and also highly receptive to the benefits of targeted supplementation.

When I give CoQ10 to treat both congestive heart failure and hypertension, it usually takes about three to six weeks for the patient to experience some form of noticeable improvement in how he or she feels, especially in the ability to breathe, exercise, and so on. Over the last fifteen years, I've also learned that healthy patients don't usually require as much CoQ10 as sicker patients. So how do I choose a dose?

Usually the blood level of CoQ10 will give me the best information regarding this process. For example, for people with very high blood pressure or severe congestive heart failure, I frequently need to drive CoQ10 levels up to 3.5mg/ml, which is approximately four to five times the normal blood level of .6 to 1mg/ml. Unfortunately, many people who use CoQ10 on a regular basis, as well as their doctors, don't know about this vital information. I've actually found that it's most essential to obtain CoQ10 blood levels for those patients who don't appear to be responding to CoQ10.

Unfortunately, some of the negative trials done on CoQ10 and congestive heart failure, in my opinion, failed to get the patient's blood levels high enough for this nutrient to do its job and make a difference. It is important to note that whether you're treating high blood pressure or any other cardiovascular condition, a simple blood level analysis can give you vital information as to whether the compound is being absorbed in the first place. Over the years, I have observed that the hydrosoluble forms of CoQ10, which will dissolve in both water and fat, are better absorbed and utilized by your body, and therefore yield higher blood levels of CoQ10 than other preparations, due to its increased bioavailability. Therefore, I prefer that my patients take the hydrosoluble CoQ10 preparations. The more bioavailable the CoQ10, the better chance it has of getting right into the tissue where it is needed.

It's my belief that CoQ10 is one of the most important medicinal discoveries of the twentieth century. After using it for more than fifteen years, and having thousands of patients take CoQ10, I've become absolutely convinced that this compound is vital for treating high blood pressure and cardiovascular disease. In fact, it would be unthinkable for me to practice cardiology without using CoQ10. It's absolutely essential for supporting the biochemistry of cardiac cells. And, because of its powerful electron-donating properties, CoQ10 can help to rescue any "tissue in need" that's been damaged by free radicals.

In my daily cardiology practice, I've been able to lower the dosages of many patients' blood pressure medications when they take CoQ10 (as in the case for Anne), and the research backs this up as well!

In one placebo-controlled, double-blind study, patients given a total of 200mg of CoQ10 supplements daily in divided doses showed reductions in both systolic and diastolic blood pressure over matched controls. In another related study published in 1994, more than 50 percent of patients with high blood pressure were able to discard at least one, and some as many as three, of their antihypertensive medications with long-term CoQ10 administration.

Now research again confirms that CoQ10 reduces both systolic and diastolic blood pressures. The researchers theorized that CoQ10 reduced oxidative stress in blood vessel tissues, which in turn resulted in lowering the resistance of the blood vessels, culminating in easier blood flow. Coenzyme Q10 also had favourable effects on carbohydrate and insulin metabolism; therefore, insulin resistance was reduced. The researchers also found that there was a decrease in adrenaline-like substances in the urine, which suggests that CoQ10 may have a hormonal effect on blood pressure lowering as well.

The most recent study of CoQ10 in blood pressure lowering (2001) involved forty-six men and thirty-seven women. In this randomized, double-blind, placebo-controlled trial of CoQ10 in isolated systolic hypertension, the mean reduction of blood pressure in the CoQ10-treated group was 17.8 ± 7.3mm Hg. Using 60mg of hydrosoluble CoQ10 twice daily over a twelve-week period, the researchers concluded that CoQ10 may be safely offered to hypertensive patients as an alternative treatment option.

Over the years, I've had overwhelming success stories with coenzyme Q10, and I've even had dozens of cases where CoQ10 made the difference between life and death. Truly, it is a remarkable compound. It is also important to note that, in this modern day of cholesterol lowering, statin drugs can cause profound CoQ10 deficiencies. In blocking cholesterol synthesis, powerful statins also block the production of coenzyme Q10, which is part of the same biochemical pathway.

I strongly recommend that anyone taking a statin drug add a "chaser" of 30mg hydrosoluble CoQ10, or 100mg of a regular CoQ10 supplement. Not only will supplemental coenzyme Q10 protect you from the side effects of statins, it will also help you maintain adequate blood levels of this important vitamin-nutrient. Although side effects of coenzyme Q10 (such as nausea, abdominal discomfort, and insomnia if taken at bedtime) are rare, it's not suggested for healthy pregnant or lactating women because both the unborn and the newborn produce sufficient quantities of the compound.

Hey, I'm Alive Again!

I've been using CoQ10 as part of my natural approach to blood pressure lowering, and the results have been truly exciting. Because hypertension is so often a silent disease, people don't actually "feel" their blood pressure coming down when I'm treating them traditionally with medication alone.

But one physical experience seems to be more universal. When people take CoQ10 for the first time, many of them report an extraordinary surge of energy. I suspect that the lower your body's CoQ10 level before you take it as a supplement, the more renewed energy you'll feel. In fact, one of my patients reported that his energy burst felt like he'd had two cups of strong coffee, but without the jittery feeling. Others have mentioned that if they take CoQ10 after eight o'clock in the evening, they find it hard to fall asleep. So if too much energy is a problem for you, I recommend you take your last dose with dinner or before eight, to avoid a possible insomnia effect.

Juggling CoQ₁₀ for the Rabbi

Many years ago I was taking care of a seventy-five-year-old rabbi with congestive heart failure. He is now eighty-eight. It was heartbreaking for me to watch him deteriorate year after year, despite the careful juggling of medications to strengthen his heartbeat (Digoxin), limit his heart's workload (nitrates), and help him get rid of excess fluid (diuretics). He was becoming an all-too-frequent patient in our cardiac intensive care unit. I was up against the wall in terms of traditional interventions; any more drugs and the rabbi would be at toxic levels. And he was too old for a heart transplant. So I had a thought. I was just beginning to have some success with CoQ₁₀ in my practice, and we had nothing to lose.

But the rabbi was a man of small stature and hardly any body fat. I found that, with his limited body mass, taking CoQ₁₀ supplements was a little too much for him. I guess you could say it was like I had put high-octane gas in the tank of a four-cylinder car with a thirty-year-old engine and over-inflated tyres. Even low doses of this wonderful nutrient made the rabbi nervous and agitated. But I didn't want to give up—he was breathing better on CoQ₁₀—so I decided to try a new approach.

I asked his wife if she could prepare her husband a couple of ounces of smoked salmon (a fish that's naturally high in CoQ₁₀) every day. She agreed, and I have to admit that even I was amazed that, for the rabbi, a breakfast of salmon and bagels every morning did the trick. After he'd spent a few months on the "smoked salmon supplement", everyone was amazed at the improvement in his energy level. He was no longer in over-drive, but he did feel like a new man. Many local doctors were equally startled. "What did you do to the rabbi?" they would call to ask. "I treated him with salmon," I responded. Later on, after the rabbi had built up a tolerance for CoQ₁₀ from the salmon, I was able to switch him over to low-dose capsules. He was now able to reap the full benefits of CoQ₁₀. But I bet he missed his morning salmon treat.

Not All Supplements Are Created Equal

CoQ₁₀ is widely available in health food stores, but most forms of it are difficult to absorb because it's such a large molecule. For blood pressure lowering, I usually recommend 60 to 120mg of the hydrosoluble form taken in divided doses over the day (four to eight of the 15mg doses, for example) to keep your blood level more consistent.

But when I first starting using CoQ₁₀ in my practice, I found that patients' responses varied. This confused me, so I started ordering blood levels on the patients who failed to respond to CoQ10. While the blood was in the lab, I sent out some of the samples of the tablets my patients were taking for assay. Many of them had bought CoQ10 on sale at various stores in the area. That's when I learned that all CoQ10 supplements are not equal.

First of all, because the Food and Drug Administration in the US does not check the quality of supplements, I found that some products claiming to contain the usual 30mg dose of CoQ10 actually had less . . . much less. In fact, one supposedly 30mg tablet contained only 1mg. That was why some of my patients weren't getting any better. The hydrosoluble forms of this remarkable nutrient, developed in 1997, are best in terms of absorption and bioavailability. Now with the better delivery system, blood levels are higher at half the cost. Be sure that whenever you purchase nutrients you check the expiration date on the bottle.

L-Carnitine

Like all superheroes, CoQ10 has a sidekick, and it's called L-carnitine. This amino-acid-like compound acts like a shuttle, bringing fatty acids into the mitochondria so they can be used for energy, and also carting away toxic by-products. In a very real sense, the mitochondria in your cells are little furnaces, CoQ10 is the generator, and L-carnitine is the fuel delivery truck.

The predominant fuel source for the heart is fat, and L-carnitine brings that fuel into the heart cells. Since L-carnitine can help your heart at the cellular level with the metabolism of fats, it can enhance the efficiency of energy within the cell. When fat is burned as fuel, toxic metabolites can build up, which can cause some reduction in blood flow. L-carnitine's magic is in supporting the removal of toxic wastes, making it an ideal nutrient for cardiovascular efficiency. I believe it is this more efficient use of energy that indirectly supports blood pressure lowering.

Research at the University of Milan suggests a profound synergistic effect between CoQ10 and L-carnitine across a wide range of cardiovascular problems. I have found the same additive effect when my patients use these two targeted nutriceuticals in combination. I especially rely on higher doses of L-carnitine when the therapeutic effect I am trying for is not achievable when using CoQ10 alone. I usually recommend 1,000 to 2,000mg of L-carnitine a day for blood pressure lowering. I like the

L-carnitine fumarate preparations that research has shown offer a slight protection to hearts that are starving for oxygen. Doctors call this state ischaemia or a deficiency of oxygen in the tissues.

I'd like to move on next to your first weekly installment of a section devoted to bringing you the latest on various food groups you'll be adding to your PAMM diet.

DIET UPDATE: SOYA AND SOYA PRODUCTS

Prized for centuries in Asia, the soya bean has finally made its way into today's Western diet. Soya is a legume, so it fits into the whole grains, legumes, nuts, and seeds group of complex carbohydrates at the foundation of the PAMM diet. Since many people aren't accustomed to using soya, I want to devote a separate section on how to incorporate it in your diet.

The modest little soya bean is a nutritional powerhouse. High in phytoestrogens (phytoestrogens are plant compounds with chemical activity similar to oestrogen), amino acids, and fibre, but low in saturated fat and cholesterol, soya beans are a great source of life-enhancing nutrition. Soya protein is one of the few plant proteins that contains all the essential amino acids and is equal in nutritional value to animal protein.

Soya is nutritious and packed with valuable constituents, including isoflavones, saponins, and phytosterols. Soya isoflavones, primarily genistein, are recognized for their antioxidant and phytoestrogenic properties. Saponins enhance immune function and bind to cholesterol to limit its absorption in your intestine. Phytosterols support healthy cholesterol and boost your immune function.

Research has repeatedly demonstrated that replacing animal protein with soya beans or soya products lowers total cholesterol without reducing the good HDL cholesterol. In addition, soya helps prevent the oxidation of LDL cholesterol and so short-circuits the atherosclerotic process. Soya may help with blood sugar control for diabetics and may also help lower risk for some of the complications of diabetes, because it has such a very low glycemic index.

In summary, soya is a valuable part of my PAMM diet to help lower your blood pressure, total cholesterol, LDL, and triglycerides, as well as to help boost those HDL levels. In one study, the combined effect of higher fibre and protein from soya lowered systolic blood pressure approximately 6mm Hg.

Soya Caveats

Although soya foods can take the place of more allergenic foods like cow's milk and eggs, some people may be allergic to soya. Those who are may be able to tolerate some soya foods but not others, or may have to avoid soya altogether.

And since the isoflavones in soya do have weak oestrogenic activity, they could have some potentially harmful hormonal effects in certain situations. While soya seems to reduce the risk of breast cancer, there is some evidence that it may exert some influence in the opposite direction, as well. For this reason and others, we don't know if high doses of soya are safe for women who have already had breast cancer. In fact, I advise women with oestrogen-dependent cancers (doctors can give you a tissue analysis report on your tumours) not to eat soya products at all.

Other groups of people who need to limit soya include those with a high Lp(a), those taking thyroid medication, and children. A July 2001 study showed that soya protein raised lipoprotein (a) or Lp(a), a recognized risk factor for heart disease. Soya has also been noted to depress thyroid function and reduce the absorption of thyroid medication, so if you're someone with thyroid considerations, you should discuss using soya products with your doctor. And I discourage the use of soya by children less than five years of age because they may develop an allergy to it, whereas this is less likely if it is introduced into their diet after the age of five, when the body is better equipped to adjust to it.

Other limitations of soya are worth mentioning here. One study of Japanese American men reported that those who ate the most tofu during midlife increased their risk of developing Alzheimer's disease by up to 2.4 times. Soya may also reduce your absorption of calcium, iron, and zinc, which shouldn't be a problem if you're taking a good multivitamin product but is noteworthy if you have a tendency toward osteoporosis or anaemia.

Despite the caveats I've mentioned, the health benefits of soya are so important that the FDA in America has allowed foods with a minimum of 6.25g of soya protein per serving to carry a cholesterol-lowering claim on their label. Studies indicate that consuming a minimum of 25g of soya protein per day will significantly reduce your cholesterol and cut your risk of cardiovascular disease. This level could easily be met with one to two servings of soya-based foods each day. For example, 4oz of tofu has 13g of cholesterol-lowering soya protein, while just 25g (¾oz) cup of soya nuts (*see page 76*) has 19g. (To learn how easy it can be to add the benefits of soya to your meals, see the box below.)

Regardless of the FDA's enthusiasm, I believe that when all is said and done, soya's limitations add up to one important bottom line for soya foods: Moderation is key! I don't recommend that anyone consume soya products on a daily basis. But four to five servings a week (the amount I have included in the PAMM diet) is a safe, conservative approach for the majority of people.

Soya Protein Values: There are eleven types of soya products that are widely available:

- *Whole soya beans,* either canned or dried, can be used like any other legume. They can be added to soups, used as the base for chilli, served as a side dish, or mashed into a spread.
- *Soya grits* are toasted, cracked soya beans and resemble coarse cornmeal. High in protein, they can be used alone as a tasty side dish or cooked with other grains like barley and cracked wheat.
- *Soya flakes* are cracked soya beans that have been crushed between rollers. Usually cooked and served as a hot cereal, soya flakes are delicious topped with cinnamon and a few potassium-rich raisins.
- *Soya milk* is made by soaking, crushing, and cooking soya beans and then straining the liquid. To make it taste more like cow's milk, manufacturers may add seaweed and malt cereals to thicken and sweeten the product. Soya milk is available plain or flavoured, and with different fat levels sweetened and unsweetened. I use soya milk in my tea and coffee and over both hot and cold cereal, as well as in breakfast smoothies and snacks. Although soya milk is not naturally high in calcium, some formulations are enriched with this mineral as well as with vitamin D.
- *Soya cheese* comes in two forms. The soft kind is a vegetarian alternative to cream cheese or sour cream. Sliceable soya cheese resembles cheddar or mozzarella. Read the labels carefully to avoid products that have high levels of sodium and fat.
- *Tofu* is a creamy white curd of soya bean that is as delicious as it is nutritious. Made by adding calcium or magnesium salt to soya milk, tofu can be added to soups, salads, desserts, and stews. There are several kinds of tofu. Extra firm is excellent for grilling and adding to stews, while soft works best for sauces and desserts. Silken tofu is generally creamier and smoother; it's wonderful in puddings, dips, sauces, and shakes. Japanese tofu yogurt works beautifully as a replacement for mayonnaise and cream cheese in your favourite recipes. Whatever type of tofu you choose, it will be packed with first-rate nutrition.

- *Tempeh* is made of cooked soya beans that are fermented with a mould. Often prepared with seeds or nuts, tempeh is easier to digest than other types of soya products. Tempeh can be stir-fried with fresh vegetables, grilled, or added to soups and chillis.
- *Miso* is a thick and salty paste of ground fermented soya beans. Most miso pastes are mixed with a grain such as barley, wheat, or rice, each providing its own distinctive flavour and colour. Miso pastes are aged from one month to three years, becoming darker and stronger the longer they ferment. White miso, aged for about one month, has a mild flavour that works well for soups, salads, and sauces. Try stirring a tablespoon into a pot of vegetable soup or a teaspoon into salad dressing. Yellow miso has a light, distinctly salty taste. Red and brown miso are strong and pungent, and are best suited for stews and braised dishes. Keep in mind that miso is very high in sodium. A single tablespoon has 600mg of sodium, about a quarter of the recommended daily intake. Use sparingly, as high levels of sodium can contribute to high blood pressure.
- *Edamame* is boiled fresh soya beans. Tender and sweet, they make a fantastic snack or side dish, packed with protein and rich in disease-fighting phytonutrients.
- *Soya protein powder* is a highly refined source that is more than 90 percent protein. Ready to eat, soya powder can be added to smoothies, oatmeal, and whole-grain side dishes.
- *Soya nuts* are the healthy alternative to chips and crisps. Make them at home to avoid unnecessary sodium. Soak dried soya beans for several hours, then roast them at 325°F/160°C/Gas mark 2½ on an olive-oil-coated biscuit tray for ten minutes. Toss occasionally while they are browning. While still warm, sprinkle them with black pepper, garlic powder, or onion powder.

Soya products are rich in magnesium and alpha-linolenic acid. You already know the benefits of magnesium; alpha-linolenic acid is an essential precursor for omega-3 fatty acids. Additionally, the phytoestrogens in soya can help alleviate a woman's menopausal symptoms. For all its health benefits, soya is a great food to have in our eight-week blood-pressure-lowering programme.

This week you have recipes to show you how to add soya to any meal. At breakfast you'll be introduced to soya smoothies, as well as oatmeal that's enriched with soya protein powder and topped with soya milk. Lunchtime meals that feature soya burgers or tofu will provide you with cholesterol-lowering nutrition that's as delicious as it is good for you. At dinner, you will enjoy vegetarian chilli made from soya beans or savour stir-fried tempeh with fresh organic Chinese vegetables.

4 Exercise, Fish, and Flax
Week 3

If you're like many of my patients, then you've probably felt the urge to skip over a chapter that recommends exercise. But don't worry! I'm not going to tell you to buy a set of weights, sign up at a gym, or schedule an hour of bone-crunching workouts daily. In fact, whatever your current level of physical activity, this will be exercise you will enjoy.

When it comes to exercise, I believe less is more. I don't recommend strenuous exercises such as jogging and running. As a doctor, I have seen way too many injuries, including strained muscles, back injuries, twisted knees, and tendonitis. The cardiology literature is studded with reports of aortic rupture, sudden death, and strokes during exercise. And long-duration runs can interfere with menstruation and contribute to osteoporosis in women.

By contrast, mild, pleasant exercise provides health benefits to the entire body without incurring any secondary problems. Research has shown that gentle, regular exercise promotes lower blood pressure. Increased activity dilates capillaries, possibly by a nitric oxide effect (see Chapter 3), thereby reducing resistance to arterial blood flow and making it easier for the heart to do its job. This easing is reflected in lower systolic and diastolic pressures.

One of the most current, large-scale studies on exercise was published in March 2001 in the *Journal of the American Medical Association*. Analysis of data from more than thirty-nine thousand healthy female professionals, aged forty-five and up, showed that light to moderate exercise, equivalent to only an hour of walking a week, lowered cardiovascular risk—even for women who were overweight, who smoked, or who had high cholesterol levels. Other research indicates that men receive similar benefits from this type of exercise as well, with added protection against prostate cancer. Walking also reduces the risk of breast and colon cancer.

Exercise also targets one of the most mysterious and silent causes of high blood pressure: insulin resistance. Remember, insulin is a hormone that helps the cells take up glucose in the bloodstream. Rising blood glucose levels signal the pancreas to release more and more insulin as needed. This concept is so essential that I'd like to expand my earlier discussion in Chapter 3, so that you can get a clear picture of what happens to the body in insulin resistance.

Receptor sites on the cells act as portals that lock on to insulin in order to transport glucose. Problems begin when a high-carbohydrate diet produces consistently high levels of glucose, thereby forcing your pancreas to work overtime to meet increasing demands for insulin. Over time, chronically high levels of insulin are believed to actually damage the receptor sites, interfering with their ability to transport glucose. This creates a number of consequences—all bad.

When insulin receptor sites can no longer function properly, your blood glucose levels stall in those high numbers, continually signalling your body to produce more and more insulin. Eventually, these continually high levels of insulin trigger the production of inflammatory chemicals that constrict blood vessels, promote clotting, and provoke arterial plaque development. Independently, each one of these factors can raise your blood pressure. In combination, they create hypertension that can be resistant to traditional pharmaceuticals. I believe that insulin resistance is the essence of the high blood pressure epidemic affecting our society today.

Fortunately, exercise helps your body to burn glucose, thwarting the cycle of insulin secretion and resistance. And, of course, the health benefits of exercise to the heart don't stop there. Exercise promotes weight loss, lowers triglyceride levels, relieves depression, improves circulation, and strengthens bones. Keep in mind that these benefits don't mean you need a £100 pair of training shoes and a personal trainer.

BENEFITS OF EXERCISE
- Reduces blood pressure
- Preserves muscle mass
- Increases metabolic rate
- Increases growth hormone secretion
- Releases stress and tension
- Relieves constipation
- Alleviates low back pain
- Improves sleep
- Enhances sexual performance
- Burns calories/reduces weight

All of the above enhance cardiovascular prevention.

There are three fundamental types of exercise—aerobic, strength-training, and flexibility—and all have a role in controlling blood pressure. Aerobic exercise increases oxygenation of the blood. Walking, cycling, dancing, and swimming provide aerobic benefits to the body. These exercises increase heart rate and cause your blood vessels to dilate, thereby bringing down your pressure. In a metanalysis of fifty-four randomized controlled trials (2,419 participants) reported in the April 2002 issue of the *Annals of Internal Medicine*, aerobic exercise reduced blood pressure in both hypertensive and normotensive persons. This very recent review in the medical literature indicates that increasing physical activity is an important component of any blood-pressure-lowering programme. To build aerobic potential, you need to work out steadily for twenty to thirty minutes at least three times weekly.

Many training programmes call for workouts at peak intensity, much like conditioning schedules for professional athletes. Maybe this works if you have Olympic ambitions, but for the rest of us it can be overwhelming, and sometimes even detrimental.

One of my patients lives by the phrase "If a little is good, then more must be better." When I suggested that she take a thirty-minute walk three times a week, she went out and bought the latest ergonomically correct training shoes, a digital pedometer, and a set of tapes to "walk away" her blood pressure problems. Less than a week later, she called the office for help. She'd developed giant blisters on both feet, and her legs ached so badly that she couldn't sleep. Instead of just thirty minutes of regular walking, she'd embarked on daily hikes that resembled the Bataan Death March. I prescribed vitamin E ointment for her blisters, as well as cool oatmeal soaks for her legs, and ordered a two-week moratorium on exercise walks. When her legs felt better, she went on shorter walks and limited her other exercise activities. Very quickly, she began to feel the physical and emotional benefits of gentle, regular exercise.

The second type of exercise that I encourage is a simple weight-training programme that will help you build muscle and strength. Such a workout can significantly reduce your insulin levels and your blood pressure, according to a study of sixteen out-of-shape men who were insulin-resistant and therefore at risk for diabetes. The men were assigned to one of two one-week programmes. The first group did aerobic exercise, while the second group followed each aerobic training session with one hour of strength training. While both groups showed reductions in insulin, blood sugar, and blood pressure, the effects in the strength-training group were significantly greater. The latter lowered their insulin level three times as much as the aerobics group, and their glucose levels and blood pressure decreased by twice as much.

Another study on strength training examined the effects of different exercises on body composition. Seventy-two men and women following the same diet were divided into two groups. One group performed thirty minutes of aerobic exercise three times a week, and the other divided the same amount of time between strength training and aerobics. Eight weeks later, the aerobic exercisers had lost three pounds of fat and half a pound of muscle, and the combination exercisers had lost ten pounds of fat and gained two pounds of muscle!

Strength-, weight-, or resistance-training exercise gradually increases your work capacity and endurance. Increasing your muscle mass through strength training has wide-ranging effects on your body—all of them good. Improved muscle tone increases oxygen delivery throughout the body, allowing the heart to do the same job with less effort. Increased strength makes it easier for the body to work, so all the thousands of physiological activities that take place are accomplished with less effort—another break for an overworked heart and circulatory system. In addition, stronger muscles mean the body can perform aerobic exercise more easily.

In my eight-week programme, you will build muscle with a series of exercises that target specific muscle groups. Some weeks you can add light weights to arms and legs as you go about your daily routine, while other weeks you can vary your workout by using your own body weight as resistance.

Flexibility, the capacity to move or bend with ease, allows us to participate more fully in an exercise programme. When your joints and muscles are tight and stiff, walking can create shin splints, and weight-training exercises can lead to spasms of the back and legs. For these reasons, stretching exercises are a crucial part of the exercise component in my natural blood-pressure-lowering programme. As with all types of exercise, stretching should be done with the same "less is more" approach. Each movement should be done slowly and evenly. Forget those high school gym classes that exhorted you to bounce during each movement. This type of quick, jerking movement can create painful strains and unnecessary soreness. Correct stretching involves holding the position just short of pain as you continue to breathe. Stretch slowly and avoid bouncing. Do not hold your breath when doing any type of exercise. Try side and neck stretches, shoulder rolls, half rolls, knee bends, and calf, hamstring, and inner-thigh stretches. The ideal warm-up uses all the same muscles that you will use when exercising. Even the smallest stretching effort will bring very big rewards.

We're going to start off this week with simple walking, but at a steady pace. If you can't remember the last time you went out for a stroll, then just start off slowly for a ten-minute walk, but keep that pace steady! This is not a stop-and-start walk, punctuated by long pauses for window shopping or snacking. I want you to start walking and keep walking. My patients report that walking to or from work is a practically effortless way to fit in exercise that can actually pay major dividends. If you drive to your job, then park some distance away and walk to your office. If you commute by bus or train, then make time to get off a stop earlier and walk the rest of the way. If you have a furry four-legged friend, go out for a walk. It's great for your dog—and, of course, for you, too!

PACE YOURSELF

Walk ten minutes every other day for one week. Then in each following week increase by increments of five or ten minutes. Within a month, you'll be taking thirty-minute strolls. Do this every other day, and you'll have a good workout routine. Five days a week is optimal. Remember, you don't have to keep up a brisk pace. The good news is that actual walking speed isn't as important as we've been led to believe. In fact, the study on women and exercise mentioned earlier found that *speed* didn't matter; it was the *length* of time women walked that was significant. Reinforcing this notion is a recent article in *Nature* reporting on a Dutch study of thirty healthy adults that showed moderate activity was actually superior to vigorous exercise for expending energy. Also, don't overdo it in summer heat. A good guideline is the 80-80 rule: Avoid exercising outdoors if the temperature is over 80 degrees or the humidity is over 80 percent. That includes avid golfers. When I was practising acute crisis cardiology, I saw at least one patient a year who'd gone into cardiac arrest on the golf course, always when the temperature and humidity were both in the 90s. Air-conditioned shopping centres are a great alternative in the heat, but pick your workout times. Before the stores open may be best if you're prone to engage in "retail therapy"—otherwise this could get very expensive!

THE RIGHT WAY TO WALK

Anyone over the age of fifteen months knows how to walk, but when you walk for exercise, you need to think about your stance and your stride. As you start out for your exercise walk, stand tall and straight. Imagine two straight lines that run from your ears, past your shoulder, and down to your hips, knees, and ankles. Look in the mirror to check your alignment. Your elbows should be bent at a 90-degree angle and your hands held in a loose fist. Push off from the ball of your foot and touch down with your heel. Your pace should be quick enough to boost cardioendurance, yet you should be able to talk without panting. Try to walk with a friend if you can.

A few years ago I investigated the effects of "active" motion (walking) and "passive" motion (exercise tables) in one hundred healthy women, who were randomly assigned to one of three experimental groups or a control group. Several of the solo walkers dropped out because they were lonely, whereas all the women assigned to the exercise tables completed the three-month study, largely motivated by the social interaction. However, while the passive exercisers (who also dieted) realized benefits in terms of weight loss, flexibility, and psychological well-being, the walkers' gains were bigger, and they got the additional bonus of improved cardiovascular conditioning. If they'd only had social support, the walkers as a group would've come out ahead.

If you can walk and maintain a conversation with ease, then try picking up your pace just a bit. Should you have any shortness of breath, chest discomfort, or arm pain with walking, you must see your doctor ASAP. Be aware of any symptoms that come up during or up to an hour after exercising. If you feel ill, stop and rest. If symptoms persist after three to five minutes of rest, seek medical attention immediately.

WARNING SIGNS THAT YOU MAY BE DOING TOO MUCH EXERCISE
- Light-headedness or dizziness
- Palpitations
- Shortness of breath (unable to carry on a conversation)
- Jaw pain
- Tingling or numbness in arms
- Tight feeling in the lungs

WALKING TIPS
- Pair up with a friend or spouse. This will help you to keep your commitment to daily exercise.
- Vary the location of your walk. Different views prevent boredom.
- Vary the speed at which you walk. Quicken the pace for five minutes, then slow down for another five minutes.
- Look for small hills on your walk to increase cardio impact.
- Change your routine. For example, as circumstances dictate, sometimes take along your dog, listen to music, or push a pram.
- Time your walk. Work up to the goal of one mile in sixteen to eighteen minutes.

DANCE DOWN YOUR BLOOD PRESSURE

I believe dancing to be one of the most underutilized exercise choices. All types of dance—whether it's folk, jazz, ballroom, rock, Latin, or your own special style—provide a wonderful cardiac workout and lift your spirit in the process. Music creates a rhythmic background that can help you to coordinate your movements, and it provides mood and atmosphere for relaxation, play, and even romance.

And dancing has great perks for your body as well as your soul. Dancing with partners can relieve isolation, promote social interaction, and build bonds between and among people. Moving rhythmically to the beat of the music can also ease muscle tension, reduce anxiety, and increase your energy level. In addition, moving creatively can allow people to express their inner feelings and open up fresh perspectives for looking at their surroundings. I guess you can tell that somewhere inside I'm more of an Astaire than a Sinatra—I love to dance! But don't do it "my way". Find your own best way to express yourself through music and movement.

If you can allow yourself to let go and just surrender to the beat and feeling of the music, then dancing can even be a great way to get over your inhibitions. I enjoy the playfulness that adults can experience through dance, and yet it can lead to some profound personal transformations, including becoming comfortable with your own body and more confident in the world. I love to dance with my wife, our children (it's a great way to play with your children, especially as they grow up), and our good friends. In fact, doing an Irish jig all by myself conjures up great memories of my childhood and my parents—I can get lost on the dance floor without even needing a partner. It's great! Maybe there are dances that have special meaning for you that way—once the body starts to move, cellular memory kicks in and you too can find yourself transported!

Dancing even allows us to express our sexuality in a socially acceptable manner. We all hold way too much tension in our hips, our pelvis, and our lower back, but dancing allows us to move our pelvis and free up some of that tension without embarrassment. And the intimacy and closeness that is part of dancing with someone special is the kind of contact that heals the heart.

In fact, you may be surprised to know that studies have actually shown that dance enhances motivation and memory, helping people feel more joy and confidence. So many feelings and emotions come up that it's virtually impossible to be negative when you commit yourself to the rhythm and melody of a song. In addition to all these benefits, dancing is also the right type of exercise to lower your blood pressure. So you may want to join a dance club instead of a health club to get yourself some ballroom exercise.

In many ways, dancing is even more convenient than walking. You don't have to worry about the weather. You can just go out with friends, join a class, or even pop in a CD of your favourite music at home and simply let yourself go. It's so easy to get the recommended fifteen to thirty minutes of daily exercise with dance. Have yourself some real fun and cash in on all those other perks at the same time!

By now you are aware of how much importance I place on regular exercise to rev up your metabolism, burn calories, build lean muscle mass, and elevate your mood. I'm not a fan of intense exercise because it ages, stresses, and injures your body. The elevated metabolic rate associated with intense exercise also skyrockets the release of free radicals. Not good.

Normally, your body can compensate for the free-radical damage that occurs with moderate exercise. But intense exercise can overwhelm your body's natural antioxidant systems. If you jog on a hot, sunny day when the air pollution level is high, the inhalation of airborne toxins creates a huge surge of free radicals that are carried along by your high metabolic rate. Combined with the free radicals produced by exercise itself, it's an unrelenting assault. Over time, such repeated influxes of free radicals set the stage for coronary artery disease. I don't want to give you the impression that exercise is bad for you. You need exercise for optimal health. Clearly, the risks of not exercising, or of exercising too little, are far greater than the risks of free-radical damage, but what I want for you is to get the best of both worlds, so to speak. That means the gains of regular, moderate exercise *and* the protection from free radicals.

Research indicates that antioxidant supplements neutralize free radicals before they can do their damage by preventing the oxidation of fats and by stabilizing cell membranes that have been broken down with exercise. I strongly suggest a quality basic antioxidant programme, such as the one I endorsed in Chapter 3.

DIET UPDATE: FISH

Eating fish provides you with incredible health benefits. Omega-3 fatty acids such as eicosapentaenoic acid (EPA) and docosahexaenoic acid (DHA) are found in fish oils. These oils stimulate the production of chemical mediators, which in turn relax the smooth muscles. In addition, fish oil stimulates the production of favourable hormones, such as prostaglandins, which have an anticlotting effect. All together, then, the omega-3s are great for blood pressure lowering and the prevention of arteriosclerosis. In addition to their relaxing effect on smooth muscle, omega-3 fatty acids help to reduce blood pressure by blocking the effects of vasoconstrictor chemical mediators that raise the blood pressure in your body.

At the June 2000 American Heart Association meeting in Reston, Virginia, researchers suggested that the effectiveness of omega-3s in reducing blood pressure in hypertensive patients depended on the dose. At 3g a day, omega-3s appear to vasodilate and reduce vasoconstrictive properties. One possible explanation is that omega-3s have some effect on nitric oxide production.

In one recent placebo-controlled trial, an average systolic reduction of 5mm Hg and a mean diastolic decrease of 3mm Hg were observed in those people taking DHA. How is it that DHA can be so effective? One of the reasons that these substances may help to prevent atherosclerosis, or narrowing of your blood vessels, is that they also have a potent triglyceride-lowering effect.

In a recent landmark decision, the Food and Drug Administration in the US reported that it would allow products containing omega-3 fatty acids to claim heart-health benefits. The FDA based that decision on the wealth of scientific evidence pointing to a correlation between omega-3 fatty acids, such as EPA and DHA, and a reduced risk of coronary artery disease. Unfortunately, the present intake of DHA in the United States is less than optimum. In a dietary study of 9,323 adults in the United States, the average daily DHA consumption was 61mg per day by women and 78mg by men—less than 35 percent of the recommended intake. And in a recent National Institutes of Health conference on essential fatty acids, sufficient evidence was presented for a recommendation of 220mg of DHA per day as an adequate intake for adults (300mg for pregnant and nursing women). Why have these agencies come out with such a strong opinion on these?

There's no doubt about it: These essential fatty acids (of which cold-water fish is a good source) have many heart-protective and cancer-preventive properties. I've mentioned the Italian study that showed an overwhelming decrease in both sudden death and all causes of death in those individuals taking only 1g of fish oil per day. I find the benefits of enjoying fish meals to be nothing short of amazing! Remember that the constituents in fish oil don't just help prevent blood from clumping and lower your triglycerides. They also help reduce excessive levels of fibrinogen (a blood protein involved in clotting) and Lp(a) while lowering your blood pressure—all of which contribute to enhancing cardiovascular health. One extremely important study showed that those individuals eating the equivalent of one fish meal a week had a 50 percent lower incidence of sudden cardiac death compared to their age- and gender- matched counterparts whose daily menus did not contain these vital oils.

The benefits of DHA and EPA go far beyond cancer and heart disease. Research also indicates that increased fish intake can help alleviate psychological problems including depression, bipolar disorder, and even suicidal tendencies. In addition, DHA is critical for the proper development of the foetal brain and extremely important in retinal development as well.

Although the side effects of fish oils are mostly abdominal upset or burping, excessive intake (more than than 6g of omega-3 fatty acids a day) may interfere with oral anticoagulants such as Coumadin (warfarin).

My recommendations? Get DHA in a pure, uncontaminated fish oil that also contains EPA. Make sure that the fish oils you purchase in health food stores have a quality control analysis profile for lipid peroxides and heavy metals—many fish oils contain excessive pollutants and metals, and some of them also are prone to rancidity. Avoid liquid fish oil packaged in bottles because these liquids tend to become rancid, even when placed in the refrigerator.

If you are a vegetarian and don't eat fish, then you need to make sure your diet contains plenty of green leafy vegetables such as spinach and mustard greens. Wheat germ, walnuts, flaxseed, and tofu contain alpha-linolenic acid, which can be converted to EPA and DHA in the body.

If you cannot find high-quality oils, perhaps the best way of taking in these precious essential fatty acids is eating healthy fish. Most fish and seafood contain at least measurable amounts of precious essential fatty acids such as the omega-3s. So the menus for my PAMM programme contain three to four servings of fish each week. But despite the wonderful health benefits, you should be aware that I have some real concerns about the purity of fish in our markets.

Fish, particularly those living in coastal waters, may be contaminated with pesticides, heavy metals, and PCBs (polychlorinated biphenyls). I'm particularly concerned about the levels of methyl mercury that have been measured in deep-sea fish such as large tuna, shark, and swordfish. Not only can methyl mercury poisoning increase your blood pressure, it can also produce neurological symptoms and provoke irregular heartbeat in adults. In children, the problems are even more insidious, producing developmental difficulties that are hard to trace and even harder to treat. And babies exposed to methyl mercury in the womb can be born with both physical and mental deficits.

The highest concentrations of pollutants and heavy-metal contaminants can be found in the dark fatty areas of the fish, usually the mid-section and tail area. I advise you to carefully trim away these parts before cooking and eating your fish. Small tuna contain less mercury than other big fish with contamination problems, but because tuna is usually eaten more frequently, the chemicals can still accumulate. Although it is high in omega-3s and widely available, I limit tuna to one serving every two months. The healthiest fish are deep-water migratory fish such as salmon, halibut, cod, and mackerel, to mention a few. However, not all fish are created equal when it comes to omega-3 content.

OMEGA-3 LEVELS IN FISH

To get omega-3s exclusively from your diet, here is how much fish you need to consume to get the recommended 900mg of EPA and DHA per day.

Fish	Omega-3 Fatty Acids g/100g of a single portion	Amount needed (oz)
Sole	0.1	32.1
Tuna (in water)	0.2	16.1
Snapper	0.2	16.1
Cod	0.3	10.7
Catfish	0.4	8.0
Trout (all but lake)	0.5	6.4
Halibut	0.6	5.4
Salmon	1.1	2.9
Albacore tuna*	1.3	2.7
Sardines	1.4	2.6
Herring	1.5	2.1
Lake trout	1.6	2.0
Mackerel	1.8	1.8
	LNA Portion (Alpha-Linolenic Acid)	Tbsp.
Flaxseed oil	12.3	1.6**

* Albacore tuna is recommended only one time every two months because of possible mercury contamination.
** The alpha-linolenic acid in flaxseed oil is converted to EPA and DHA in the body. Approximately 3–6 percent of LNA (omega-3) is converted to EPA, and 1.9–3.8 percent is converted to DHA. Therefore, the amount listed is only an average measurement.

As I've mentioned, omega-3 fatty acids are also available in fish oil capsules. In 1996, the American Heart Association recommended fish oil capsules only for people with very high triglyceride levels. In the years that have followed, new evidence for the benefits of omega-3s caused the association to expand its recommendation to include anyone with heart disease. So if you don't eat at least three or four fish meals a week, then supplement with 1,000mg of fish oil daily. If you have high blood pressure, use at least 2g per day; go up to 3g if your blood pressure is not coming down.

SUPPLEMENT UPDATE: FLAXSEED/LINSEED

The ancient Egyptians valued flaxseed (or linseed as it is also known) for its natural healing properties, and yet it's taken us until now to discover its health benefits. Studies have reported that flaxseed can lower cholesterol, heal eczema, and prevent gallstones. Research also suggests that flaxseed may affect coronary artery disease by preventing the inflammatory reactions that lead to arterial blockage by plaque formation.

Flaxseed is rich in essential fatty acids. Our bodies need EFAs to make hormones and other essential compounds. EFAs protect cell membranes throughout your body, assisting with the transport of health-promoting nutrients and putting up barriers against toxic agents. Unfortunately, your body can't produce enough of its own EFAs to meet the demand, so you need to supplement EFAs in your daily meals. For this reason I've included flaxseed, which is high in alpha-linolenic acid (ALA), a precursor of the omega-3 fatty acids. Flaxseed is also an EFA option on the PAMM programme for those of you who are allergic to fish or just don't care to eat it.

Under ideal circumstances, your body can metabolize alpha-linolenic acid into EPA and DHA, but some people's bodies may not be as efficient at the conversion process because of a natural lack of necessary enzymes or because the conversion reaction is blocked by stress, alcohol, ageing, and other factors. Still, I encourage the daily use of flaxseed. In addition to alpha-linolenic acid, flaxseed is loaded with fibre and provides many other important health benefits. Flaxseeds have more fibre than oats, plus they are high in lignan, a fibre compound that has been shown to have remarkable immune-enhancing activities and perhaps can help prevent cancer.

GROUND-UP FLAXSEED IS BETTER THAN FLAXSEED OIL
Use a coffee grinder to make your own. Sprinkle on cereals, soya shakes, and salads, or try my recipe: 1 Tbsp. ground flaxseed mixed with 240ml. of soya milk. Makes a great shake in your blender!

Flaxseed: A Bonus for Blood Pressure Lowering

With flaxseed, you access the two key types of essential fatty acid, EPA and DHA, so it's a good omega-3 source that's also great-tasting. Flax contains approximately 19 percent activated omega-6s and 48 percent alpha-linolenic acid (an omega-3 precursor) by weight.

When ALA is converted to EPA and DHA, inflammation potential in the body is decreased. And because one of the biggest culprits lurking in the shadows behind increased blood pressure is an inflamed blood vessel, flaxseed's anti-inflammatory effect can have a favourable impact on blood pressure lowering. In fact, should you elect to join me in taking flaxseed for blood pressure lowering, you'll also be rewarded with healthier skin, lower cholesterol levels, improved digestion, and a cleaner bowel. The last of those results in less energy drain on your liver—the most important filter in the body. Remember that whenever your liver is breezing along, working at its optimum level of functioning, your LDL cholesterol goes down and your HDL level climbs.

There are two basic forms of flaxseed, and I use both of them in the meal plans that I've developed. *Ground flaxseed* has a crunchy, nutty flavour and can be sprinkled on your cereal, cottage cheese, or yogurt, or even mixed into a morning shake (it's a real treat with soya milk). *Flaxseed oil* can be mixed with other oils, herbs, garlic, and lemon for a delicious yet nutritionally awesome salad dressing.

Unlike olive oil, you can't cook with flaxseed oil, because heating destroys its health benefits. Both ground flaxseed and flaxseed oil tend to go rancid fairly quickly, so store whole flaxseed in an airtight container in your freezer and grind only what you need for each meal. Purchase whole flaxseed in small quantities, and be sure to use it up within three months.

Choose flaxseed oil in an opaque bottle and keep it refrigerated but not frozen. If the oil develops a strong paint-like odour, that's your signal that it's gone bad and no longer offers cardioprotection.

On my eight-week programme, I add 2 Tbsp. of flaxseed daily, either as oil or as ground meal. I prefer the ground seed because it's a two-for-one-deal: It contains lots of fibre and lignans, as well as those health-promoting EFAs for an added perk. You can also take flaxseed oil in capsules, but you'll need fourteen of them to equal 1 Tbsp. of oil. These nutritional superstars offer numerous health benefits throughout the body.

FLAXSEED OIL AND LINSEED OIL: AN IMPORTANT CAUTION
Flaxseed oil is also known as linseed oil. However, industrial linseed oil, found in paint shops, has poisonous additives, and this product is *never* to be used internally.

---

5 I'm All Stressed Out
Week 4

Here we are, in the fourth week of my blood-pressure-lowering pro-gramme. It's a good time to introduce an element often overlooked by many cardiologists—your emotional and spiritual health. Excessive stress, anxiety, and unresolved anger can trigger a fundamental and very protec-tive biological mechanism known as the fight-or-flight response.

This preprogrammed and unconscious physical response to a perceived threat entails a multi-organ chain of events that include physical and chemical changes. When we are faced with a perceived threat, whether it be running away from a hungry lion, meeting a pressing deadline, or deal-ing with a difficult teenager, our sympathetic nervous system goes into overdrive, flooding our body with stress chemicals such as the cate-cholamines adrenaline and noradrenaline. These chemicals produce a sharp rise in blood pressure, heart rate, oxygen consumption, and blood flow to the muscles.

These changes heighten our senses and mental focus and bolster our physical strength in the face of serious challenges. I'll bet you've all heard of cases where a man or woman has accomplished a superhuman feat, such as lifting a car, to save a loved one. This is fight-or-flight at its very best. This biological mechanism helped early humans survive a savage, primi-tive world and was absolutely essential to the survival of our species back when we had to outrun a woolly mammoth. But the problem is that in our modern urban civilization, this type of whole-body response to stress is the kind of physiological overkill that's linked to a host of physical disor-ders, from lowered immunity and infections to an increase in stroke, hypertension, and heart disease.

The fight-or-flight response involves these physiological changes, or adaptations, to prepare the body to fight for survival or escape from the situation. Blood is shunted to organs essential for self-defence and the mobilization of physical strength.
   Blood is shunted away from some areas:
* the gastrointestinal system, shutting down digestion (a low-priority function)
* the capillaries of the skin, to reduce bleeding in case of injury
   Blood is shunted to other centres of action:
* the eyes, for visual acuity
* the brain, for mental clarity and decision making
* skeletal muscles in the arms, legs, hands, and feet
* the heart, to increase the volume of blood ejected with each heartbeat
* the liver, to mobilize glucose for energy

Each day we face many challenges, both big and small. And each time we run the risk that our body will jump headlong into crisis mode: a process that pours out stress hormones that can literally kill us! It's this same cascade of chemical events that starts to surge when you're under chronic daily stress. Take the morning traffic jam. Your digestive system slows; you become aware of your palms sweating; you may experience generalized perspiration; and your muscles tense and tighten as your mind and body become involved in a physiological response that has no physical outlet or release. You are trapped at the wheel, at your desk, or wherever, with your juices in high gear and your body stuck in place.

We need to learn how to comfortably adapt to the wide range of issues that face us each day. We must try to avoid the harmful impact emotional stress can have on all aspects of our health.

For example, it is important that we not overlook the crucial role that emotions play in the development of high blood pressure. Emotions such as anger, hostility, and rage can be lethal. I reported on one case where a decorated World War II soldier ruptured his aorta during an episode of intense anger. This gentleman, whom I'll call Bill, had never had any known hypertension. In fact, he'd been checked often when donating blood to the Red Cross, and his blood pressure had always been fine.

What was his big stressor? Well, Bill was a nursing-home administrator. One day the facility's owner insisted that he fire his best nurse. Bill didn't agree with that decision, and a verbal argument ensued. He defended his nurse as if she had been one of his platoon leaders. Ultimately, however, he lost the argument; he had to surrender the issue to the nursing home owner's demands. Bill was upset and infuriated. Immediately following this confrontation, the nursing home owner asked Bill to drive him to the airport to catch a flight.

So there Bill was, trapped in a situation where he now had to do a favour for a man who had overpowered him—a man who had forced him to betray a trusted employee. Bill was confronted with a fight-or-flight situation in which he couldn't win the battle and he was also unable to flee. Just before driving to the airport, Bill's blood pressure soared so high that his aorta ruptured. Luckily, he got to a hospital and into emergency surgery, so he lived to tell his story.

To many, both doctors and patients alike, seething anger and rage represent the dark side of our personality, the part that tends to be denied or suppressed. Getting in touch with these powerful hidden emotions and becoming aware of their contribution to high blood pressure is critical in helping patients reverse this problem. This week I'm going to introduce to you a technique that will help your body. The key is to be productive without being self-destructive. Relaxation responses are counter-efforts by the body to reverse the unhealthy developments produced by acute and chronic stress reactions.

RELAXATION THERAPIES: IT *IS* ALL IN YOUR HEAD

Relaxation is characterized by an absence of physical, mental, and emotional tension—in direct contrast to the fight-or-flight response. You may not be aware that sometimes your heart essentially goes into combat when you're startled. Many of us tune out our bodies, not realizing that symptoms such as high blood pressure, chest discomfort, or shortness of breath are an indication that the heart is struggling. Relaxation can reduce levels of the stress hormones adrenaline and cortisol. It helps to bring increased heart rate, faster respiration, increased muscle tension, and higher blood pressure—all normal involuntary responses—down to more reasonable levels.

Herbert Benson, a Harvard-trained cardiologist, developed Relaxation Response, a quiet form of meditation, in 1975 to help his patients relax both mind and body while enhancing their sense of physical and mental well-being. Benson found that Relaxation Response could be successfully practised in combination with conventional medical therapy. I often advise my patients to try Benson's meditation or other relaxation techniques such as guided imagery, visualization, deep breathing, prayer, or listening to music, to name a few, whether they think they need them or not. A form of this Relaxation Response will be discussed later in this chapter. Interestingly, after doing some relaxation exercises, many patients report back that they had no idea how stressed they were. It's only after they have learned to let go that they have a point of reference for seeing just how much tension they were containing.

In this chapter, I give you an example of a guided imagery process that's particularly crafted to help you to relax your body and even your circulation. In any imagery exercise, it's essential to use several key techniques so that your body will connect with the process. First of all, images are important. In addition, the process should help you to reframe your experience— looking at a negative situation from a more positive perspective instead of struggling against it or trying to change it. Cognitive-behavioural therapies are about challenging your belief system. The old adage about seeing your glass as half full rather than half empty is a good example of reframing. When something happens to you, don't look at yourself as a victim of circumstance. You can talk yourself into stress . . . but you can also talk yourself out of it. The next time you're stressing out, just ask yourself, "Is it worth dying for?" In most instances, I think you'll decide that it's not.

You'll be engaging your right brain for this exercise, and we now have interesting research that shows healing is accomplished through the right brain. Your unconscious mind responds to pictures, sound, metaphors, and biological images, but it also knows when it's being tricked, so true statements are necessarily part of a health-promoting guided-imagery dialogue. You've probably heard of athletes using this technique to picture themselves crossing that finish line, making that basket, sinking that putt, or scoring that goal. Now you can try it to drop that blood pressure.

Try this exercise, and use it as a guide to make up your own personalized scripts if you choose. Be creative. The more personal the images that you select, the more likely it is that your body will respond. If you have a microphone and tape recorder, you can "talk" to your unconscious in your own voice, and play it back to relax. If not, you can get great relaxation and imagery tapes from my colleague Belleruth Naparstek (www.healthjourneys.com).

HAND-WARMING EXERCISE

This hand-warming imagery exercise is a great intervention for your high blood pressure. Be sure to find a quiet place where you won't be disturbed for twenty to thirty minutes. Turn down the lights, burn a candle if you wish, get comfy and play back your recording (See previous page).

As your mind becomes clearer and clearer, feel it becoming more and more alert . . . Somewhere deep inside of you . . . a brilliant light begins to glow. Sense this happening . . . The light grows brighter and more intense . . . This is the body–mind communication centre . . . Breathe into it . . . Energize it with your breath . . . The light is powerful and penetrating . . . a beam begins to grow out of the light . . . The beam shines into the aura of your hands and feet . . .

As you deepen your relaxation . . . feel . . . as you . . . breathe with the next few breaths . . . Let a picture come to your mind of your aorta, the blood vessel that leads out from your heart . . . This big, muscular blood vessel is much like the trunk of a beautiful tree . . . growing from the top of your heart . . . See the branches that lead off the aorta and up into your shoulders . . . These branches of blood vessels travel down the interior of your arm muscles . . . In your mind's eye, this may resemble the branches of a weeping willow tree . . . The branches divide again at your elbow and move down each side of your inner arm . . . past the pulse points at your wrists . . . into the palm of each hand . . . In your imagination, maybe now you can see that circle of blood vessels in the palm of each hand, much like a warm, golden red sunset in each hand . . . leading off from each circular sun ray . . . branches of smaller vessels guide the pulsing flow of warmth into each of your fingers . . . all the way to your fingertips . . . Can you hear the sound of the pulsing flow of warmth?

As you look even more clearly at this network of tiny blood vessels in your fingertips . . . within each one is a layer of fine strands of muscle, entwining the vessel in a circular fashion . . . As your relaxation deepens . . . you might scan your body . . . getting more relaxed . . . getting more comfortable . . . find that best position right now . . . The muscle fibres of your blood vessels also are relaxing . . . As they relax their hug around each vessel . . . they are able to get a bit larger . . . and more warm blood flows into them . . . This warmth . . . radiates . . . from the blood vessels and shines . . . all the way . . . to the surface of your fingers . . . Feel that warmth increasing as the size of the blood vessels increases in your fingers . . .

You might let yourself imagine for a few moments what happens to the bloodflow into your fingers when you are feeling anxious, afraid, or threatened . . . The muscle fibres tighten their grip around the blood vessels . . . The vessels are squeezed down to a smaller diameter, and less and less blood is allowed to flow into your fingertips . . . You can feel them getting cooler by the moment . . . The moisture in your hands also increases and evaporation further decreases your hand temperature . . .

Now begin to change your image . . . Focus on the way you want to respond when you are next faced with feeling anxious or afraid . . . Use this as an opportunity to focus on your smooth, quiet breathing . . . Return to a feeling of peace and calm . . . Take all the time you need to allow the warmth to return to your hands . . . enjoy the true feeling of accomplishment that comes with knowing what is happening to your body . . . You can change events with your relaxation and imagery skills . . .

Take a few energizing breaths as you come back to full awareness of the room . . . Know that whatever is right for you at this time is unfolding just as it should . . . know that you have done your best, regardless of the outcome . . .

Modified from Achterberg, Dossey, Kolkmeier, *Rituals of Healing; Using Imagery for Health and Wellness* (New York: Bantam, 1994).

The key to the relaxation response lies in our brain wave activity. There are four different types of wave:

Beta waves: associated with daily conscious activity, or "waking state"
Delta waves: prominent during sleep and dreams
Theta waves: dominant in withdrawn, dream-like state
Alpha waves: elucidate states of deep physical relaxation and psychological peace; the mind is peaceful yet alert

Some of you may prefer meditation to guided imagery. Meditation is another concentrated relaxation exercise that promotes the emergence of both alpha and theta waves, a sign of physical and emotional peace and balance. Studies have shown that when the brain is emitting alpha and theta waves, the body increases its production of mood-lightening neurotransmitters such as serotonin. We have research documenting the blood-pressure-lowering effect of meditation practices, which include prayer and relaxation. In fact, the American Medical Association now recommends that people with borderline hypertension try meditation as a first-line approach, before medication, to lower their blood pressure.

Meditation is a simple kind of mind–body technique involving quiet contemplation to induce a state of mental and physical balance. Most schools of meditation began centuries ago in China, India, or Japan. In the West, interest in meditation began only in the 1960s and focused largely on the health benefits rather than the spiritual aspects of the practice. Studies have shown that meditation lowers levels of stress hormones and improves immunity. In addition, the regular practice of meditation lowers your risk of heart disease in a number of ways. Meditation is a relaxation technique that improves blood circulation and calms your heart rate, blood pressure, and breathing, reducing the energy drain on vital organs—including your heart.

There are three major types of meditation, all of which can be helpful, depending on your personal preference. *Mindfulness meditation* acknowledges the impact of events and circumstances on emotions. As thoughts come up, they're released, emptying the mind to induce a state of peace. *Breath meditation* focuses the attention, using conscious, slow, deep breathing to calm and relax the mind and body. *Transcendental meditation*, known as TM, involves the repetition of a word or sound, which is referred to as a mantra, to focus the attention inward. Most of the research done on the benefits of meditation have explored the use of TM.

TWENTY MINUTES A DAY THAT CAN CHANGE YOUR LIFE

This week I want you to set aside just twenty minutes each day to start your exploration into these life-saving relaxation strategies. You can choose from simple relaxation training and meditation, or you can select the qigong exercises that follow this section. You don't need any expensive equipment, lessons, or gurus. All that's required is your time, your interest, and a quiet location. Then in each of the following four weeks I'll be introducing you to more forms of relaxation therapies that will include massage, music therapy, yoga, and body-oriented therapies.

Whatever type of relaxation technique you practise, start by dressing comfortably in loose trousers and shirt. Find a quiet, comfortable place where you won't be disturbed, and sit down on a chair or a pillow on the floor. Keeping your back straight, close your eyes, and breathe deeply.

Meditation can be done at any time of the day, but choose a moment that provides the least stress or distraction. Meditation practice involves a brief relaxation process to bring you into a state of quiet reflection. Try the following instructions to see the impact that a twenty-minute meditation can have on your emotional and physical health.

RELAXATION/MEDITATION PROCESS

As you begin to quiet yourself, bring your awareness into your body, relaxing tightened muscles. Start at your head, opening your mouth wide and scrunching your face. Slow down your breathing, inhaling to the count of three through your nose and slowly exhaling to the count of three through your mouth. Slowly tilt your head to the right side, then to the left. Raise your shoulders, then lower them gradually. Take your time rolling them forward and then back again. Put your arms out to the side and shake them loose; open and close your fist and wiggle your fingers; shake out your legs, flex your ankles, and do a few ankle circles clockwise, then anti-clockwise.

Now, just sit with yourself for a while with eyes closed, allowing your mind to empty itself of the thoughts and concerns of the day. If it helps you to use a mantra, repeat that word to yourself in your mind. A mantra could include phrases such as "om", "shalom", "the Lord is my shepherd", or "hail Mary full of grace". Thoughts may drift into and out of your mind. That's normal. Neither judge them nor attend to them—just simply push them away like a big fluffy cloud. If it helps, picture a big, round balloon. Mentally blow your distracting thoughts into the balloon and watch them drift up, up, and away. Allow any images that come forth to be there with you now. They too may drift through your consciousness and float away. Stay with this process as long as you're comfortable, allowing your mind to have empty spaces. Welcome the sacred emptiness without any thoughts, and know that you are truly resting your spirit, your heart, and your soul.

As you feel ready, slowly, slowly come back to the room, back to your body. Notice how you feel. Gently, gently open your eyes, feeling how relaxed and calm you are.

I have found the most common problem that people experience when they first try a relaxation therapy such as guided imagery or meditation is a fear that somehow they're not doing it right. Keep in mind that this is not a test or a challenge to overcome. Just the fact you have made the commitment to set aside time for meditation means that you are indeed doing it right. You have made the right, healthy choice.

One of my patients with resistant hypertension was eager to cooperate with the nutritional and supplement programme. Helen agreed that my approach to exercise made her feel stronger within just a few weeks. But when I introduced the concept of meditation, she just lost it! "My mother has Alzheimer's, my son is dropping out of college, and my company is laying off people in my department," she said. "How can sitting in a room and saying the same stupid word over and over solve my problems?"

Of course it can't solve your very real problems, but meditation can allow your mind and body a retreat from the fight-or-flight mode, assuaging the physical changes of stress. What Helen did find was that achieving a relaxed state assisted her with problem solving in her waking state, just as was suggested in the research literature. It also helped her body to regroup its resources and better cope with real-life issues and concerns.

I have a lot of people in my practice whose lifestyles are particularly intense. Many others struggle with anxiety disorders, and many of their symptoms are cardiac in nature: racing or irregular heartbeat, light-headedness, chest tightness or pain, elevated blood pressure. Relaxation has been demonstrated to profoundly lessen these symptoms, but often extremely tense or anxious people just get more tense and anxious if I ask them to try techniques that involve sitting quietly. For them, movement therapies, such as t'ai chi and qigong, are more effective.

Check this out with yourself, too. You know yourself best, so if starting with a "moving meditation" has more appeal for you, then read on to my next discussion.

Or if you try relaxation, imagery, and meditation practices for several days but find that you're feeling more restless, annoyed, and irritated than relaxed, then try one of my personal favourites in the relaxation technique department: qigong.

QIGONG: ANCIENT CHINESE SECRET REVEALED

I often recommend that my patients investigate a form of relaxation therapy that combines slow, rhythmic movement and deep breathing, such as t'ai chi or qigong. I've been interested in various types of healing bodywork over the years, but more recently I've had amazing personal experiences with qigong.

Qigong combines two concepts: *qi* (also known as *chi*), the vital energy, and *gong*, the skill of mobilizing or working with the *qi*. You can think of qigong as cultivating the life force within you and tapping into your body's energy system. There are hundreds of types of qigong methods, but generally qigong practice involves deep breathing and soft, deliberate movements, as well as meditation and guided imagery.

I have no doubt that *qi* exists and can be worked with, because I have felt the results in my own body. Clinical and experimental data also demonstrate that qigong can have a positive impact on various organs and body systems. Once you begin to experience your body's *qi*, you'll be able to help heal yourself of the effects of chronic stress, as well as regain lost vitality and vigour. When you experience your *qi*, you'll not only reduce stress and lower your blood pressure, you'll also magnify the inner peace that Dr. Roger Jahnke, a qigong master, refers to as the "healer within". I wholeheartedly agree!

The History and Science

Qigong owes its roots to the martial arts, but the intention of this meditation exercise is to keep your body in harmony rather than to train for self-defence. Chinese doctors believe that qigong can help a wide range of health problems, and the scientific studies back them up.

In 1993, researchers released results of a thirty-year study with a group of 242 hypertensive patients. All the subjects were placed on medication, but the experimental group practised qigong for thirty minutes twice a day as well. The results were impressive: The mortality rate was 25.4 percent in the qigong group and 40.8 percent for the controls. The rate of stroke, one of the most serious consequences of hypertension, was lower in the group that practised qigong. Researchers also reported that over the years of the study, blood pressure levels of the qigong group stabilized, while those of the study participants on drugs alone increased. Interestingly, drug dosage for the qigong group actually decreased, and for 30 percent of the group, drugs could be eliminated. The drug dosage for the control group increased.

Other studies reported the frequent practice of qigong to be associated with lowering of cholesterol levels and increased circulation to the brain. It's also been suggested that qigong increases the flow of the lymphatic system, improving immunity. In addition, qigong can relieve pain, probably by increasing the release of endorphins, your body's own natural painkillers, and by enhancing your flexibility.

There are literally thousands of qigong forms. Some offer relatively simple movements to teach better breathing techniques, while more complex exercises are aimed at experiencing the *qi*, or flow of energy. Any of these forms and interpretations can have a favourable effect on heart rate and blood pressure. To get you started, I'll describe two of my favourite qigong exercises. You can elect to incorporate these into the twenty minutes a day that you've set aside for meditation.

Qigong Exercise 1

The following exercise is one that I learned from Roger Jahnke, author of a book entitled *The Healer Within*. I attended his workshop on qigong at Omega, a holistic conference centre in Rhinebeck, New York, in July 2001. This is a great exercise for relaxation of the whole body.

- Start by placing your feet about two feet apart. Bend your knees lightly. Slowly inhale.
- With your arms at your sides, gently bring your arms up, palms facing forward.
- Spread your fingers as you raise your arms, elevating your heels off the floor as you shift your weight up onto your toes, bringing your eyes to gaze up toward the sky with the motion, gradually stretching your hands over your head.
- Now exhale slowly as you turn your hands over and bring your arms slowly back down to your sides, rocking your weight from your toes back onto your heels.
- Repeat this movement without pausing, seven to ten times.
- Remember the breath: inhale as you extend upward, exhale as you come down to the floor again.

Many of you may feel your own *qi* or life force as a vibrational, electromagnetic kind of energy in your hands. If you do feel your *qi*, then I encourage you to keep working with it and allow yourself the experience of feeling it.

Qigong Exercise 2

Another qigong exercise that I enjoy is one that I learned from Luke Chan at a December 2001 conference on psychoneuoroimmunology, a field of medicine that addresses how the mind affects the body and the immune system. Luke advises me that this simple exercise is a well-kept secret that's been handed down for generations, but you need strong legs for this one.

- Stand facing a wall, feet together.
- With your nose, forehead, and feet close to the wall, bend your knees slightly and tilt your pelvis forward. Inhale.
- Lean in, bringing your nose in to almost touch the wall.
- Slowly, lower your legs into a full squatting posture, keeping your nose as close to the wall as possible until you reach your final point of stretch, keeping your heels on the ground.
- Hold the position and lift with your waist and legs, not your shoulders, exhaling on your ascent.
- Gradually come back to standing, pulling your face away from the wall, as you straighten and align your back.
- Repeat two to four times, and try to add one repetition a day until you reach ten cycles daily.

Luke Chan recommends doing this exercise for one hundred days consecutively. It's great for strengthening the legs and stretching the low back. It has helped me to ease a lot of the back tension that I experience from old sports injuries.

If you're a beginner, you may want to keep your feet a few inches apart, standing about six inches away from the wall. As you improve your physical condition, you can bring your feet closer together and your body closer to the wall.

This week, you can practise meditation and alternate it with qigong exercises, or you can choose either one.

DIET UPDATE: FIGS AND RAISINS

Go Fig-ure

One of nature's oldest foods, figs are a great source of fibre, potassium, calcium, and iron. They're especially rich in magnesium, which, you'll recall, is the cardinal mineral for supporting favourable blood pressure. Dried or diced into small cubes, figs can add sweetness and nutrition to cereals, salads, and whole-grain side dishes.

Depending on the season, you might see four or five varieties of figs.

There are black Mission figs, which have black skins and yellow seeds; Kadota figs, with their green coat and purple seeds; Calimyrna, a large yellowish green variety; and Smyrna, a fig grown in Turkey. While fresh figs are available for only a very short time in the market, dried figs can be found all year. Health food stores are your best bet for finding organic figs, as well as their sister fruit, dates.

Rockin' Raisins

Organic raisins are a good source of fibre and iron. They also contain small amounts of calcium and potassium, great minerals for blood pressure lowering. I advise my patients who are low in iron, and even those who are anaemic, to use raisins as a natural iron source. Raisins are also an excellent source of quercetin, the antioxidant that seems to protect the hearts of fifty million French people from the consequences of their high-fat diet.

But there is a caveat to raisins: They're high in sugar and calories, so use them sparingly unless you're iron-deficient. Add a tablespoon of raisins to hot and cold cereal, or stir them into a salad or a side dish of hearty whole grains.

SUPPLEMENT UPDATE: L-ARGININE

L-arginine is an amino acid with an uncanny ability to offset the damaging effects of high cholesterol. Research has shown that L-arginine relieves coronary artery spasm and reduces blood pressure by enhancing the synthesis of nitric oxide in the cells that line the blood vessels, as we discussed in Chapter 3.

In rats, the oral administration of L-arginine reduced salt-dependent increases in blood pressure. In a small human study, high dietary intake of L-arginine was associated with significantly lower blood pressure—an average drop of 6mm Hg in systolic blood pressure and 5mm Hg in diastolic blood pressure. In a study of renal transplant and hemodialysis patients, the oral administration of high-dose L-arginine (9–18g) was well tolerated and had a favourable impact on systolic and diastolic blood pressure.

L-arginine can even retard the development of heart disease, including hardening of the arteries, by reducing plaque build-up in vessels. This multi-talented amino acid may also help reduce male impotence caused by poor circulation, beef up immune response, and encourage wound healing.

The average American diet contains about 5g of L-arginine, but most of that is found in the fatty red meat you're omitting on the PAMM programme, so you'll need to be knowledgeable about other ways to secure a good dietary intake of this nutrient.

While nuts, seafood, and eggs are even better food sources of L-arginine than red meats, you need to ingest 6 to 9g a day to get the cardioprotective effects. The problem is that in order to get this amount from your diet alone, you'd need to eat half a pound of tuna or two pounds of tofu each day. That's hardly a realistic serving size! So this week in your blood pressure lowering programme, I am adding 1,000mg of supplemental L-arginine twice a day to your programme.

CIRCULATORY BENEFITS OF L-ARGININE
- Lowers blood pressure
- Supports healthy blood flow
- Stabilizes angina
- Reduces pain of claudication (leg pain due to poor circulation)
- Improves symptoms of Raynaud's syndrome
- Relieves congestive heart failure
- Reduces blood platelet stickiness
- Helps overcome impotence

EXERCISE UPDATE: FLEXIBILITY

We all know what it means to be a flexible person in terms of adjusting easily to meet change in everyday situations. But flexibility also relates to the mobility or range of motion of your joints and back. The degree of flexibility you have in a particular joint is related to the length of the muscle that services it and the muscle's ability to stretch. Shortened muscles tend to be tighter, while long muscles have fuller, more natural movement. Flexible muscles are far less likely to become sprained or injured during exercise. Daily activity is a critical part of my natural blood-pressure-lowering programme, so it's important that you learn to avoid muscle cramps and spasms that can interfere with regular exercise.

Promoting flexibility also keeps your muscles comfortable and relaxed, relieving tensions that can lead to headaches and back pain. Finally, pliable muscles contribute to the strength and energy that let you meet the physical and mental challenges of daily life.

How Flexible Are You?

Before you start flexibility exercises, you need to establish where you are in terms of your existing range of motion. That way you can identify all the areas where your muscles tend to be on the tight and tense side. Try these three tests to get a baseline reading on your flexibility. Then at the end of the week take the tests again to gauge how far you have come.

Flexibility Test 1: Lower Body

- Sit on a straight chair with your back straight.
- Leaving one foot on the floor, raise the other leg parallel to the floor.
- If you can raise the leg to the thigh without straightening your leg, shifting your position on the chair, or raising your other foot, then your lower body enjoys a healthy range of motion. If not, then the exercises that follow will improve strength and mobility.

Flexibility Test 2: Upper Body

- Reach over your shoulder and behind your back with your right hand and stretch down toward your waist.
- Slip your left hand behind your back and, reaching up toward your neck, try to touch or overlap the fingers of both hands.
- If there is a gap of over a few inches, then flexibility exercises will help to make this a smooth and easy stretch.

Flexibility Exercise 3: Overall

- Sit on the floor with legs outstretched and your feet resting against a box or coffee table leg.
- See how far you're able to reach. This will give you a guide to your flexibility.
- Don't be surprised if you can't even reach the box or table with your fingertips. After a week of regular flexibility workouts, you may well be able to stretch up to nine inches past the edge of the box or table.

Flexibility Guide
Excellent ..... 8–9 inches past box
Very good ...5–8 inches past box
Fair ....1–5 inches past box
Poor..............Cannot reach box

Stretching It Out

Muscles are naturally more flexible after they've been warmed up. A five-minute hot shower can relax muscles, relieving chronic pain and stiffness. After your morning shower try doing at least two of these wonderful flexibility exercises each day, just to keep limber. Remember not to hold your breath. Breathe evenly, exhaling on any effort.

Exercise 1: Thigh Stretch

- Lie face-down on the floor with your legs outstretched.
- Bend your right leg up to touch the back of your thighs and buttocks.
- Grab your toes with your right hand.
- Pull slowly, feeling the stretch through the thigh.
- Hold for a count of four, then slowly release.
- Repeat with your left leg.

Exercise 2: Hamstring Stretch

- Lie on your back with right knee bent and right foot flat on the floor.
- Keep your left leg stretched out flat on the floor.
- Straighten your right leg as high as you can go, holding the back of your leg with both hands; feel the stretch through the back of the leg.
- Hold for a count of three, then slowly lower leg to the floor.
- Repeat with your left leg.

Exercise 3: Shoulder Stretch

- Sit cross-legged on the floor with your back nice and straight.
- Lean forward a bit and clasp hands behind your back.
- Without hunching your shoulders, pull your arms back and upward.

- Hold for a count of three.
- Release slowly and repeat.
- If you can't clasp your hands together, then hold one end of a towel in each hand as you pull up and back.

6 Triple A: Asparagus, Avocado, and Anger
Week 5

Last week we completed the four pillars of my blood-pressure-lowering programme. You're now on the PAMM diet, taking a broad spectrum of nutritional supplements, incorporating exercise into your daily routine, and appreciating the connection between your emotions and your blood pressure. If you've been following the menus and guidelines, then you've probably shed a few pounds and are starting to feel a renewed sense of energy. In the next four weeks, you'll continue to expand upon my basic programme, adding new ideas about nutrition, supplements, exercise, and mind–body components that will enhance and increase your control over your own health.

DIET UPDATE 1: ASPARAGUS

Long, green, and elegant as they are, asparagus aren't just beautiful and delicious; they also deliver a first-rate package of nutrients. These crunchy spears contain protein, fibre, vitamin C, folic acid, and beta-carotene. They also are an excellent source of glutathione, a valued nutrient with both antioxidant and anticancer properties.

Dark green asparagus offers your best nutritional value, while the more expensive white asparagus has far less antioxidant value. So it may not be easy being green, but it's your best buy in the asparagus depart-ment, and luckily the green stalks are easy to find. And, by the way, keep your asparagus cold and crispy to retain its vitamin content. Frozen asparagus has a nutritional value similar to that of fresh, but not the same satisfying fresh crunch. Your best bet on frozen is to store fresh organic asparagus in your own freezer bags after they've been washed and towel-dried.

For a quick and easy way to prepare these green babies, check out my own personal recipe. It's even a hit at our summer-time family barbecues. For best results in terms of crunch and nutrition, just be careful not to overcook asparagus.

DR. SINATRA'S QUICK AND EASY ASPARAGUS PREPARATION
Place fresh asparagus in a pot with water to cover. Bring to a simmer over medium heat and cook for about five minutes; don't boil. Avoid overcooking. Drain off water (or save it to use as a nutritious base for soup). Sprinkle asparagus sparingly with garlic salt, squeeze on a bit of fresh lemon juice, drizzle with extra-virgin olive oil, and enjoy!

DIET UPDATE 2: AVOCADOS

Although avocados are high in fat, their fat is the heart-healthy monounsaturated kind, offering invaluable antioxidant and anti-inflammatory protection. Avocados are equally rich in vitamin E, folic acid, vitamin B6, and pantothenic acid. Their creamy rich flesh is also a great source of essential minerals and fats, especially alpha-linolenic acid. In addition to containing health-promoting doses of iron, copper, and magnesium, avocados offer you 60 percent more potassium than bananas. And that's not all!

The avocado's benefits go on to include glutathione, the anticarcinogenic antioxidant, as well as a healthy supply of cholesterol-lowering beta-sitosterols. That's quite a nutritional payload! Just toss a few cubes of avocado into your salads, tuck a few slices into your sandwiches on wholemeal pittas, or mash some up with tomatoes to dab on raw vegetables. Don't let your fear of this healthy fat prevent you from including this wonderful food in your diet. Now you understand why avocados are such a perfect PAMM food!

SUPPLEMENT UPDATE: GRAPESEED EXTRACT

Grapeseed extract is an interesting nutriceutical. The technical term for its active ingredient is oligomeric proanthocyanidin (OPC). OPCs are complex chemicals including polyphenols, which are found in fresh fruits, vegetables, pine bark, cherries, plums, and blueberries, with the highest concentration occurring in grapeseed. OPCs are so highly bioavailable that they are taken up by all the tissues. They not only get inside the bloodstream rapidly, but also penetrate brain cells because they're transported across the "blood brain barrier" easily. Grapeseed extract has extraordinary health benefits when used in doses of 150 to 300mg daily.

First of all, it's a superior antioxidant with free-radical-scavenging activity as well as potent anti-inflammatory activity. Grapeseed extract improves the elasticity of venous structures and is great for stabilizing varicose veins. It also improves the integrity of the arteries and improves blood vessel elasticity. Because it acts like an ACE inhibitor, this OPC also lowers blood pressure. Some researchers also speculate that grapeseed extract reduces blood pressure via vasodilation, by enhancing the production of nitric oxide.

In one study using Concord grapes, researchers reported that their various chemical compounds, including proanthocyanidins, promote improvement in cardiovascular function. In another study performed by researchers at the University of California, Davis, the flavonoids found in grapeseed extract helped increase blood flow, resulting in better control of blood pressure. Yet other research has shown that grapeseed extract can inhibit the oxidation of LDL and also prevent clumping of platelets. This is one nutrient that has multiple cardiovascular benefits. It certainly has a place in my natural blood-pressure-lowering programme.

EXERCISE UPDATE: STRENGTH TRAINING

Seventy percent of people over sixty-five can't lift a gallon of milk above their shoulder, so it's clear that we all need to be aware of maintaining physical strength as we age. That's where strength training— exercises that focus on toning particular muscle groups—comes in. A crucial partner to cardiovascular fitness, strength training involves the use of weights and resistance.

Light weights can be added to your routine body movements to force your muscles to contract against resistance, helping to gradually increase muscle mass, strength, and tone. Stronger muscles not only translate into a firmer, more toned body but also extract oxygen and glucose from your blood more efficiently than flabby muscles. And whenever an organ or muscle can metabolize oxygen and nutrients more effectively, your cardiovascular system hums along with less stress and strain. So exercise and strength training are no-brainers when it comes to better blood pressure dynamics.

In addition to better oxygen utilization, the enhanced glucose metabolism benefits of exercise and strength training mean your insulin secretion is more stable, tackling yet another risk factor for higher blood pressure. My advocacy of weight training does not mean that I am in favour of bench-pressing a hundred pounds every morning before breakfast. Far from it! Working out with heavy weights is the last thing I would recommend to people with high blood pressure.

Less Is More

The strain of lifting heavy weights can raise your blood pressure to dangerous levels and has been linked to several cases of sudden fatal heart attacks. In fact, isometric weight lifting, which involves holding your breath and straining while you lift a heavy weight, should not be tackled by anyone who has a cardiac concern, including high blood pressure. Other less obvious forms of isometric exercises include water skiing, where the arms are held in a state of tension, pulling on the tow rope; moving a refrigerator; or pushing a car. These activities create an increase in intrathoracic pressure (pressure within the chest cavity), which squeezes down on the heart and raises pressure inside its chambers.

Cardiologists advise isotonic exercises—those that involve breathing through the effort of lifting a light weight (under five pounds) held away from the body. I have a "less is more" approach when it comes to weight training. Instead of investing in gut-busting barbells, I advise you to buy two-to-three-pound weights. You can select the barbell shapes because they are easy to grip, or try the leather type that have Velcro straps for more versatility—you can attach these to your arms and/or ankles when you go out for your daily walk. Light ankle weights can also be worn as you go about your chores around the house. These tricks can help you to build muscle in your arms, legs, and thighs while you're doing everyday activities. Start off using weights for up to thirty minutes, and gradually work your way up to an hour a day. It won't add a minute to your daily to-do list, but your body will show the benefits with more energy and greater strength. You'll notice that over time, less effort is required for simple tasks, which in itself can lower your blood pressure.

MIND–BODY UPDATE: ANGER MANAGEMENT

Anger is a perfectly natural emotion that we all feel in day-to-day situations. Ever have a car pull right out in front of you, so that you have to swerve to avoid disaster? Or have a car cut a corner only to splash mud all over your new dress or suit right before that big interview? Or have someone cut in front of you in line after you've been waiting and waiting? Or hurry through rush-hour crowds only to watch your train just pulling away from the station? Or miss that big putt in an important golf game? You get the picture.

These are situations that we all find stressful and unpleasant, and to feel angry is a natural response. But how you express and handle that anger is what determines its impact on your blood pressure and your overall health.

No Shortage of Advice

Much has been written about anger management. Some experts suggest staying calm and trying to roll with the punches. Others recommend that you express anger in a kind of "let it all out" approach. But I think these strategies miss the main point.

Anger in and of itself is not an inherently ugly or bad emotion. It's what you do with it that can be adaptive, maladaptive, or even harmful. You see, to live in a social environment, we need to be able to control our anger. So, early in our lives we are sanctioned or even shamed if we display anger, especially when it's displayed in aggressive behaviour. It doesn't take us long to send those feelings underground, disowning them in order to see ourselves as "good."

But angry feelings aren't necessarily bad, and there's an energy in anger that, when properly channelled, can be transformed into a powerful healing force. The first step is recognizing and acknowledging your feelings. As a cardiologist, I frequently see patients like Rob, a man whose blood pressure is impacted by the lack of connection between his head and his heart.

At forty-four years of age, Rob would have been considered successful by anyone's standards. He had a good income, a fine home, a loving family, and a very prestigious job. But his blood pressure was frightening! At readings like 220/110, his hypertension had defied control with traditional diet and drug programmes. Looking at Rob sitting across from me,

I would have to have been blind not to notice his jaw clenched with tension.

I was frustrated and deeply concerned about Rob, so I elected to put him through the paces with some equipment I had purchased that was an offshoot of NASA technology. My computer-based cardioimpedance system was developed from equipment used to test the effects of weightlessness on the cardiodynamics of astronauts. NASA was careful to screen their astronauts to see if their hearts could take the stress of living in space.

The space-age impedance equipment was adapted to perform psychophysiological stress tests on the cardiovascular system that were developed by cardiologist Robert Eliot, author of a book called *Is It Worth Dying For?* This scientific evaluation allowed me the opportunity to give Rob an emotional stress test. I could use my computer to measure the effect of anger on his blood pressure and other cardiodynamic parameters by having him frustrated by simple exercises, such as counting backward by sevens and trying to beat the computer at a game of car racing.

I also asked Rob some pretty personal questions about his life while his hands were plunged into ice-cold water up to his mid forearm. In a reasonably calm person in the same situation, I'd expect about a 5 to 10mm Hg rise in systolic blood pressure, and maybe a little increase in diastolic pressure, too, just from the vasoconstricting effect of the cold water. What were Rob's numbers? Off the charts! He went up 15 to 20mm Hg on both his systolic and diastolic readings, especially when he spoke about his work and personal relationships. During our session, his blood pressure had risen to a very dangerous 240/125, even though he looked like Cool Hand Luke on the outside! I was astonished to see what Rob's unexpressed feelings were doing to his body. There is actually a name that has been coined to describe this phenomenon: "hot reactivity".

There was little doubt about it: Rob was a "hot reactor". Though he appeared the picture of composure, his cardiovascular system was in overdrive. My suspicion was now a certainty: The root cause of Rob's hypertension was his internalized anger, and no drug or diet would have much of an impact until he dealt with the issues that were consuming him.

When I asked him gently if he was aware of how much anger he had inside, Rob began to cry. He confided to me that this was the first time anyone had recognized his "secret" and with it, his personal pain and suffering. I made arrangements for Rob to see a psychotherapist who understood the links between physical health and unexpressed emotional issues. Six months later Rob's blood pressure was almost normal.

Rob's type of long-term, simmering-but-hidden anger feeds a constant flow of stress hormones in the body that constrict blood vessels, render platelets sticky, and even provoke heart palpitations or chest discomfort. Unresolved, unexpressed anger can be a real Achilles' heel for the cardio-vascular system. It places an undesirable burden on the heart by increasing the resistance in blood vessels. It's no wonder Rob's blood pressure resisted change until we worked on his unresolved anger.

And though this case that I've shared with you involves a man, it surely doesn't mean that women are off the hook in this regard. I have had similar scenarios with women in my practice, one of which comes to mind immediately.

I first met Joyce in the accident and emergency room in full-blown cardiac arrest. For three days she had been in a state of rage. She had been deeply wounded. Her husband of thirty years had been unfaithful, and when she'd discovered it, her feelings of heartbreak and betrayal found their expression in unrelenting, seething anger. Her blood pressure was sky high, and her heart finally gave way; she had a heart attack.

We would later find out that Joyce had normal coronary arteries. There were no blockages, but the anger that had taken her hostage had almost killed her.

HOW ANGRY AM I?
To gauge your hidden anger levels, try taking this little test:
• Do I ever give people dirty looks?
• Do I ever strike out verbally or physically?
• Am I sarcastic with others?
• Do I sometimes flare my nostrils when I'm annoyed?
• Do I become so impatient I find myself interrupting people?
    If you answer yes to two or more questions several times a week, unresolved anger could be driving up your blood pressure.

Living daily with suppressed rage or anger is unhealthy for you and those around you. Burying and denying feelings is a poor solution. Over the past decade I've found that men and women who hide their emotions are at the greatest risk of developing high blood pressure and heart disease. This week you're going to start working on anger management strategies with exercises I've developed with my own patients.

Exercise 1: Go Fly a Kite

Spend some time outdoors doing something you enjoy, such as browsing through flea markets, flying a kite, walking your dog, puttering in the garden, or playing catch with your son or daughter. I've found that the combination of spending time out of doors and taking the time to do something you really enjoy can have a more profound effect on your blood pressure than powerful medications.

Being with your pet dog, cat, or bird can also have enormous benefits. Research has shown that the simple stroking of a dog's fur can cause remarkable blood pressure lowering. But there is an even greater realization that occurs with just being in the simple space of an animal that gives you unconditional love. As a cardiologist, I've always tracked the survival rate of people who have suffered a heart attack. It is four to five times greater for those who come home from the hospital to a loving pet than for those who come home to a lonely house. The unconditional love of a dog or any other pet creates a calmness and tranquillity that can transcend your blood pressure.

The love an animal gives you can lift your spirits, taking you away from darkness and despair. I often bring my chow, Chewie, to my surgery. Chewie accompanies me when I see new or established office patients. Although I always ask permission from a new patient to bring Chewie into the room, it's a rare occurrence where the patient forbids it. As a doctor, I find that some patients can literally drain your energy, while others can help empower your healing ability. One of the worst things a doctor can do is carry any anger, resentment, or hostility from one patient into the next room. Whenever I confront that situation, I use my dog as my therapist, and I'll pet her as I talk to the patient who is draining my energy. The love I feel from my pet helps me just let the negative energy go. When I head into the next room, I have a renewed sense of self and an exciting willingness and enthusiasm to meet with my next patient. Pets can indeed give you a simple spiritual experience.

Speaking of spirituality, you also need to put time aside for spiritual experiences, even if it means scheduling them on your busy calendar. Sometimes the pressures of family life and work commitments create a daily field of obligations to others that results in deep-seated resentments and spiritual exhaustion. Many of us are reluctant to take time away from our busy lives. We've become so accustomed to meeting professional and personal demands that the idea of taking time to just be with ourselves actually feels foreign.

For some people, I get around this issue by actually writing down "personal time" on my prescription pad, so they'll take my advice more seriously. I've even become very specific, prescribing golf, fishing, and walking on the beach. Once they have taken the time for themselves, they return to tell me that they can't believe how good they feel—and they are amazed at how their stress levels and blood pressure numbers start to go down.

Exercise 2: The Message Is the Massage

When your blood pressure is high, massage is a necessity, not a luxury. In addition to lowering your heart rate and blood pressure, a good massage will relax your muscles, promote general circulation, and help to detoxify your body. Bodywork can help to heal your emotional scars, as well as release stored emotions that can block healing energy.

Doctors have recognized for centuries that touch is essential for growth, healing, and well-being. Research studies have demonstrated the benefits of bodywork for relief of pain, anxiety, and depression as well as the promotion of a healthy immune system. Add a touch of aromatherapy to your session and just feel your body unwind.

There are over eighty different schools of massage and other forms of bodywork for you to choose from, but popular styles include the following:

- *Swedish massage* is the traditional Western bodywork based on conventional ideas of anatomy and physiology. You lie unclothed under a sheet on a padded table. The massage consists of a combination of long gliding strokes, friction, and kneading. Working to direct blood flow to the heart, Swedish massage has been shown to relieve tension, improve circulation, and loosen stiff joints.
- *Shiatsu* is a form of massage that originated in Japan. Using firm finger pressure at individual spots on the body, the goal of shiatsu is to increase circulation of the vital energy, or *qi*. In Eastern medicine it is believed that *qi* flows through invisible channels in

your body. During the session, you lie on a padded mat on the floor with the therapist seated beside you. It is a stronger massage than Swedish massage but can be very effective in dissipating chronic muscular tension.

- *Neuromuscular massage* provides deep body work of muscles, tendons, ligaments, and nerves. The goal is to increase blood flow and release spasms of muscular tension known as trigger points.
- *Rolfing* is more invasive and involves deep tissue work in order to work out tension and restructure the musculoskeletal system. Therapists apply pressure firm enough that you may experience discomfort. "Getting Rolfed" means completing ten sessions, each focused on a different part of your body. Rolfing is particularly helpful for releasing repressed emotions.
- *Reiki* is an energy work technique in which healing energy is believed to be channelled through the hands of a Reiki-trained therapist. Some researchers believe that Reiki promotes the release of endorphins, the body's natural painkillers. During a Reiki session you lie fully clothed on a padded table; the practitioner starts by "scanning" your body for areas of blocked energy. As trouble spots are identified, the Reiki practitioner places a hand lightly over these areas. This gentle touch lasts five to twenty minutes, with the entire session running sixty to ninety minutes. Reiki massage is believed to reduce stress, improve concentration, and relieve pain. Many people who are overweight have issues about having their bodies seen, let alone touched. Some older people may be hesitant about disrobing for a massage. Reiki is especially good for anyone who's a little queasy about bodywork because you keep your clothes on while the practitioner works with your energy field, applying soft touch and often no touch at all.

My local hospital even offers a reasonably affordable course for couples to learn how to massage one another to promote health, relaxation, and closeness. So see what's available in your area, and rest assured that whatever type(s) of massage you decide to try, this kind of energy work can bring down your blood pressure.

Even if you don't follow any other mind–body advice this week, take the time to schedule a Reiki session or a massage. Many of my patients start with a traditional Swedish massage. As they recognize the health benefits of bodywork, they look into other forms, such as Rolfing, in order to focus on specific problems. And remember that all forms of massage can also help to detoxify your body by mobilizing lymphatic blood flow, so rest and drink plenty of water afterward. This in itself will assist blood pressure lowering.

Exercise 3: The Power of Tears

Sadness often lurks just beneath the surface of anger. From a very young age, many of us are urged to hide our own sadness. We may have been constantly admonished not to cry, with words such as "Big boys don't cry" or "Stop your crying right now, or I'll give you something to cry about!" Ugh! I shudder just to think of how parents inadvertently deny the true feelings of their own children. And as a society, we try to mask sadness with antidepressants.

Ever feel a "blocked cry"? It's often that lump or tightness in your throat that just won't go away. Sometimes it comes up when your feelings have just been hurt, following a personal injustice. But a good cry is exactly what the body needs. Deep sobs allow anger and stress to be released. Crying frees your heart of muscle tension that can push up your blood pressure. The deep sobs of a good cry can increase the flow of oxygen to your brain, releasing chemicals that relax your body—part of the reason you feel calmer after an episode of stress-relieving tears.

Even more important, when you release emotional tension with tears, you lower your circulating levels of cortisol and adrenaline, two hormones that raise your risk of hypertension and heart disease. We have such strong prohibitions against crying in our society that you may be woefully out of practice. To help you get started, rent a tearjerker movie, such as *Beaches, Little Women,* or whatever moves you. The emotional release of crying when young Beth dies in *Little Women* will affect your entire body. (My wife cries every time she watches them try to resuscitate E.T. or when Sally Field's character loses her daughter in *Steel Magnolias.* For me, I lose it when Rudy keeps on trying to make it as a football player.)

Try these three mind–body exercises on different days during this week. Choose the right time for each one. For example, rent a tearjerker video for an evening at home; playing catch with a child is a great weekend activity; just being with your pet can help you unwind after a tough day at work; or schedule a massage. It's important to use these exercises when it feels most comfortable for you. Trying to fit them in when other demands are present will only raise your stress levels, not to mention your blood pressure.

7 Will Legumes, Mushrooms, Garlic, and Yoga Help Lower My Blood Pressure? Week 6

This week I am going to give you some more nutrition basics so you'll understand why the food selections on the PAMM diet are so good for your blood pressure, your heart, and your overall health.

DIET UPDATE 1: WHOLE GRAINS, LEGUMES, NUTS, AND SEEDS

Whole grains, legumes, nuts, and seeds are the foundation of my PAMM diet. These foods provide complex carbohydrates, fibre, protein, and precious vitamins and minerals. Remember that complex carbohydrates are "slow burners"—they are converted into blood sugar very slowly. This stabilizes your blood sugar, helping you avoid insulin resistance.

Whole grains are an important source of fibre, B vitamins, and minerals. At my health food shop in Manchester, Connecticut, the chefs use a variety of grains that include spelt, amaranth, bulgur, quinoa, and barley in our organic lunches.

Spelt flour makes a hearty, chewy bread that many of our customers enjoy, particularly when they wash it down with barley vegetable soup. Spelt is a low-glycemic-index relative of wheat that originated in Southeast Asia. This tasty grain is rich in soluble fibre and can be used in breads, and pastas, and as a breakfast cereal.

Amaranth is a sweet, hardy grain that was prized by the Aztecs in Mexico. It is rich in minerals such as iron, copper, and magnesium, and is best when mixed with coarser grains such as brown rice or spelt. Sandy's crab cakes, using amaranth as a base, are a big hit on Fridays. (See the recipe section of this book.)

Bulgur is produced when whole-wheat kernels are steamed, dried, and cracked into bits. Treated in this manner, the grains offer an excellent source of fibre and niacin. Unlike other hearty grains, bulgur is so easy to cook! All you need to do is soak it in hot water, drain, and enjoy. With its hearty flavour and texture, bulgur can be eaten as a breakfast cereal or used in place of rice in pilaf and salad recipes.

Quinoa is a high-protein grain that delivers a terrific nutritional payload of B vitamins and minerals. Mild and sweet-tasting, quinoa can be substituted for rice in your favourite recipes such as paella or rice pudding. As quinoa cooks, its outer coating splits open to form a little tail, much like the tip of a bean sprout. While the cooked grain has a soft texture, the little tail retains a delightful crunch.

Barley is a food of the ancient world, found in countries as diverse as Scotland and Ethiopia. Like oats, barley is high in cholesterol-lowering soluble fibre. Barley has a good source of a number of minerals, including iron, manganese, and phosphorous. Creamy and mild, barley can be used in soups, in pilafs, and even as a breakfast cereal. For maximum nutrition, look for barley that hasn't had its vitamin- and mineral-rich hull removed. You can find this type of barley in health food shops. In general, supermarkets only stock pearled barley, a grain that's lost much of its nutritional benefits in processing.

It's fun to be innovative with grains. They can even be used as leftovers, accompanied by a cold tossed salad with raw veggies, tofu cubes, and dressing.

Grains also are great-tasting with nutritious nuts and seeds, a fantastic source of healthy fat, protein, and fibre.

Nuts and seeds provide a host of key minerals such as magnesium, potassium, calcium, zinc, iron, and copper. When combined with organic dried cranberries, raisins, and dates, magnesium-rich nuts and seeds are part of a perfect recipe for lowering one's blood pressure. Many nuts are rich in vitamin E and phytosterols, which help to maintain normal cholesterol levels when consumed as part of the PAMM diet. You just can't go wrong with nuts.

Practically any type of nut or seed has specialized nutritious qualities. For example, almonds are rich in vitamin E and high in phytosterols. Sesame seeds provide a great source of calcium. Pistachio nuts are potent in vitamin B₆ and exceptionally high in phytosterols. Pine nuts are packed with phytosterols, while Brazil nuts have the highest selenium content of any food. In fact, just one ounce of Brazil nuts will serve you up about 800mcg of selenium. Supplementing selenium, by the way, is one of the best ways to detoxify the body of mercury, a heavy metal that can wreak havoc on your cardiovascular system. Selenium is also one of the most important nutrients in the prevention of tumours.

Nuts are also high in healthy fats. Most of the fat in nuts and seeds is unsaturated or monounsaturated. Almonds, hazelnuts, macadamia nuts, peanuts (which are actually legumes), pecans, and pistachios are all rich in health monounsaturated fats. Peanuts are especially high in vitamin E and contain great sources of L-arginine, which will support the production of nitric oxide, a blood-pressure-lowering chemical that you are now familiar with.

NUT AND SEED TIPS
- Choose raw, organic, unsalted nuts as often as possible. Avoid the honey-roasted varieties, as they just add empty calories.
- Sprinkle nuts and seeds on just about anything: yogurt, cereals, soups, salads, and especially cooked grain dishes.
- Use nuts and seeds as a convenience food. They can be a tasty snack, or even a meal for that matter.

DIET UPDATE 2: LEGUMES

A recent study published in the *Archives of Internal Medicine* in 2001 demonstrated a significant relationship between legume intake and risk of coronary heart disease. Those patients eating four or more legume foods per week had a 22 percent lower risk of coronary heart disease than those eating less than one legume food a week.

A study that followed a total of 9,332 men and women without any previous history of heart disease over 19 years looked at the frequency of legume intake and how it was a significant factor in the risk of coronary heart disease. Researchers observed that a diet rich in legumes, which are high in protein and soluble fibre, was associated with lower blood pressure levels. In this rather large study, people with more frequent legume intake had, on average, a lower systolic blood pressure. In addition, they had lower levels of total cholesterol, less diabetes, and a lower body mass index than their counterparts who consumed less legumes. Since legumes are generally low in sodium and rich in minerals such as potassium, calcium, and magnesium, they are perfect foods for lowering blood pressure.

As part of my PAMM diet, I recommend that you eat legumes, a food group that includes a large variety of beans (chickpeas, lentils, navy beans, kidney beans, etc.), on a daily basis. Remember that when you eat beans with whole grains, nuts, or seeds, you are getting a complete protein meal, containing the nine essential amino acids. Legumes are an excellent source of fibre, both soluble and insoluble. Foods with insoluble fibre will speed up the transit of foods through the bowel, so your body can't absorb as much fat and sugar from them. This not only reduces your cholesterol levels but also protects you from soaring blood sugar. All this adds up to helping normalize your blood pressure, preventing insulin resistance, and preventing heart disease.

DIET UPDATE 3: MUSHROOMS

Low in calories and fat free, and yet rich in B vitamins and calcium, mushrooms have been long valued for the flavour they add to cuisines throughout the world. In recent years, scientists in China and Japan have identified remarkable health properties in mushrooms that can help combat a range of problems, including heart disease, cancer, and liver disorders.

The delicious shiitake mushroom is an invaluable source of eight amino acids, thiamin, riboflavin, niacin, and fibre as well as ergosterol (an unsaturated hydrocarbon of the sterol group that is converted by sunlight into vitamin D). Shiitake mushrooms also contain lentinan, a polysaccharide that appears to help block tumour growth, lower blood pressure, and reduce cholesterol levels.

In addition, shiitake mushrooms contain lentinula edodesmycelium (LEM), a compound that may be helpful in the prevention and treatment of cancer, heart disease, high blood pressure, and hepatitis. Another substance in shiitake mushrooms, eritadenine, is thought to reduce cholesterol and fat levels by encouraging their exit from the body. Shiitake mushrooms have been shown to enhance the activity of natural killer cells, the body's first white blood cells to the rescue in defence against cancer cells and viruses. Currently these mighty mushrooms are used in conjunction with traditional chemotherapy in China and Japan.

Shiitake mushrooms are probably one of the most delicious nutritional aids that I've discovered. You can use them fresh or dried in stir-fry dishes, soups, salads, omelettes, and whole-grain side dishes. One of my favourite dishes is shiitakes with garlic and artichokes. (See recipes.)

The Myth of the Dancing Mushroom

In the past ten years, Japanese scientists have found an even more potent disease fighter in the maitake mushroom. *Maitake* means "dancing mushroom" because, according to folklore, when people found them they danced for joy, both because of the mushroom's flavour and because of its health-enhancing properties. The chemical structure of the maitake mushroom contains beta-glucan derivatives, important nutrients for cellular immunity.

Ongoing research demonstrates that maitake mushrooms can improve insulin sensitivity, thereby reducing problems of insulin resistance. Preliminary studies indicate that maitake mushrooms may also lower your cholesterol and triglyceride levels as well as your blood pressure. Dried maitake mushrooms can be found in well-stocked health food shops, but to preserve their health benefits, take care not to overheat them.

You can rehydrate mushrooms in hot, rather than boiling, water, and add them to soups and bean dishes that are already cooked. Don't discard the soaking liquid, though, because this liquid contains valuable nutrients—just add it to your soup base for extra nutrition. Maitake can also be taken as a supplement. You can go to your health food shop to purchase this or obtain it from mail order outlets or via the Internet.

SUPPLEMENT UPDATE: GARLIC

The health benefits of garlic have been known for centuries. Doctors in ancient Greece, Rome, China, and Japan used garlic to fight life-threatening illnesses such as typhus, plague, and cholera. Garlic contains immune-enhancing properties that combat twenty-three different kinds of bacteria, including salmonella, and at least sixty-one different types of fungi, including candida. As long ago as the late nineteenth century, the great French scientist Louis Pasteur investigated garlic's antibacterial properties. During World War I, doctors on the front lines used garlic juice to treat the wounded to prevent infection.

Garlic contains a complex variety of sulfa-containing compounds, including allicin, alliin, ajoene, and other constituents. In fact, you'd need a Ph.D. in botany to even know how to pronounce their names. Intact cells of garlic contain an odourless, sulfa-containing amino acid derivative known as alliin. When garlic is crushed or bruised, alliin comes into contact with alliinase, which converts alliin to allicin. It is allicin that has the potent antibacterial properties. Most researchers agree that allicin and its derivatives are the active constituents of garlic, yielding its medicinal qualities.

Although the cardiovascular literature is hesitant to endorse the routine use of garlic for treating cardiovascular disease, there is good evidence to show that just ½ to 1 clove of garlic per day can reduce your cholesterol by 9 percent. Other research also suggests blood-pressure-lowering effects. Garlic worked especially well with one of my patients, Richard, a man in his late fifties whose hypertension was well controlled by diet and several of the supplements that I had recommended, including garlic. Richard felt so terrific, in fact, that he decided to discontinue his garlic when his blood pressure had stabilized at 138/80. Unfortunately, after going off his garlic his blood pressure shot up to 170/95 in only two months. Needless to say, he opted to go back on the 1,000 mg/day of organic garlic capsules, and his pressure normalized again.

How does it work so well? Garlic has an ACE-inhibiting quality (you'll recall that ACE inhibitors are a class of antihypertensive drugs) that helps to lower blood pressure. Experimental studies have shown a blood-pressure-lowering effect in both rats and humans. In addition, garlic reduces stickiness, therefore lowering your risk of developing clots.

Note that you can get too much of a blood-thinning effect if you overdose on garlic, or if you take it with a lot of other products with similar anticoagulant properties. Case reports in the cardiovascular literature have described bleeding episodes in garlic-loving people who were ingesting doses that averaged over four cloves a day. And one person I was treating was taking multiple supplements including ginkgo biloba, fish oils, and garlic, which have blood-thinning capabilities. When he reported that the bleeding persisted for over several hours after he had cut himself shaving, I advised him to stop the garlic, as there was a risk of serious haemorrhage should he be in a traumatic accident or need emergency surgery. Because of its potent blood-thinning activity, garlic should not be used by patients taking oral anti-coagulants, such as aspirin or Coumadin (warfarin), or injectable agents such as heparin.

Aside from the negative effects that garlic odour from your breath and body can have on your social life, garlic is a very safe herb to take in moderate amounts. It causes few adverse effects, but ingesting five or more cloves daily may result in heartburn, flatulence, and other GI disturbances. Despite these minor disadvantages, the health benefits of garlic are extraordinary and a must for anyone trying to lower their blood pressure. In fact, if you do get a good blood-pressure-lowering effect with garlic, then I suggest that you do not stop taking the herb if you are within the safe guidelines below.

For optimum benefits I recommend using one-half to a whole clove of raw garlic each day, but because this may seriously affect your social life, I suggest you try adding garlic supplements to your list of nutriceuticals. For blood pressure control, take capsules that provide between 500 and 1,000mg of garlic a day. Look for coated softgel capsules that can pass undigested through the stomach and be broken down in the large intestine, yet provide full absorption of allicin.

Garlic and other herbs such as hawthorn (500–1,500mg), green tea (50–100mg), ginger (25–50mg), and even *Coleus forskohii* root extract (125–250mg/day) are safe to use in the management of high blood pressure. However, you need to exercise caution when taking herbs or herbal blends. For example, one of my patients took a Chinese herbal remedy with ginseng that skyrocketed his blood pressure. Thinking the cause of this rise was stress, I asked him what was going on in his life. He told me about this new herbal blend that he'd started taking to decrease fatigue that his friend told him about. I immediately told him to stop this remedy, and one week later his blood pressure returned to normal. It is so important to understand what you are putting in your mouth. I have seen so many patients who have had negative reactions from taking herbs. And while I'm on the subject of bad reactions from herbs, please do not use ephedra for weight loss or as an energy booster. Many cardiovascular-related deaths have occurred with this herb, including stroke from soaring blood pressure.

EXERCISE UPDATE: YOGA

This week I want you to experience the enhanced physical strength and inner peace that the practice of yoga can bring. There are both physical and mental components to yoga, so in this sixth week of my blood-pressure-lowering programme, I'm adding yoga for exercise and spiritual renewal. Since research has shown that the practice of yoga low-ers blood pressure, this, like qigong, should be considered as part of your own individualized programme.

Yoga is an ancient Sanskrit word meaning "union"—a perfect descrip-tion of an approach to precious harmony between mind and body. There are six distinct schools of yoga, but the type known as hatha yoga is the most popular in the West. Hatha yoga is a seamless blend of exercise, meditation, and breathing techniques to help the body achieve the nat-ural balance that is the essence of good health.

Breathing exercises, known as *pranayama*, help the mind to focus for deep relaxation. Slow, deep breathing patterns improve respiratory health and increase lung capacity. We all tend to take breathing for granted—an autonomic response that we don't think about. Stress and tension cause us to take shallow or irregular breaths. Learning to pay attention to breath-ing, especially during stressful situations, will help you to stay calm and relaxed and keep your blood pressure under control.

Posture is equally important for yoga-based breathing control. When you slouch, the ribcage presses down on the diaphragm, causing respira-tion to be limited to just the upper chest. This type of breathing forces the heart to work harder. The exercises or poses, called *asanas*, balance and stretch your body, increasing flexibility, improving circulation, and pro-moting relaxation. Advanced or power yoga can actually cause discomfort and raise your blood pressure, but the simpler positions of beginning-level yoga are far better for people with hypertension.

Dhyana, the meditational component of yoga, improves concentration and relieves mental stress. All three yoga components—breathing, postures, and meditation—work synergistically with one another. Studies have shown that yoga produces a reduction of alpha brain wave activity, indi-cating greater relaxation and focus.

Research has demonstrated that yoga improves strength and flexibility, decreases blood pressure, and relieves anxiety. Yoga also helps restore function to people with arthritis and has been helpful for chronic pain that failed to respond to traditional methods of physical therapy and med-ication. Experts believe that stretching the muscles and ligaments in the yoga poses relieves the spasms that are part of the pain cycle.

This week I want you to include these yoga *asanas* as part of your exer-cise commitment. Alternate muscle-stretching *asanas* with twenty-to-thirty-minute walks. For example, on Monday you might choose to do the yoga exercises, followed by a walk on Tuesday, weather permitting. Then do yoga on Wednesday, walking on Thursday, and so on. Those of you with treadmills will enjoy the most flexibility in your daily exercise.

Yoga Exercise 1: Corpse Pose

Lie on your back, legs slightly apart, arms by your side with palms up. Consciously relax each part of your body, starting at your feet. Wiggle your toes and gently flex your ankles. Breathe comfortably. Shake out the tension in your arms, then your legs. Roll your neck from side to side to relieve shoulder tension. Stay in this position for ten minutes, but try not to fall asleep.

Yoga Exercise 2: Bound Ankle Pose

Sit on the floor with the soles of your feet touching each other. Grab your ankles and slowly pull them toward your body. Bend over until your back is like a flat table, parallel with the floor. Then gently try to push your thighs down toward the floor using the gentle pressure from your elbow. Exhale as you bend. Make sure you don't hold your breath during the exercise. Hold for a few seconds.

Yoga Exercise 3: Knee-Up Pose

Stand straight and lift your right leg up, bending the knee and pulling the leg toward your chest with your arms. Flex your ankle down and take two deep breaths, exhaling fully each time. Switch to the left leg and repeat slowly. Do the exercise three times with each leg.

Yoga Exercise 4: Child's Pose

While kneeling on the floor, with your arms to the side, sit back on your heels. Keeping your buttocks as close to your heels as you can, exhale and then stretch your torso forward and down until you can rest your forehead on the floor. Breathe in and out as you enjoy the gentle stretch. Hold for one to two minutes.

MIND–BODY UPDATE: YOGIC BREATHING AND MEDITATION

In your emotional update this week, I want you to experience the mental clarity and inner peace that yogic meditation can bring. During a yoga meditation session, the mind can stop racing and begin to look inward. The goal is to empty the conscious mind and step back from routine prob-lems of family, work, friends, finances, and health issues, including your concerns over your blood pressure.

Start your yoga meditation by finding a comfortable position. You want to be completely relaxed but still awake. There is no single correct posi-tion. Try sitting on the floor with your back against the wall and legs outstretched, cross-legged on a pillow, or sitting in a chair with your feet on the floor and your back fully supported. Whatever position feels best is the right position for you.

Again, I want to remind you that your environment is important for successful meditation. The room should be very private and quiet, the temperature neither too warm nor too cold. I find that soft light and incense help to encourage a state of relaxation. Dress in comfortable, loose pants and top and take off your shoes. If your feet tend to get cold, wear soft cotton socks without tight elastic.

Once you settle into your meditation space, begin relaxation with breathing exercises. The yogic breathing techniques encourage breathing deeply through the nostrils. Inhaling fully stretches the chest and fills the lungs. Exhaling fully cleanses the lungs and helps to eliminate toxins. Yogic breathing helps you bridge the conscious voluntary mind and the involuntary state of deep relaxation. It helps eliminate intrusive thoughts and feelings, replacing them with a softer, contemplative focus.

As you do the yogic breathing exercises, pay attention to your posture. If you tend to slump, the ribcage will press down on the diaphragm. As a result, respiration will be limited to the upper chest, negating the benefits of yogic breathing. During meditation, straighten and pull back your shoulders to bring oxygen to the bottom, middle, and top of your lungs. Now let's try some easy-to-learn exercises.

Yogic Breathing Exercise 1

Sitting cross-legged on the floor, place your right hand on your abdomen and your left hand at the base of your ribcage. Breathe in deeply, feeling your chest and abdomen expand. As you exhale slowly through the nose, feel your lungs empty completely. Avoid holding your breath between inhaling and exhaling. Repeat five times.

Yogic Breathing Exercise 2

Again sitting cross-legged on the floor with your eyes closed, hold one nostril closed with the thumb and breathe in deeply as you mentally count to four, visualizing each number as it passes. Release your nostril, hold your other nostril closed, and exhale slowly to the count of four, visualizing the numbers. Don't rush; let each number fade away effortlessly. Repeat three times.

Yogic Meditation Exercise 1

For this exercise you will need a meditation object. Select the object of your choice, such as a perfect flower, a flickering candle, a glass of water, or something that has very special meaning for you, and place it about three feet in front of you. If you are sitting on a chair, place the object on a desk or dining room table. If you are sitting on the floor, the meditation object should be on a low table (like a coffee table) to keep it at eye level. Stare at the object for sixty seconds, trying not to blink too often. Then close your eyes and visualize the object that you've selected at a spot between your eyebrows. Hold this image for at least thirty seconds. Relax, and repeat three times.

Yoga Meditation Exercise 2

In your comfortable meditation position, repeat a word or mantra each time you inhale or exhale. Select a word or phrase that has positive meaning for you, such as "shalom" or "the Lord is my shepherd", or use the traditional yoga mantra "om". Spend at least five minutes doing this.

These breathing and meditation exercises should last for at least twenty minutes per session. If you like the way you feel after these yoga exercises, you may want to look into classes in your vicinity to explore this life-giving discipline.

8 Beverages and Biofeedback, Hawthorn and Happiness Week 7

This week I'd like to take a look at beverages on the PAMM plan. As we move into the final two weeks of the programme, I hope that you have been keeping yourself well hydrated with six to eight glasses of water a day, which will also help to keep detoxifying you from the processed foods and hidden salt that you used to eat. I just can't emphasize enough the importance of water for your health. If necessary, we can live for weeks without food, but we can survive only a few days without water. It's essential for every organ process and every cell function. If you want to perk up the taste of fresh water, try adding a slice of lemon or lime, especially during those warmer summer months.

DIET UPDATE 1: YOUR BEST BETS IN THE BEVERAGE DEPARTMENT

You know, sometimes people can be doing pretty well with their meal plans, cutting back on fats and carbohydrates, and adding all the healthy food selections that I've been reviewing with you. But when they get thirsty or want to wash down that healthy meal, they make a poor choice for their liquid nourishment. So we need to review the good drink selections and the not-so-healthy ones so you can stay on target with blood pressure lowering, weight loss, and good nutrition.

It *Can* Be Easy Being Green

For additional benefits, occasionally you can try substituting a few cups of decaffeinated green tea for plain water. This fragrant beverage has terrific antioxidant properties. Research has shown that green tea supports healthy blood pressure by supporting weight loss. It also helps to stop the oxidation of LDL cholesterol (in fact, one study showed green tea to be more effective against LDL oxidation than vitamin E), cuts your risk of skin cancer, and promotes wound healing. And green tea is particularly effective for doing combat with those dangerous free radicals.

Green tea is one of the three forms of tea derived from the *Camellia sinensis* plant. After harvesting, green tea (an absolute favourite in Japan) is dried without fermenting. Black tea, popular in Western countries, is first fermented heavily, then dried. Many people in China prefer oolong tea, which is lightly fermented. All three forms of tea contain a form of antioxidant known as catechins, but green tea has the highest levels.

In the wintertime, there's just about nothing that's more comforting than wrapping your hands around a hot mug of tea. Inhale the fragrant steam as you drink, and think about the wonderful antioxidants flooding through your body, protecting your cells. In the summer, you can make up a cool, refreshing jug of decaffeinated iced green tea and drink it throughout the day. Note that because there is some caffeine in regular green tea, it can interrupt your sleep. That's why I recommend decaffeinated green tea.

Battle of the Brews

Coffee, like alcohol, should be regarded as a drug rather than a food. The high amounts of caffeine found in coffee, chocolate, and many soft drinks can stimulate the brain, relax small airways in the lungs (bronchioles), and raise your stress hormone levels. Many studies have looked at the role of caffeine in health and disease, but so far the results have been inconclusive. In the short term, studies have shown that caffeine can at least temporarily raise your blood pressure by a few points.

I've observed higher resting pulses, irregular heartbeat, insomnia, and chronic gastric reflux in patients with heavy caffeine habits. But once I've convinced them to limit their coffee to one cup a day, the symptoms usually vanish. Coffee can cause a host of problems and has minimal medicinal value. My preference is tea!

Coffee has about three times the caffeine that you'll find in a single cup of black or green tea, so I recommend that you restrict your coffee to one cup daily. For committed coffee drinkers, this will feel like a punishment.

So, to avoid going into coffee withdrawal, decide which time of day your body most craves its caffeine fix. Some of my patients find that splitting the single serving into a half cup at breakfast and another half cup in the afternoon satisfies their caffeine habit. However, I would like to convert you to tea.

There's another reason why drinking tea could be better for you than you thought. Much has been made of COX-2 (cyclo-oxygenase-2) inhibitors such as Celebrex (celecoxib) and Vioxx (rofecoxib), which provide pain relief for arthritis and other inflammatory conditions, but did you know that the natural quercetin in tea can also act as a COX-2 inhibitor? And it has all of the upside with none of the downside of the drugs. The latest findings about medications such as Celebrex and Vioxx—that there is a possible link between synthetic COX-2 inhibitors and increased risk of heart attack, and that the drugs can cause gastrointestinal bleeding—may make you think twice about their safety. This is not the case with the natural versions of COX-2 inhibitors, like the quercetin in tea. Not only does it help combat cancer, but it also helps protect against heart disease.

These are just a few compelling reasons for taking a new look at tea, a healthy alternative that has about half the caffeine of coffee. So tomorrow morning, think twice before you go to brew that pot of coffee. You'll do your body a big favour by skipping the coffee and sipping some tea instead.

Avoid Soft Drinks and Fruit Juices

I'm also strict when it comes to diet drinks. It goes without saying that regular sugar-filled soft drinks are banned completely from my programme, but diet drinks are too. They tend to be high in caffeine, unhealthy colourings, dyes, and phosphoric acid, all of which make blood pressure harder to control.

While fruit juices are great sources of vitamins and bioflavonoids, unfortunately they're high in the glycemic-index department. Rich in natural sugars and devoid of the fibre you'll find in whole fruits, they can spike your blood sugar, precipitously evoking excessive insulin surges that threaten blood pressure control. With the exception of lemon juice in salads, I avoid processed fruit juices entirely. If, however, you want to "juice" for yourself, I encourage you to make juices from your own fresh veggies and add a little fruit juice for a touch of sweetness.

My Hard Line on the Hard Stuff

When it comes to alcoholic beverages, I draw a hard line. Beer, wine, and spirits are metabolized into aldehydes, highly irritating compounds that accelerate the ageing of membranes. So unless you want to speed up the ageing process, you need to slow down on your alcohol intake. Also, be advised that your body will metabolize the sugars in wine and beer in just the same way that it does any other carbohydrate. That means calories and pushing the envelope on insulin resistance. Alcohol restriction for only three weeks reduced systolic blood pressure while improving heart rate variability in Japanese men, as reported in the *American Journal of Hypertension* in 2002. Thirty-three Japanese male volunteers who were all habitual drinkers reduced their consumption by at least one-half. The daytime systolic blood pressure was significantly lower in the reduced-alcohol period when compared to their usual drinking habits. Thus, a reduction in alcohol is another must intervention for blood pressure lowering.

However, wine contains a variety of polyphenols and other powerful antioxidants, which can help combat free radicals and prevent the oxidation of LDL cholesterol. Polyphenols also have remarkable anti-ageing and anti-allergy properties. All these health-promoting benefits are the driving force behind the so-called French paradox—the fact that French men and women eat a diet high in saturated fat and white flour, yet have one of the lowest rates of heart disease in the world.

It almost doesn't seem fair, does it? Why are they so unaffected by their diet of pâtés, butter, and cream? Many researchers have suggested that it's the red wine that the French drink at lunch and dinner that may counteract the fat in those fabulous French meals. Further studies point to the quercetin content of the wine they drink as the key cardioprotective ingredient.

For example, one study showed that just one to two glasses of red wine before dinner prevented the oxidation of cholesterol that can promote plaque build-up. And while a Dutch study identified quercetin as the most health-promoting ingredient in your *vino*, it also suggested that there are other quercetin sources that are easier on your liver, and lower in calories.

Remember the Dutch study: Men, aged sixty-five to eighty-five, who ate onions, green apples, and green tea (foods high in quercetin) had lower death rates. So if you're interested in taking advantage of quercetin's antioxidant and cardioprotective perks, then choose foods that are naturally high in this nutrient, such as apples and onions, and avoid the problems of heavy wine intake. And remember—while the French may have a lower incidence of coronary artery disease (second only to the Japanese) they also have one of the highest rates of cirrhosis of the liver in the world. So drink your wine in moderation!

Once the eight-week plan is over, I allow my hypertensive patients two to three glasses of wine per week. Red wines are a better choice because they also contain slightly more antioxidant polyphenols than white wines.

DIET UPDATE 2: SWEETENERS

Unfortunately, artificial sweeteners just aren't a good substitute for white sugar. While the good news is that they don't rocket your blood glucose levels, artificial sweeteners do carry their own health drawbacks, so I believe that switching to these chemicals will simply exchange one set of problems for another.

In 1970, the FDA in the US removed all cyclamates from supermarket shelves because laboratory studies with rodents linked the artificial sweeteners to a higher incidence of cancer. Cyclamates were also banned in the UK, but are now provisionally permitted again. Less than a decade later, some experts petitioned the government to do the same with saccharin because it seemed to cause bladder cancer in rats. In more recent years, there have been disturbing reports about aspartame. The FDA has been deluged with complaints from consumers claiming that aspartame produced headaches, mood swings, memory loss, and seizures. And dedicated dieters were appalled to find that both aspartame and saccharin were actually shown to increase appetite.

To satisfy your sweet tooth, I recommend very small amounts of honey. Long valued for its therapeutic benefits, honey was cherished by the ancient Egyptians for its medicinal properties. The Romans thought so highly of the amber syrup that they sometimes paid their taxes in honey rather than gold. Honey is much sweeter than sugar, so a little goes a long way. As we near the end of our eight weeks together, I am confident that your diet, high in antioxidants and fibre, won't be damaged by small amounts of honey. You've been working very hard to follow a healthier diet, setting time aside for both mental and physical exercises, and taking a full schedule of supplements. You've earned the right to drizzle a bit of honey on your cereal, in your tea or coffee, or on your soya smoothies.

Quick tip: Starting to eat local honey four to six weeks before hay fever season begins is a great way to desensitize a highly allergic person to tree pollen and grains. Just add ½ teaspoon to your favourite dish or drink!

SUPPLEMENT UPDATE: HAWTHORN

Hawthorn is a herb with established cardiovascular benefits and I use it frequently in my practice with excellent results. The hawthorn shrub's leaves, berries, and blossoms contain valuable flavonoids and proantho-cyanidins that offer you strong antioxidant properties. European doctors often prescribe hawthorn as a substitute for digitalis, one of the most commonly ordered medications for improving contractibility in a weak-ened heart. Hawthorn dilates blood vessels, bringing blood to the heart, and improves your heart's ability to pump more effectively by strengthening its force of contraction. So, like digitalis, Hawthorn enhances coronary cir-culation and increases cardiac energy levels.

In animals, hawthorn increases coronary blood flow while decreasing arterial blood pressure. Studies have shown that this increase in coronary blood flow also helps to prevent angina, a symptom resulting from a tem-porary lack of oxygen to the heart muscle. Besides having properties similar to digitalis and nitrates, Hawthorn also acts like an ACE inhibitor, and can lower your blood pressure by assuaging blood vessel constriction. In the body, angiotensin II is a natural substance that narrows blood ves-sels, causing pressure to rise. ACE inhibitors block the formation of angiotensin-converting enzyme (ACE), the enzyme responsible for creat-ing angiotensin II.

I recommend one 500mg hawthorn capsule two to three times a day, but *only* for those not taking digitalis products (Lanoxin/Lanoxin-PG [digoxin] or Digicaps). If you're already taking other antihypertensive medications, such as calcium channel blockers, beta blockers, or ACE inhibitors, check with your doctor before adding hawthorn to your daily supplement programme. I especially like hawthorn in combination with coenzyme Q10 and L-carnitine for congestive heart failure, as these three nutrients complement one another, helping to relieve the shortness of breath that plagues many people with CHF.

EXERCISE UPDATE: UPPER-BODY STRENGTH

As you grow older, the strength in your arms and chest declines more rapidly than your lower-body fitness. You see, the everyday activity of walking around at home, at work, or during leisure activities keeps your lower extremities active, at least at a minimum level. By contrast, most adult men and women rarely lift their arms above their heads or require their shoulder muscles to do much more than an occasional shrug. For many of us, using a hair dryer is as close to upper-body work as we get— if we still have enough hair left on our heads! So this week I want to get you back to using your upper body, and learning some exercises to add into your programme that will make it easy for you to do so.

This week's exercise tips are important because a programme of light exercise for the large muscles in your chest, back, and shoulders can actually promote the blood flow to your heart without making any major oxygen demands that will push up your blood pressure. (And speaking of push-ups, that's an isometric exercise that's *not* recommended for anyone with hypertension.) Upper-body workouts are beneficial for your overall health and essential for people with hypertension.

Your exercise sessions should begin, as always, with a good warm-up, paying special attention to the muscle groups that you plan to focus on. To increase your shoulder flexibility, just do ten forward shoulder rolls gently. Raise your shoulders up toward your ears and rotate up and around in a circular motion. Take your time and be sure to do each exercise smoothly without jerking your arms abruptly. Then repeat, rolling your shoulders in a backward rotation.

Upper Body Warm-up

Lie on your back on the floor with your arms at your sides, your knees bent, and your feet flat on the floor. Inhaling, slowly swing your arms back over your head, feeling the stretch. Gently bring your arms over your head, then cross your bent arms over your chest and lower them slowly as you exhale until they rest on your upper body. Hold for a count of five, breathe in again slowly, then bring your arms to your sides as you exhale. Repeat three times.

Exercise 1: Bent Arm Fly for Chest and Shoulder Muscles

Lie on the floor with two- or three-pound weights in your hands, elbows bent on the floor, hands touching one another over your chest. This is the resting position. Inhale slowly. As you start your next natural exhale, slowly raise your arms until they are straight up in the air; hold momentarily. As you inhale again, slowly lower the weights back down with your arms outstretched until your hands touch the floor; you will feel a gentle pull in your chest. Enjoy the stretch in your upper body as your lungs fill with air. Bring your hands, with dumbbells, back to the resting position, centred over your chest, as you exhale. Repeat four to ten times as your strength and comfort allow.

Exercise 2: Upper Back Muscles and Shoulders

To strengthen the muscles in your back and shoulders, bend over, rest one hand on a chair, and hold a three-pound dumbbell in the other. Lift the weight to the shoulder and then extend your arm down again. Repeat four times, then switch to the other arm.

MIND–BODY UPDATE: BIOFEEDBACK

Biofeedback is a mind–body approach that uses equipment to measure physiological responses—heart rate, body temperature, and muscle tension—and allows a person to observe what's going on with his or her body. While you may feel somewhat sceptical about this practice, researchers have proven that individuals who were "fed back" information about their involuntary responses, such as blood pressure, could learn to alter them.

Early in the twentieth century, psychologist Edmund Jacobson developed and introduced the concept of "progressive relaxation" to help his patients assuage their anxiety by relaxing muscle groups and the mind. But it wasn't until the 1940s that we had the technology, and the curiosity, to use medical equipment to measure autonomic functions of the body, such as digestion, brain activity, and muscle tension. Researchers exploring the health impact of yoga found that master practitioners could indeed regulate brain and metabolic activity. This serendipitous discovery led to the concept of biofeedback, a self-regulatory technique to help people consciously manage physical problems (such as high blood pressure) with their mind, rather than through medication.

With the help of a well-trained biofeedback therapist you can learn to manage critical aspects of the autonomic nervous system. During a typical biofeedback therapy session, sensors taped to your skin monitor muscle tension, heart rate, and skin temperature. A compact machine, about the size of a breadbin, converts the sensor readings into audible beeps or visual flashes of light. As you practise relaxation techniques, the sounds or lights tell you how effective your efforts are.

For example, if you are having back spasms, the light signal slows and eventually stops flashing as your muscles relax. Over time your body gradually learns the process of gearing itself down to a desired level. The eventual goal is that you will be able to get the same results without the biofeedback equipment. This intervention has afforded relief to people with a variety of problems from tension headaches, heart rate irregularities, and asthma to chronic anxiety that's been resistant to medication. Biofeedback gives you the opportunity to learn how to use the mind–body connection to relax and alleviate their symptoms, including high blood pressure that's due to stress.

A good friend of ours, Susan, is a spa nurse. Well trained in the art and technology of biofeedback, she uses her personal and professional skills at a beautiful oceanside location at Gurney's Inn in Montauk, New York, and reports phenomenal success in using this approach with her spa attendees. Often, just one or two sessions during their stay gives them phenomenal feedback about themselves and their bodies. Susan has observed that there can be immediate results once her clients use her biofeedback equipment to make their *own* mind–body connection. "For many," she says, "it's a revelation!" Quite a few have written to her after going home to tell her that learning how to work with their own bodies has made a big difference in their health concerns, especially hypertension. And we have research to back up Susan's confidence in this method.

In 2001, researchers at the College of Nursing at the University of Florida at Gainesville conducted a study to determine the effectiveness of biofeedback in the treatment of essential hypertension. They performed a metanalysis of the previous biofeedback research from adult randomized clinical trials—a good research methodology. When they compared biofeedback with both active control and inactive control, both biofeedback and active control treatments reduced systolic and diastolic blood pressures. But only biofeedback with related cognitive therapy (i.e., addressing the client's belief system and his or her thinking about stress, conflict, etc.) and relaxation training showed a significantly greater reduction in both systolic (6.7mm Hg) and diastolic (4.8mm Hg) pressures.

I find that those of my patients who are into numbers, such as engineers, mathematicians, accountants, and so forth, really appreciate biofeedback because it gives them information in a form they can relate to and understand. Biofeedback isn't "fuzzy maths"; it's real data that you can sink your teeth into.

This week, I encourage you to consider adding biofeedback techniques to your mind–body exercises. Your best bet is to try one or more biofeedback sessions with a trained professional, but I do realize that some of you may not have access to or can't afford a formal biofeedback session with the equipment. If so, then use any of the techniques we've worked on for the past few weeks, such as relaxation and imagery, meditation, qigong, or yoga, to get in touch with the tension or stress that you feel as you start your session.

At the end of the twenty-to-thirty-minute session, evaluate the impact of your intervention by noting how you feel in terms of muscle tension. You can use your pulse before and after as a general guide, or get feedback from any at-home blood pressure device you may have. It's to your advantage to vary your personal daily programme to keep yourself interested and to give yourself insight into which mind–body exercises produce the greatest benefits for your body.

The long-term goal of this eight-week programme is for you to become familiar with several exercises and mind–body activities so that you can stay on a lifestyle programme that's as multi-faceted and as interesting as you are. And remember that in the nurses' study, the cognitive component made a contribution to the success of biofeedback. So, if you cannot work with a biofeedback professional and a psychotherapist, then try discussing and challenging your personal way of looking at the world, problem solving, and responding to stress, with the help of a significant other whom you trust to give you some honest feedback and to make suggestions for change. Such feedback can also uplift our spirits.

MIND–BODY UPDATE 2: DON'T WORRY, BE HAPPY

Did you know that, in general, happy people live longer than people who aren't happy? If you suspected that this might be true, research now proves you right!

It's true that depression and pessimism typically shorten people's lives.

I've advised you about depression but I want to emphasize the similar role of attitude. If you know that you're on the pessimistic side, you must understand how important it is to your health that you change your mind-set. Beliefs and expectations can eventually affect every cell in your body. And negativity is a toxic commodity for the people you live and work with, too.

A study reported in the *Mayo Clinic Proceedings* looked at measurements of optimism and pessimism as a risk factor for death. The researchers looked at 839 patients over a thirty-year period. All of their subjects completed an often-utilized psychological assessment tool called the Minnesota Multiphasic Personality Inventory, or MMPI for short. Of the 839 patients studied, 124 were classified as optimistic, 197 were pessimistic, and 518 were mixed.

After the data was analyzed, those who were more pessimistic had a 19 percent increase in the risk of mortality. Clearly, seeing your cup as half full instead of half empty has a dividend if you want to live longer. But how can you refill your cup? Are there ways to develop a more optimistic mind-set?

One way to become less pessimistic is to practise some mind–body therapies recommended in this book. Regular practice of relaxation techniques such as yoga, t'ai chi, prayer, and qigong can help you to achieve higher levels of calmness and tranquillity. Using the mind to connect with and soothe the body can actually shift your worldview as well as lower your blood pressure.

You're never too old to try a new trick. The elderly, in particular, have realized true longevity benefits when they replace their negative thoughts of "feeling old" with positive ones about the grace, respect, and generational identity associated with being a true elder, such as was appreciated by Native Americans. When this transition occurs, a more youthful vitality begins to emerge.

So, whether you're a self-acknowledged negativist (if you're not sure, ask the people who live and work with you) or a generally optimistic person who struggles to stay upbeat, take my advice: If you find yourself feeling blue, down in the dumps, downright toxic, or just old, *don't just lie there feeling stuck!* Consider trying any of the mind–body techniques, which can raise your spirits and give you a new outlook on life.

Next week we'll be looking at my final nutrition and mind–body recommendations for your personal programme, as well as some tips to help you stay on the plan as a total lifestyle change.

9   Healing in the New Millennium
Week 8

By now you're well on your way! You're on the complete PAMM diet, exercising, trying new mind–body techniques, and taking targeted nutritional supplements including:

1. A diverse multivitamin and mineral supplement with suggested A, C, and E doses.
2. 60–120mg hydrosoluble coenzyme Q_{10}
3. 1,000–2,000mg L-carnitine
4. 400–800mg magnesium
5. 2 g omega-3 fish oil
6. 1–2 Tbsp. crushed flaxseed/linseed
7. 2 g L-arginine
8. 150–300mg grapeseed extract
9. 500–1,000mg organic garlic
10. 500–1,000mg hawthorn

At this point, we're done with the diet updates. Take a good deep breath and lean back in your chair. Give yourself a mental pat on the back. If you've stayed on the plan, then you have all the information that you'll need to make good food selections and understand why the wholesome foods you are choosing will be so good for your overall health and your blood pressure. You're more physically active now, so in this last week I just want to make things simple for you. You've worked hard to get to this point, and you should be as proud of yourself as I am of you.

My primary concern now is that you have a few more pointers to help you stay with this diet for the rest of your life. It's important that you know how to make good food selections when you dine out, that you stay on track during your holiday, and that you're savvy about how to grab healthy food on the run. I will be briefly addressing these areas. And now that your legs are in shape from walking, qigong, and yoga, you'll be getting one last set of exercises to strengthen your legs a little more, so you'll feel like jumping out of bed each morning. Music is one last but simple addition to your daily life that can add rhythm to your daily chores and exercise sessions or soothe the soul during quiet times such as meditation, reflection, or reading.

To start off, though, let's look at one last supplement that a lot of people ask me about: DHEA. I've saved this one for last, but not because it's the best. I've waited until now because I wanted you to see how much more energized and relaxed you would feel by changing over to the PAMM diet and doing your physical exercise routines and your mind–body sessions. For those of you who still feel that your body needs a little something more, DHEA is an option, but read about it first to see if you're someone who might benefit from it, and then think it over for yourself.

SUPPLEMENT UPDATE: DHEA

DHEA (dehydroepiandrosterone) is a steroid hormone, the precursor of eighteen different essential hormones in your body. It's one of those critical compounds whose levels fall as we age. In animal studies, DHEA intake was correlated with increased life span, reduced body fat, and lowered incidence of degenerative diseases. Other studies indicated that DHEA might enhance immunity as well as improve energy and sense of well-being. I find it intriguing that DHEA levels will fall when stress levels (serum cortisol) rise, which may be a clue as to why we're all more vulnerable to becoming sick with a cold, flu, sore throat, or what-have-you when we're going through periods of severe emotional distress.

Remember that DHEA is a hormone, and hormones are potent chemicals, but I do endorse DHEA under certain circumstances and conditions. One study, for example, showed low levels of DHEA to be a heart attack risk factor for men under the age of fifty. I feel particularly confident when I recommend this hormone precursor to those who have documented low serum levels of it because it can bring them back to a normal range. And we have research to suggest that, among other things, DHEA improves your sleep patterns and affords you higher levels of energy.

One study showed improved physical and psychological well-being for both men and women aged forty to seventy who took either 50mg of DHEA or placebo. Researchers did not observe improvement in lipid and cholesterol panels in the DHEA group, as they had anticipated; however, that group's increased blood levels of DHEA were associated with improved mood, sleep, and ability to relax. And because improving these three parameters is important for supporting balanced blood pressure, there may be a place for DHEA in treating hypertension.

The mechanism by which DHEA enhances the well-being of men and women is not clear. Perhaps it is DHEA's effect on the central nervous system that brings about the improved physical and psychological well-being reported by the study participants. Improved sexual function may also make a contribution; in one study of ageing men with erectile dysfunction the administration of 50mg of DHEA seemed to show a benefit, especially in those with high blood pressure.

Who Should Take DHEA?

DHEA is prescribed for both men and women and has been shown to improve energy and libido in women. Despite its promising benefits, DHEA is a powerful steroid similar to oestrogen, progesterone, and testosterone, all of which the body produces. For this reason, I do not recommend DHEA for everyone. I strongly discourage the use of DHEA by any male with an enlarged prostate or prostate cancer, as this may exacerbate the problem. If you're a woman with a positive family history of ovarian or breast cancer or have other high-risk factors for these diseases, you should not take DHEA, as it could increase your risk. And DHEA can have a masculinizing effect on women when taken in high doses—women taking 50 to 100mg of DHEA daily have reported an increase in facial hair, oily skin, and even acne. So before you start taking the DHEA supplements (only available on prescription in the UK), exercise caution—it's a potent compound.

But you may want to consider DHEA if you feel that you're exhausted. My patients, many of them executives, come to me complaining that they're constantly strung out, burned out, or struggling with sleeplessness. This state of exhaustion is in and of itself a risk factor for heart disease, especially for men. And I have some patients who want to try DHEA for its anti-ageing effects.

The first thing to do if you're considering DHEA—for blood pressure lowering or any other reason—is to have your doctor order a blood test to determine your present DHEA level. Only if it's apparent that your serum level is low should you take DHEA, and even then, only in low doses under the supervision of a doctor. Ask your doctor to write a prescription for pharmaceutical-grade DHEA to be taken sublingually (under the tongue). (Note that in the UK, prescription of DHEA is at your doctor's discretion, and in some other countries DHEA is not available.) Generally, I advise that men take a daily dose of 12.5 to 25mg, and for women 5 to 10mg is usually enough to help enhance libido.

I don't take DHEA regularly myself, but I do supplement it during my vulnerable month: May. You see, where I live in the Connecticut Valley, the pollen is fierce in May, and my allergies drain me and my *qi* or life force. Even though I try to travel somewhere else or stay inside when I'm at home, I feel incredibly exhausted as my immune system battles the onslaught of pollen. Our cars are covered with the green dust, my dogs bring it into the house, and we all take it into our homes and offices on our shoes, our clothes, and our hair. I feel totally overwhelmed. My chest tightens, I have difficulty breathing, and I'm sleepless for weeks. These last few years, I've started taking DHEA in April, and continued with it as long as I feel exhausted. It does seem to assuage my symptoms. Once June comes, I discontinue this hormone and save it for next year.

In a nutshell, if you are suffering from hypertension, exhaustion, or a lack of energy with some difficulty sleeping, low-dose DHEA under the supervision of your doctor may give you additional support in improving your quality of life. Over time, it may even help to lower your blood pressure numbers.

DIET UPDATE 3: CABBAGE, THE BEST ANTICANCER FOOD

With all the nutritional benefits that it offers, I just don't think that cabbage gets the respect it deserves. It's rich in vitamin C and an excellent source of cancer-fighting compounds known as indoles.

In the supermarkets you can usually find three types of cabbage. *Green cabbage* is the most ubiquitous form of this important vegetable. Look for firm heads with dark green outer leaves. The darker the leaves, the more nutrients it contains. Shredded thinly, cabbage can be used in salads, lightly sautéed as a side dish, or added to soups and stews.

Red cabbage is bursting with proanthocyanidins, those powerful anti-oxidants that protect you against free radicals in your body. And did you know that just 100g (3½oz) of red cabbage contains 100 percent of the RDA for vitamin C? You'll notice that red cabbage has a slightly tougher texture than green cabbage, so you will need to shred it very finely when you're eating it raw. It's terrific when mixed in a salad with other dark greens, adding great colour and crunch. Red cabbage is equally delicious when stir-fried with other vegetables, and can even be added to soups and stews.

Savoy cabbage is a very pretty vegetable and has loose ruffled leaves. A good source of beta-carotene (the other types of cabbage lack this nutrient), savoy cabbage has a mild taste and texture that's perfect for fresh, sweet salads. Any type of cabbage contains lots of fibre, and remember, fibre is a must for blood pressure lowering.

EXERCISE UPDATE: LOWER-BODY EXERCISE

Strong muscles in your legs and hips give you the power you need to get around, and strengthening your legs not only increases your body's capacity for work and play, but improves the health of the hip, knee, and ankle joints, protecting you from joint damage and painful muscle strains. So in this last week of my programme I want to give you three exercises to work your lower body.

You'll be learning isotonic exercises, which use the weight of your body to provide resistance through the range of motion of a muscle. Hold for a count of three, to allow for full contraction of the muscle, and then gently release; don't rise too quickly, with a jerky movement, as it can lead to injury, and don't hold for too long, since this can cause a slight rise in your blood pressure.

The Squat

Stand straight with your feet about twelve inches apart, placing your hands on your hips. Exhaling on the effort, slowly lower yourself as though you are going to sit down in a chair. Keep your head up and your eyes looking forward while you lower your body, leaning forward at the waist. Breathe. Don't lock your knees; just allow your thigh muscles to do all the work while you hold for a count of three. Gently straighten back up to standing. Repeat four times.

The Lunge

Stand with your left leg in front of your right and bent, and place one hand on your hip while resting the other on the back of a chair. Bend both knees, and slowly lower your body as far as you can. Hold for a count of three. Your right heel will naturally rise off the floor. Push off with the balls of your feet and return to the original position. Repeat four times, then switch sides and repeat with the other leg.

Leg Lifts

Lie on the floor on your left side, with your knees slightly bent and your head resting on your outstretched left arm. Raise your right leg until your right foot reaches the height of your shoulder, then slowly lower your leg back down. Repeat this three times. Lie on your other side and perform the same movement.

MIND–BODY UPDATE: MUSIC THERAPY

Not only does music soothe the savage breast, it can be another useful tool to lower your blood pressure. Studies have shown music improves mental focus, promotes healing, and improves mood. Different types of music generate a wide range of emotions and physical responses. Research indicates that, depending on the tempo and the tone, music can alter your heart rate, your breathing, and your blood pressure. Relaxing music has been shown to lower levels of the hormone cortisol, which rises naturally with stress. Equally promising, music stimulates the release of endorphins, the body's natural mood lifters.

Music can focus attention away from painful or upsetting situations. Doctors are using music to distract patients from the pain of dentistry, childbirth, and surgical procedures. A study published in *Psychosomatic Medicine* reported that listening to music of their choice helped eye surgery patients keep their blood pressure normal both before and after surgery. In this eighth week, I want you to start using music to create a health-enhancing environment in your life. For soothing the heart, I recommend music with a tempo ranging from 60 to 120 beats per minute—that's the usual range of the human heart rate. Bach's Brandenburg Concertos and slower pieces by Mozart are my personal favourites, as well as *The Planets* (Holst).

You can also open your mind and taste to different types of music.

Listen to jazz, symphonies, popular show tunes, chamber music, songs from other cultures. Turn on the radio and actively listen, noting the names and artists that you enjoy most for light activity, reading, exercising, and so on. Personalize tapes for different moods: soothing for anxious times, or upbeat when depression seems to weigh you down. Use music to create a positive environment in your home and your work environment. Slip a tape or CD in your car stereo to destress your commute or lighten your mood while transporting children and running errands.

STAYING ON THE PROGRAMME WHEN YOU'RE ON THE MOVE

I know that we've given you a lot of recipes for healthy meals that you can prepare at home. Many of the lunch selections can be easily packed and taken to work. But let's be realistic. We are a society on the move, so I'd like to give you some additional pointers on how to make healthy food selections when you're dining out for business or for pleasure, or on long car trips.

Table for Two: Me and My Diet

Eating in restaurants isn't as challenging as you might think. As I pointed out, eating Mediterranean doesn't mean loading up at your favourite Italian restaurant, but by now you know how to make some healthy selections. First of all, don't be afraid to ask the waiter how various dishes are prepared before you decide. You know the no-no's: salt, bad fats, gravies, butter, and preservatives. For instance, as healthy as some Chinese dishes may be, you're not on the PAMM plan if they're using MSG in your favourite restaurant, and you can check that out on the phone before you go. Remember, MSG is monosodium glutamate, so it can't be good for your blood pressure. There are many Asian restaurants that don't use this chemical, though, so don't lose heart!

If you are in an Italian or Greek restaurant, try to find some of the dishes you've become familiar with on the PAMM diet, but be careful to ask how they're prepared. There may be more fats, oils, and salt than there is in the recipes you've been provided with in this book. Avoid steak restaurants unless they have a few fish selections, and remember that salads are always a safe bet. Whether you're running out of the office for lunch or dining out for a special occasion, most restaurants will have a few salads to choose from, or even a full salad bar. You can top your salad with chicken, shrimp, fish, nuts, seeds, or tofu for protein.

Japanese dining offers you a variety of dishes in addition to the raw fish that it's so well known for. Strips of lean pork, chicken, or beef can be cooked on a hot grill right at your table—an exciting way to have an occasional meat dish. Other dishes, like soups and appetizers, are also light and appealing, and there's always fresh fruit for dessert.

And don't forget your supplements. I recommend prepacking your vitamins and nutrients in individual doses inside plastic bags so that you can keep a stash on hand in your handbag, briefcase, office desk drawer, or locker. During cooler months, you can even stow a bag or two in your glove compartment. At first preplanning may feel awkward, but eventually it will become second nature. If you find yourself dining out on the spur of the moment, then you'll have your supplements within easy reach. And remember it's best to take your supplements after meals.

Food on the Run

Sometimes when I'm on a road trip, it can be miles and miles between restaurants, and even then, the pickings can be slim! On a recent trip to Colorado we found ourselves on the road in a rental car with no supplies of healthy food. Eventually what we did was find a good-sized supermarket with a big produce department and a well-stocked salad bar. We filled our bags with bottled water, yogurt, plastic boxes brimming with fresh salad ingredients that included chickpeas and beans, fresh-cut melons (watermelon, cantaloupe, and honeydew), nuts, and trail mix (diced fruit, seeds, nuts and cereal). We even found a place to park for lunch with a vista of the Rockies! All in all, a much healthier meal and more ambiance than we had thought we were going to be able to find. So when you travel, be creative, and keep your eyes open. And when you have the luxury of packing ahead for a trip, you can have even better selections. The secret to eating on the run, or even preparing a quick meal at home, is to keep it fresh and simple, yet colourful, appetizing, and delicious.

By now you've probably developed some of your own meal shortcuts, such as having trail mix and health bars within easy reach at home. Just be sure you've checked those ingredient labels: not all "health foods" are really healthy. Many health bars, for example, are loaded with trans fatty acids and should not be consumed.

Holiday Time

Most of us are not looking for the kind of travel stressors associated with those Chevy Chase holiday movies. And now that you have some tips on dining out and keeping on schedule with your supplements, it should be fairly simple for you to follow the PAMM diet when you're holidaying. But one thing that can be hard for me when I travel is getting in my exercise routine. I always bring my tracksuit and training shoes along, and I advise you to do the same. Many full-service hotels have exercise rooms, and you can catch up on the news while you walk on the treadmill, cycle, or lift a few light weights.

But accommodation along your path may not have such facilities. I get around that by working some walking into my holiday days as often as I can. Walk the halls of the airports while waiting for your flight; park your car farther from your destination and take in your surroundings as you walk to where you're going. I've had a real kick out of some of the pricier hotels in Europe that advertise dogs you can walk while enjoying your stay. Smart marketing!

Many of these holiday activities may not be the same calorie-burning, cardiovascular workouts that you are used to, but they will help you maintain your flexibility and keep you thinking about exercise. Let's face it, friends, anything is better than nothing! Remember to bring along your mind–body therapies, too. My wife loves to pack a scented candle for our room, as well as one or two of her favourite tapes or CDs and a small portable player.

TRY A SPA

One way to take control of your blood pressure, reduce stress, decrease your waistline, and lighten your spirits is to consider a spa experience. If your budget allows you to splurge, try one of these healthy adventures. Over the next several years, I believe that spas are going to be meccas for much needed health education, counselling, alternative methodologies, and other health strategies that are simply not available in hospitals today. My first spa experience made me a believer in health education. In 1984 I lectured at Canyon Ranch in Tucson, Arizona. During this weeklong experience, I lost five pounds while nurturing my body at the same time. I had a very positive experience and learned some new alternative therapies to complement my traditional training.

Back home on the East Coast, in 1988 I discovered Gurney's Inn, a jewel of a seaside resort in Montauk, New York. There I wrote two of my books, *Lose to Win* and *Optimum Health*. The spa experience at Gurney's and other places like it can certainly change your life. The programmes are designed to educate, rejuvenate, and nurture guests. Another spa that I visited recently is the Cuisinart Health and Wellness Program in Anguilla, British West Indies. Taking Control the Cuisinart Way is an innovative ten-day retreat conducted monthly at a beautiful Caribbean beachfront resort. The wellness programme combines nutrition, exercise, body pampering, and therapeutic and medical guidance to help clients participate in and take control of their total well-being.

At a holistic health spa you're likely to find skilled, caring professionals, including exercise physiologists, nutritionists, registered nurses, personal trainers, yoga instructors, and licensed massage therapists. In addition to serving a healthy menu of nutritional, high-fibre cuisine, such facilities often provide nutritional seminars offering information on weight loss and other healthy approaches to eating.

One of the advantages of a spa is that the guests eat properly, exercise, and relax while learning progressive methods for healing for both mind and body. Many of us need to get started under professional guidance. For me, my Canyon Ranch experience several years ago re-emphasized and supported my interest in complementary healing modalities.

When you engage in a total spa experience, you nurture your body from the physical, biochemical, and psychological points of view. The key is to experience these mind-and-body-oriented therapies and then take the knowledge back home. Learning how to eat healthily is another bonus of the spa programme. Gurney's Inn offers Mediterranean-like cuisine, and Cuisinart offers organically and hydroponically grown fruits and vegetables. Eating properly, engaging in exercise, and utilizing the mind–body techniques offered at these holistic spas can be the perfect jump-start in helping to lower your blood pressure. And the wisdom gained will certainly enrich your life.

If you'd rather spend your money on other things when you travel, then improvise. You can follow my wife's tips to create a quiet time with soothing music and fragrances in your hotel room. Making time for a warm bath and a couples massage is another great way to unwind and feel connected. Just pack a bottle of almond oil or even your favourite body cream, and you and your partner can take turns massaging each other into a state of deep relaxation. And if you're travelling with small children, you'll be amazed at how a massage can help them fall asleep in a strange bed. Even our older children respond to foot massages during family-centred time, and it makes us all feel more connected as well as more relaxed.

Staying on this plan to lower your blood pressure isn't going to be as difficult as you may think, and soon you'll even begin to realize that it can add quality to your life. And hopefully, with your blood pressure down where it should be, you'll also be gaining some "quantity" to your years.

10 Tomorrow Is the First Day of the Rest of Your Life

We've now completed the last week of the eight-week programme. To paraphrase Winston Churchill, this is not the end, but the end of the beginning. May it be so for you. Your diet is now rich in life-giving antioxidants and your body feels renewed strength and energy from these few weeks of walking and strength training. You understand the critical link between physical and mental health and have learned to use a wide range of stress reduction strategies to protect both your body and your mind. I am so proud of all the work you have done and deeply honoured that you have come along with me for this healing journey. But before we end our time together, I do want to share with you one last story about a woman named Pat.

A CASE OF THE HYPERTENSIVE BLUES SUCCESSFULLY TREATED WITH ALTERNATIVES

Pat, aged forty-six, came to see me in November 1998 for an alternative approach for blood pressure lowering. Although she had been advised that her blood pressure was in the borderline-to-high range (140s–150s/ lower 90s), Pat wasn't yet convinced that she needed to sign up for blood-pressure-lowering medications, as her doctor so strongly recommended. Her intuition told her that she'd be in for a host of possible side effects. But Pat was also concerned about her family history. Her father had died at age sixty-six from a heart attack, and her mother had high blood pressure. She knew the risks she was facing.

Pat was serious when she told me that she'd inherited a "bad set of genes", as if it were a bad hand that had been dealt her at a high-stakes poker game. But a family history of hypertension can mean more than genetics. We learn value and belief systems from our families, and in a way we "inherit" attitudes and behaviours such as how we eat, how we view the world, how we deal or don't deal with stress and anger, whether we exercise, or whether we use alcohol and cigarettes.

Pat had decided to take control of her high blood pressure, starting with a lifestyle change that would set her apart from her hypertensive relatives. She was in total agreement when I suggested the PAMM diet and a walking programme. She was even enthusiastic about taking nutritional supplements, so I started her right off on a multivitamin/ multimineral formula, coenzyme Q10, magnesium, and calcium. I ordered another round of blood work, looking for the newest identified risk factors: fibrinogen, ferritin (iron storage), homocysteine, Lp(a), and a cholesterol analysis.

With her blood work in my hands, I could give her better feedback about her personal risk for further cardiac problems. Luckily, she had an HDL level of 75, affording her excellent protection against plaque development. And her fibrinogen, ferritin, and homocysteine levels were all well within normal limits. From November 1998 until April 2001 Pat continued to follow her new lifestyle, adding in more supplements: grapeseed extract, fish oils, hawthorn, and garlic.

Pat was delighted. She'd lost weight, and her blood pressure had come down to a health-promoting 120/80. But then she got overconfident. You see, Pat felt so good about herself that she backslid a bit on her programme. We all know how easy that can be—a little of the wrong food here and a little there, skipping your exercise one day and then the next, and before you know it, you're off the track, off the programme . . . and unfortunately back where you started.

At her last evaluation in October 2001, Pat had gained back five pounds, and her blood pressure had crept up to 140/88. But she took notice! When I saw her that day, she recommitted herself to get back on track, lose a little weight, and exercise more. Maybe you can see yourself in Pat. Although her family history was not ideal, her low homocysteine, fibrinogen, and cholesterol along with her high HDL allowed me to incorporate lifestyle changes over a gradual period of time so that Pat could find these changes acceptable; it was a programme she could live with, as we say. Some of you may need to take far more drastic measures if your blood pressure has been higher or if you have failed to respond to the treatment plan you've been on, whatever that may be.

But the bottom line is the same for all of us. Once on a healthy plan, like the eight-week programme you've just learned in this book, you need to stay on track or you will backslide. If you catch yourself feeling a little overconfident, or as though you're "over the hump", and you return to your old ways of eating and living, then your weight and your blood pressure will also creep back up to where they had been. My best advice is to get as many other people as you can in your household, extended family, or group of friends to do this programme with you so that you can support one another, especially should one of you fall off track.

CONGRATULATIONS FOR RECOGNIZING THE MEDICINE OF THE FUTURE

And there's another lesson from Pat's story. Like many patients I see in my surgery on a day-to-day basis, she was hungry for information about alternative ways to take care of her blood pressure, her heart, and her overall health. And if you have just finished this book, then I know that you too have been on that same search. You're all part of a larger trend in health care, and it's one that mainstream medicine will likely be taking more note of.

Massive numbers of patients are consulting alternative practitioners and frequenting health food shops in record numbers. We now have an enormous industry of complementary approaches completely outside the mainstream of the medical community. While some doctors are comfortable supporting their patients' integration of these therapies alongside their traditional ones, others are not, and some are even hostile. But the real problem is that there are still very few doctors who practise integrative medicine in their own surgeries, even if they may be taking supplements and the like at home. Reflecting on the whole situation, I can't help but see the image of Nero fiddling while Rome burns.

For those doctors reading this book, I would ask you to consider questions that I have all too often asked myself these last few years:

- Whose responsibility is it to examine all the therapeutic options that have the potential to reduce risk and ease human suffering?

- Who is best to partner with individual patients in their quest to take charge of their health and well-being?
- Who is better qualified than the highly trained medical professional to test the efficacy and safety of alternative and complementary therapies under strict review, protecting people from quackery, charlatans, and snake oil?
- Once empowered with the knowledge of a wide variety of healing modalities, who is better able to provide patients with the best possible care?

It's my feeling that it is conventional doctors, grounded in orthodox, mainstream, and scientific approaches, who are the best placed to incorporate alternative approaches for their patients. For those of you who are not doctors, I hope that this will be the first of many books you will be able to find that have been written on the subject of complementary medicine by well-trained doctors.

As we embark into the twenty-first century, medicine is poised on the edge of a major transformation. Our old models of waiting for the body to break down before attempting to fix it are no longer viable in terms of both economic cost and the cost of human suffering. It is now obvious that the alternative involves a shift away from crisis-and-disease medicine toward prevention and health-promoting measures that strengthen and support the body.

There are many reasons for the increase in popularity of alternative methods in healing, including patient dissatisfaction with the side effects of pharmaceuticals, and the fact that conventional medicine has all too often become impersonal, relying on high-tech methodologies and time-limited surgery visits. In this day and age, it's my belief that people are looking for orthodox doctors to consider complementary approaches in healing. It's my hope that my fellow doctors reading this book will listen to the cry of the public and incorporate safe and natural methodologies in their own practices. Remember, we all swore to do no harm as we took the Hippocratic oath.

More than seventy years ago, Dr. Francis Peabody wrote in the *Journal of the American Medical Association*: "Disease is never exactly the same as disease in an experimental animal, for in man the disease at once affects and is affected by what we call the emotional life. Thus, the doctor who attempts to take care of a patient while he neglects this factor is as unscientific as the investigator who neglects to control all the conditions that may affect his experiment. The good doctor knows his patient through and through, and his knowledge is sought daily. Time, sympathy, and understanding must be lavishly dispensed, but the reward is to be found in the personal bond that forms a greater satisfaction in the practice of medicine. One of the essential qualities of the clinician is interest in humanity, for the secret of the care of the patient *is caring for the patient*."

My practice of medicine has been personally affected by Dr. Peabody's last line: "The secret of the care of the patient *is caring for the patient*." Patients really want their doctor to see their suffering and help them search for a better quality of living. Forgive me for this moment on the soapbox, but it's my belief that as doctors become more willing to use alternative and complementary therapies, together we can and will improve quality of life and begin to reduce some of the human suffering we have seen around us in this new millennium. This paradigm shift that's slowly being forced onto our medical system is really the only logical and ethical thing to follow.

It is my hope that this book has been a paradigm shift for you, the reader, to realize that there are many more approaches to treating your blood pressure than you had imagined, and that many of them are as close as your own home and kitchen. Now your real adventure begins, because living a healthy lifestyle in a fast-food-oriented, fast-paced society so often presents challenges. To help you stay well, search out support where you live. Join a yoga class, find a meditation centre, and make friends with the owner of your local health food shop. Spend time with family and friends who share your beliefs about the importance of diet and exercise for good health. Share your new knowledge with people whose lifestyle is damaging their health. If you can pass on what you've learned, then you can make a real difference in your own community.

Remember, treating your high blood pressure is not just about taking pharmaceuticals. In reality, it's a total lifestyle change and commitment. If you are up to the challenge and want to maintain the vitality and vigour of your youth, follow this eight-week approach. It really works. If you put your whole heart into becoming well, you will heal. Be well on your own journey. I wish you many blessings as you try to stay on the path to a lower blood pressure—and a healthier and longer life.

Part Two

1,500-Calorie Meal Plan (Women)

WEEK ONE

Day One

Calories: 1,480　　　　　　　Sodium: 1,240mg
Calories from Fat: 290　　　　Total Carbohydrate: 237g
Total Fat: 32g　　　　　　　Dietary Fibre: 33g
Saturated Fat: 5g　　　　　　Sugars: 103g
Cholesterol: 135mg　　　　　Protein: 74g
% of Calories from Carbohydrate/Protein/Fat: 61/19/19

WEEK ONE

Day Two

Calories: 1,490　　　　　　　Sodium: 990mg
Calories from Fat: 610　　　　Total Carbohydrate: 166g
Total Fat: 68g　　　　　　　Dietary Fibre: 35g
Saturated Fat: 11g　　　　　　Sugars: 43g
Cholesterol: 75mg　　　　　　Protein: 72g
% of Calories from Carbohydrate/Protein/Fat: 42/18/39

WEEK ONE

Day Three

Calories: 1,500　　　　　　　Sodium: 490mg
Calories from Fat: 460　　　　Total Carbohydrate: 202g
Total Fat: 52g　　　　　　　Dietary Fibre: 40g
Saturated Fat: 8g　　　　　　Sugars: 86g
Cholesterol: 120mg　　　　　Protein: 74g
% of Calories from Carbohydrate/Protein/Fat: 52/19/30

WEEK ONE

Day Four

Calories: 1,490

Calories from Fat: 480

Total Fat: 53g

Saturated Fat: 9g

Cholesterol: 485mg

Sodium: 770mg

Total Carbohydrate: 183g

Dietary Fibre: 46g

Sugars: 69g

Protein: 88g

% of Calories from Carbohydrate/Protein/Fat: 47/22/31

WEEK ONE

Day Five

Calories: 1,520

Calories from Fat: 470

Total Fat: 52g

Saturated Fat: 7g

Cholesterol: 150mg

Sodium: 1,040mg

Total Carbohydrate: 196g

Dietary Fibre: 37g

Sugars: 77g

Protein: 87g

% of Calories from Carbohydrate/Protein/Fat: 49/22/29

WEEK ONE

Day Six

Calories: 1,470

Calories from Fat: 555

Total Fat: 62g

Saturated Fat: 11g

Cholesterol: 585mg

Sodium: 1,090mg

Total Carbohydrate: 158g

Dietary Fibre: 22g

Sugars: 86g

Protein: 83g

% of Calories from Carbohydrate/Protein/Fat: 39/27/34

WEEK ONE

Day Seven

Calories: 1,450

Calories from Fat: 340

Total Fat: 38g

Saturated Fat: 7g

Cholesterol: 325mg

Sodium: 1,030mg

Total Carbohydrate: 221g

Dietary Fibre: 41g

Sugars: 94g

Protein: 72g

% of Calories from Carbohydrate/Protein/Fat: 58/19/22

WEEK TWO

Day One

Calories: 1,510	Sodium: 1,520mg
Calories from Fat: 400	Total Carbohydrate: 211g
Total Fat: 44g	Dietary Fibre: 27g
Saturated Fat: 7g	Sugars: 84g
Cholesterol: 110mg	Protein: 85g

% of Calories from Carbohydrate/Protein/Fat: 53/22/25

WEEK TWO

Day Two

Calories: 1,490	Sodium: 1,260mg
Calories from Fat: 360	Total Carbohydrate: 234g
Total Fat: 41g	Dietary Fibre: 26g
Saturated Fat: 7g	Sugars: 99g
Cholesterol: 5mg	Protein: 56g

% of Calories from Carbohydrate/Protein/Fat: 61/15/24

WEEK TWO

Day Three

Calories: 1,500	Sodium: 1,120mg
Calories from Fat: 540	Total Carbohydrate: 182g
Total Fat: 60g	Dietary Fibre: 39g
Saturated Fat: 8g	Sugars: 67g
Cholesterol: 80mg	Protein: 75g

% of Calories from Carbohydrate/Protein/Fat: 46/19/35

WEEK TWO

Day Four

Calories: 1,520	Sodium: 880mg
Calories from Fat: 360	Total Carbohydrate: 209g
Total Fat: 40g	Dietary Fibre: 43g
Saturated Fat: 7g	Sugars: 84g
Cholesterol: 145mg	Protein: 99g

% of Calories from Carbohydrate/Protein/Fat: 52/25/23

WEEK TWO

Day Five

Calories: 1,460	Sodium: 1,240mg
Calories from Fat: 330	Total Carbohydrate: 213g
Total Fat: 37g	Dietary Fibre: 36g
Saturated Fat: 6g	Sugars: 82g
Cholesterol: 460mg	Protein: 78g

% of Calories from Carbohydrate/Protein/Fat: 57/21/22

WEEK TWO

Day Six

Calories: 1,500	Sodium: 1,210mg
Calories from Fat: 520	Total Carbohydrate: 183g
Total Fat: 58g	Dietary Fibre: 24g
Saturated Fat: 11g	Sugars: 93g
Cholesterol: 330mg	Protein: 79g

% of Calories from Carbohydrate/Protein/Fat: 47/20/33

WEEK TWO

Day Seven

Calories: 1,440	Sodium: 1,840mg
Calories from Fat: 290	Total Carbohydrate: 243g
Total Fat: 32g	Dietary Fibre: 36g
Saturated Fat: 5g	Sugars: 125g
Cholesterol: 50mg	Protein: 63g

% of Calories from Carbohydrate/Protein/Fat: 63/16/19

WEEK THREE

Day One

Calories: 1,450	Sodium: 620mg
Calories from Fat: 490	Total Carbohydrate: 197g
Total Fat: 55g	Dietary Fibre: 36g
Saturated Fat: 7g	Sugars: 87g
Cholesterol: 60mg	Protein: 61g

% of Calories from Carbohydrate/Protein/Fat: 52/16/32

WEEK THREE

Day Two

Calories: 1,420   Sodium: 1,030mg
Calories from Fat: 380   Total Carbohydrate: 187g
Total Fat: 42g   Dietary Fibre: 35g
Saturated Fat: 6g   Sugars: 76g
Cholesterol: 205mg   Protein: 89g
% of Calories from Carbohydrate/Protein/Fat: 50/24/26

WEEK THREE

Day Three

Calories: 1,500   Sodium: 1,370mg
Calories from Fat: 450   Total Carbohydrate: 205g
Total Fat: 50g   Dietary Fibre: 36g
Saturated Fat: 9g   Sugars: 79g
Cholesterol: 515mg   Protein: 77g
% of Calories from Carbohydrate/Protein/Fat: 52/20/28

WEEK THREE

Day Four

Calories: 1,470   Sodium: 850mg
Calories from Fat: 260   Total Carbohydrate: 241g
Total Fat: 29g   Dietary Fibre: 41g
Saturated Fat: 5g   Sugars: 121g
Cholesterol: 220mg   Protein: 81g
% of Calories from Carbohydrate/Protein/Fat: 62/21/17

WEEK THREE

Day Five

Calories: 1,440   Sodium: 680mg
Calories from Fat: 390   Total Carbohydrate: 181g
Total Fat: 43g   Dietary Fibre: 34g
Saturated Fat: 7g   Sugars: 88g
Cholesterol: 85mg   Protein: 91g
% of Calories from Carbohydrate/Protein/Fat: 49/25/26

WEEK THREE

Day Six

Calories: 1,500
Calories from Fat: 390
Total Fat: 44g
Saturated Fat: 8g
Cholesterol: 525mg

Sodium: 1,180mg
Total Carbohydrate: 207g
Dietary Fibre: 35g
Sugars: 91g
Protein: 87g

% of Calories from Carbohydrate/Protein/Fat: 53/22/25

WEEK THREE

Day Seven

Calories: 1,470
Calories from Fat: 380
Total Fat: 42g
Saturated Fat: 8g
Cholesterol: 60mg

Sodium: 1,120mg
Total Carbohydrate: 212g
Dietary Fibre: 43g
Sugars: 66g
Protein: 76g

% of Calories from Carbohydrate/Protein/Fat: 55/20/25

WEEK FOUR

Day One

Calories: 1,440
Calories from Fat: 420
Total Fat: 47g
Saturated Fat: 7g
Cholesterol: 80mg

Sodium: 770mg
Total Carbohydrate: 201g
Dietary Fibre: 31g
Sugars: 87g
Protein: 71g

% of Calories from Carbohydrate/Protein/Fat: 53/19/28

WEEK FOUR

Day Two

Calories: 1,420
Calories from Fat: 440
Total Fat: 49g
Saturated Fat: 9g
Cholesterol: 40mg

Sodium: 960mg
Total Carbohydrate: 184g
Dietary Fibre: 25g
Sugars: 101g
Protein: 73g

% of Calories from Carbohydrate/Protein/Fat: 50/20/30

WEEK FOUR

Day Three
Calories: 1,430
Calories from Fat: 430
Total Fat: 48g
Saturated Fat: 12g
Cholesterol: 515mg
Sodium: 1,180mg
Total Carbohydrate: 184g
Dietary Fibre: 39g
Sugars: 85g
Protein: 78g
% of Calories from Carbohydrate/Protein/Fat: 50/21/29

WEEK FOUR

Day Four
Calories: 1,430
Calories from Fat: 430
Total Fat: 48g
Saturated Fat: 9g
Cholesterol: 155mg
Sodium: 970mg
Total Carbohydrate: 176g
Dietary Fibre: 38g
Sugars: 69g
Protein: 92g
% of Calories from Carbohydrate/Protein/Fat: 47/25/29

WEEK FOUR

Day Five
Calories: 1,450
Calories from Fat: 520
Total Fat: 57g
Saturated Fat: 9g
Cholesterol: 310mg
Sodium: 1,090mg
Total Carbohydrate: 179g
Dietary Fibre: 27g
Sugars: 83g
Protein: 72g
% of Calories from Carbohydrate/Protein/Fat: 47/19/34

WEEK FOUR

Day Six
Calories: 1,500
Calories from Fat: 320
Total Fat: 36g
Saturated Fat: 7g
Cholesterol: 650mg
Sodium: 710mg
Total Carbohydrate: 219g
Dietary Fibre: 37g
Sugars: 85g
Protein: 91g
% of Calories from Carbohydrate/Protein/Fat: 56/23/20

WEEK FOUR

Day Seven

Calories: 1,410

Sodium: 1,260mg

Calories from Fat: 410

Total Carbohydrate: 200g

Total Fat: 46g

Dietary Fibre: 31g

Saturated Fat: 11g

Sugars: 104g

Cholesterol: 105mg

Protein: 67g

% of Calories from Carbohydrate/Protein/Fat: 54/18/28

WEEK FIVE

Day One

Calories: 1,480

Sodium: 1,220mg

Calories from Fat: 290

Total Carbohydrate: 234g

Total Fat: 32g

Dietary Fibre: 24g

Saturated Fat: 6g

Sugars: 113g

Cholesterol: 90mg

Protein: 80g

% of Calories from Carbohydrate/Protein/Fat: 60/21/19

WEEK FIVE

Day Two

Calories: 1,460

Sodium: 1,660mg

Calories from Fat: 410

Total Carbohydrate: 201g

Total Fat: 45g

Dietary Fibre: 37g

Saturated Fat: 9g

Sugars: 90g

Cholesterol: 495mg

Protein: 81g

% of Calories from Carbohydrate/Protein/Fat: 52/21/27

WEEK FIVE

Day Three

Calories: 1,420

Sodium: 710mg

Calories from Fat: 370

Total Carbohydrate: 211g

Total Fat: 41g

Dietary Fibre: 34g

Saturated Fat: 6g

Sugars: 92g

Cholesterol: 70mg

Protein: 67g

% of Calories from Carbohydrate/Protein/Fat: 57/18/25

WEEK FIVE

Day Four

Calories: 1,470
Calories from Fat: 300
Total Fat: 34g
Saturated Fat: 7g
Cholesterol: 75mg

Sodium: 1,180mg
Total Carbohydrate: 233g
Dietary Fibre: 57g
Sugars: 77g
Protein: 79g

% of Calories from Carbohydrate/Protein/Fat: 60/20/20

WEEK FIVE

Day Five

Calories: 1,470
Calories from Fat: 370
Total Fat: 41g
Saturated Fat: 8g
Cholesterol: 280mg

Sodium: 1,310mg
Total Carbohydrate: 198g
Dietary Fibre: 56g
Sugars: 50g
Protein: 93g

% of Calories from Carbohydrate/Protein/Fat: 52/24/24

WEEK FIVE

Day Six

Calories: 1,530
Calories from Fat: 510
Total Fat: 57g
Saturated Fat: 9g
Cholesterol: 310mg

Sodium: 870mg
Total Carbohydrate: 181g
Dietary Fibre: 28g
Sugars: 83g
Protein: 85g

% of Calories from Carbohydrate/Protein/Fat: 46/22/32

WEEK FIVE

Day Seven

Calories: 1,430
Calories from Fat: 430
Total Fat: 47g
Saturated Fat: 6g
Cholesterol: 65mg

Sodium: 1,410mg
Total Carbohydrate: 212g
Dietary Fibre: 35g
Sugars: 105g
Protein: 66g

% of Calories from Carbohydrate/Protein/Fat: 55/17/28

WEEK SIX

Day One

Calories: 1,490

Calories from Fat: 490

Total Fat: 54g

Saturated Fat: 8g

Cholesterol: 75mg

Sodium: 910mg

Total Carbohydrate: 205g

Dietary Fibre: 41g

Sugars: 64g

Protein: 65g

% of Calories from Carbohydrate/Protein/Fat: 52/17/31

WEEK SIX

Day Two

Calories: 1,440

Calories from Fat: 300

Total Fat: 33g

Saturated Fat: 5g

Cholesterol: 125mg

Sodium: 1,160mg

Total Carbohydrate: 224g

Dietary Fibre: 40g

Sugars: 92g

Protein: 78g

% of Calories from Carbohydrate/Protein/Fat: 60/21/20

WEEK SIX

Day Three

Calories: 1,420

Calories from Fat: 450

Total Fat: 49g

Saturated Fat: 7g

Cholesterol: 90mg

Sodium: 1,130mg

Total Carbohydrate: 206g

Dietary Fibre: 28g

Sugars: 76g

Protein: 59g

% of Calories from Carbohydrate/Protein/Fat: 55/16/30

WEEK SIX

Day Four

Calories: 1,480

Calories from Fat: 450

Total Fat: 50g

Saturated Fat: 9g

Cholesterol: 490mg

Sodium: 1,010mg

Total Carbohydrate: 187g

Dietary Fibre: 32g

Sugars: 77g

Protein: 83g

% of Calories from Carbohydrate/Protein/Fat: 49/22/30

WEEK SIX

Day Five

Calories: 1,520
Calories from Fat: 470
Total Fat: 52g
Saturated Fat: 10g
Cholesterol: 575mg

Sodium: 1,130mg
Total Carbohydrate: 192g
Dietary Fibre: 30g
Sugars: 60g
Protein: 88g

% of Calories from Carbohydrate/Protein/Fat: 48/22/29

WEEK SIX

Day Six

Calories: 1,440
Calories from Fat: 430
Total Fat: 48g
Saturated Fat: 6g
Cholesterol: 75mg

Sodium: 550mg
Total Carbohydrate: 201g
Dietary Fibre: 54g
Sugars: 95g
Protein: 71g

% of Calories from Carbohydrate/Protein/Fat: 53/19/28

WEEK SIX

Day Seven

Calories: 1,510
Calories from Fat: 400
Total Fat: 44g
Saturated Fat: 6g
Cholesterol: 25mg

Sodium: 600mg
Total Carbohydrate: 223g
Dietary Fibre: 32g
Sugars: 99g
Protein: 68g

% of Calories from Carbohydrate/Protein/Fat: 57/17/26

WEEK SEVEN

Day One

Calories: 1,460
Calories from Fat: 410
Total Fat: 45g
Saturated Fat: 8g
Cholesterol: 135mg

Sodium: 770mg
Total Carbohydrate: 197g
Dietary Fibre: 24g
Sugars: 109g
Protein: 82g

% of Calories from Carbohydrate/Protein/Fat: 52/22/27

WEEK SEVEN

Day Two

Calories: 1,480

Calories from Fat: 360

Total Fat: 40g

Saturated Fat: 7g

Cholesterol: 115mg

Sodium: 1,060mg

Total Carbohydrate: 249g

Dietary Fibre: 28g

Sugars: 106g

Protein: 53g

% of Calories from Carbohydrate/Protein/Fat: 63/14/23

WEEK SEVEN

Day Three

Calories: 1,460

Calories from Fat: 320

Total Fat: 36g

Saturated Fat: 8g

Cholesterol: 660mg

Sodium: 1,390mg

Total Carbohydrate: 196g

Dietary Fibre: 32g

Sugars: 109g

Protein: 97g

% of Calories from Carbohydrate/Protein/Fat: 52/26/22

WEEK SEVEN

Day Four

Calories: 1,450

Calories from Fat: 360

Total Fat: 42g

Saturated Fat: 7g

Cholesterol: 120mg

Sodium: 380mg

Total Carbohydrate: 198g

Dietary Fibre: 31g

Sugars: 100g

Protein: 87g

% of Calories from Carbohydrate/Protein/Fat: 52/23/24

WEEK SEVEN

Day Five

Calories: 1,440

Calories from Fat: 330

Total Fat: 37g

Saturated Fat: 4g

Cholesterol: 0

Sodium: 930mg

Total Carbohydrate: 257g

Dietary Fibre: 54g

Sugars: 106g

Protein: 58g

% of Calories from Carbohydrate/Protein/Fat: 65/15/21

WEEK SEVEN

Day Six

Calories: 1,480

Calories from Fat: 460

Total Fat: 51g

Saturated Fat: 8g

Cholesterol: 265mg

Sodium: 680mg

Total Carbohydrate: 183g

Dietary Fibre: 41g

Sugars: 80g

Protein: 81g

% of Calories from Carbohydrate/Protein/Fat: 48/21/30

WEEK SEVEN

Day Seven

Calories: 1,410

Calories from Fat: 330

Total Fat: 37g

Saturated Fat: 8g

Cholesterol: 160mg

Sodium: 590mg

Total Carbohydrate: 207g

Dietary Fibre: 31g

Sugars: 101g

Protein: 79g

% of Calories from Carbohydrate/Protein/Fat: 56/21/23

WEEK EIGHT

Day One

Calories: 1,420

Calories from Fat: 350

Total Fat: 38g

Saturated Fat: 5g

Cholesterol: 85mg

Sodium: 830mg

Total Carbohydrate: 218g

Dietary Fibre: 32g

Sugars: 99g

Protein: 73g

% of Calories from Carbohydrate/Protein/Fat: 58/19/23

WEEK EIGHT

Day Two

Calories: 1,440

Calories from Fat: 530

Total Fat: 59g

Saturated Fat: 10g

Cholesterol: 100mg

Sodium: 390mg

Total Carbohydrate: 175g

Dietary Fibre: 32g

Sugars: 85g

Protein: 68g

% of Calories from Carbohydrate/Protein/Fat: 47/18/35

WEEK EIGHT

Day Three

Calories: 1,490
Calories from Fat: 360
Total Fat: 40g
Saturated Fat: 7g
Cholesterol: 65mg

Sodium: 1,180mg
Total Carbohydrate: 233g
Dietary Fibre: 28g
Sugars: 84g
Protein: 67g

% of Calories from Carbohydrate/Protein/Fat: 60/17/23

WEEK EIGHT

Day Four

Calories: 1,510
Calories from Fat: 430
Total Fat: 48g
Saturated Fat: 10g
Cholesterol: 115mg

Sodium: 1,940mg
Total Carbohydrate: 206g
Dietary Fibre: 35g
Sugars: 102g
Protein: 79g

% of Calories from Carbohydrate/Protein/Fat: 52/20/28

WEEK EIGHT

Day Five

Calories: 1,500
Calories from Fat: 460
Total Fat: 51g
Saturated Fat: 12g
Cholesterol: 380mg

Sodium: 1,130mg
Total Carbohydrate: 180g
Dietary Fibre: 32g
Sugars: 96g
Protein: 99g

% of Calories from Carbohydrate/Protein/Fat: 46/25/29

WEEK EIGHT

Day Six

Calories: 1,480
Calories from Fat: 420
Total Fat: 47g
Saturated Fat: 6g
Cholesterol: 275mg

Sodium: 910mg
Total Carbohydrate: 224g
Dietary Fibre: 40g
Sugars: 113g
Protein: 59g

% of Calories from Carbohydrate/Protein/Fat: 58/15/27

WEEK EIGHT

Day Seven

Calories: 1,450   Sodium: 840mg

Calories from Fat: 440   Total Carbohydrate: 207g

Total Fat: 48g   Dietary Fibre: 36g

Saturated Fat: 6g   Sugars: 78g

Cholesterol: 75mg   Protein: 62g

% of Calories from Carbohydrate/Protein/Fat: 55/16/29

See page 281 for information on measurements

1,500-CALORIE DAILY PLAN: WEEK 1

(* denotes recipes)

Day 1

Breakfast: *225g (8oz) cooked oatmeal (not instant packages) with 1 Tbsp. raisins; 125ml (4fl oz) skimmed or plain soya milk; 1 cup tea or coffee (decaffeinated is best)*

Lunch: *60g (2oz) canned no-salt-added or fresh cooked salmon in a wholemeal pitta with lettuce, tomato, and onion seasoned with lemon juice and 1 tsp. olive oil; 1 apple*

Snack: *1 Apricot Oatmeal Bar**

Dinner: *1 serving Steamed Mussels*; 1 cup steamed broccoli; 1 medium baked potato with 2 Tbsp. fat-free plain yogurt; ¼ melon*

Day 2

Breakfast: *2 slices wholemeal toast; 2 Tbsp. soya nut butter; ¼ of a melon; 1 cup coffee or tea*

Lunch: *1 serving Grilled Rosemary Chicken Breast*; large bowl tossed salad with 2 Tbsp. Flaxseed Dressing*; 100g (3½oz) strawberries*

Dinner: *1 serving Wholemeal Pasta with Aubergine Tomato Sauce*; 1 serving Spinach and Tomato Salad**

Day 3

Breakfast: *50g (1¾oz) unsweetened shredded wheat, 2 tsp. walnuts, 3 Tbsp. raisins, 125ml (4fl oz) cup skimmed or soya milk; 1 cup coffee or tea*

Snack: *1 orange*

Lunch: *1 serving Vegetable Soup*; large bowl tossed salad with 2 Tbsp. Flaxseed Dressing*; 1 Apricot Oatmeal Bar**

Dinner: *1 serving Roast Pork Tenderloin with Rosemary and Garlic*; large bowl tossed salad with Ginger Flaxseed Dressing*; 1 serving Lentils with Garlic and Tomatoes*; 60g (2oz) raspberries with 120g (4oz) fat-free plain yogurt and 2 tsp. honey*

Day 4
Breakfast:　2 scrambled eggs prepared with 2 Tbsp. skimmed milk; 1 slice wholemeal toast with 1 tsp. light margarine (with no trans fatty acids); ¼ melon; 1 cup coffee or tea

Lunch:　1 serving Tempeh Chilli*; large bowl tossed salad with Ginger Flaxseed Dressing*; 1 apple

Dinner:　1 serving Roast Salmon*; 1 serving Spinach with Pine Nuts and Garlic*; 1 serving Chickpea Salad with Rosemary*; 1 peach

Day 5
Breakfast:　2 slices wholemeal toast with 2 Tbsp. unsalted natural peanut butter and 1 Tbsp. all fruit preserves; 1 cup coffee or tea

Snack:　1 pear

Lunch:　1 serving Chickpea and Chicory Soup*; 125g (4½oz) steamed broccoli; 125g (4½oz) strawberries; 25g (¾oz) walnuts

Dinner:　150g (5oz) sliced roast turkey breast with rocket and 25g (¾oz) sun-dried oil-packed tomatoes (drained) stuffed in a wholemeal pitta; 1 piece Carrot Cake*

Day 6
Breakfast:　2-egg omelette made with 2 Tbsp. skimmed milk, 25g (1oz) mushrooms, and 1 slice soya cheese; 1 piece whole-grain toast with 1 tsp. light margarine; 240ml (8fl oz) calcium-fortified orange juice; 1 cup coffee or tea

Lunch:　½ of a 180g (6oz) can low-sodium water-packed tuna, drained and seasoned with lemon juice; 2 cups tossed salad with 2 Tbsp. Flaxseed Dressing*; 2 rye crisp crackers; 1 apple

Dinner:　1 serving Turkey Meatloaf*; 1 serving Grilled Courgettes*; large bowl of tossed salad with Ginger Flaxseed Dressing*; 1 piece Carrot Cake*

Day 7
Breakfast:　2 slices wholemeal French toast made with 1 egg and 2 Tbsp. skimmed milk and seasoned with cinnamon; 50g (1½oz) unsweetened apple sauce; 240ml (8fl oz) calcium-fortified orange juice; 1 cup coffee or tea

Lunch:　1 serving Chicken Vegetable Soup*; 4 wholemeal crackers; 1 Apricot Oatmeal Bar*

Dinner:　1 serving Pasta à la Sinatra*; large bowl of tossed salad with 2 Tbsp. Ginger Flaxseed Dressing*; 75g (2½oz) red grapes and 100g (3oz) strawberries

DAILY PLAN: WEEK 2

Day 1
Breakfast:　Fruit Smoothie*

Lunch:　1 serving Stir-Fried Tofu and Vegetables*; 1 orange

Dinner: *1 serving Breaded Sole or Flounder*; 1 serving Spinach and Tomato Salad; 1 small baked sweet potato; 170g (5½oz) blueberries with 120g (4oz) fat-free plain yogurt and 1 tsp. honey*

Supplements: *A good multivitamin/mineral supplement containing all the essential vitamins and minerals is recommended with the suggested doses below. The supplement should contain natural carotenoids, flavonoids, and vitamin E with gamma-tocopherol, as well as some grapeseed, lutein, alpha-lipoic acid, lycopene in combination with full vitamin B support, and minerals such as magnesium, selenium, and chromium, to mention a few. Suggested doses for the Sinatra Foundation Programme include the following:*

- *10,000 units (6,000µg) of mixed carotenoids with beta-carotene, or 2,500 units (750µg retinol) of vitamin A with 7,500 units (4,500µg) of mixed carotenoids with beta-carotene*
- *Vitamin C in divided doses of 200–400mg/day*
- *Vitamin E 200–400 IU with some gamma-tocopherol*
- *Magnesium 400–800mg/day*
- *Calcium 250–1,000mg/day*
- *CoQ10 15–30mg 4 times daily*
- *L-carnitine fumarate 250–500mg 4 times daily*

Each week we will build on this programme. Remember to take supplements with meals in divided dosages.

Day 2

Breakfast: *225g (8oz) oatmeal enriched with 1 Tbsp. soya powder; 125ml (4fl oz) plain soya or skimmed milk; 240ml (8fl oz) calcium-fortified orange juice; 1 cup coffee or tea*

Lunch: *1 serving Tofu, Tomato, and Black Olive Salad*; 1 small wholemeal roll; 1 apple*

Dinner: *1 serving Tempeh and Stir-Fried Vegetables*; 90g (3oz) diced pineapple with 120g (4oz) fat-free plain yogurt and 1 tsp. honey*

Supplements: *Sinatra Foundation Programme (see dosages above)*

Day 3

Breakfast: *½ medium grapefruit; 2 slices soya cheese tucked into a wholemeal pitta and toasted in the grill/oven; 1 cup coffee or tea*

Lunch: *1 serving Antiguan Black Bean Soup*; 4 wholemeal crackers; large bowl tossed salad with 2 Tbsp. Flaxseed Dressing*; 75g (2½oz) grapes*

Snack: *75g (2½oz) baby carrots with 2 Tbsp. Hummus**

Dinner: *1 serving Grilled Rosemary Chicken Breast*; 1 serving Spinach with Pine Nuts and Garlic*; 1 medium tomato, sliced, and 4 black olives; 1 apple*

Supplements: *Sinatra Foundation Programme*

Day 4

Breakfast: *125g (4½oz) low-sodium low-fat cottage cheese with 170g (5½oz) melon cubes and 2 tsp. chopped walnuts; 1 cup coffee or tea*

Lunch: *60g (2oz) sliced roast turkey breast on 2 slices wholemeal bread with lettuce, tomato, and 2 tsp. light soya-based mayonnaise; 1 serving Bean Salad*; 1 apple*

Snack: *1 Peanut Butter Biscuit*; 240ml (8fl oz) plain soya or skimmed milk*

Dinner: *1 serving Roast Pork Tenderloin with Mustard*; 1 small baked potato with 1 tsp. light margarine; 1 serving Grilled Courgettes*; 1 medium tomato, chopped and mixed with fresh basil; 180g (6oz) strawberries with 120ml (4fl oz) fat-free plain yogurt and 1 tsp. honey*

Supplements: *Sinatra Foundation Programme*

Day 5

Breakfast: *1 poached egg on 1 slice wholemeal toast; 180g (6oz) strawberries or 150g (5oz) organic blueberries; 240ml (8fl oz) calcium-fortified orange juice; 1 cup coffee or tea*

Lunch: *Soya burger on a wholemeal roll with sliced tomato and onion; 1 serving Pinto Bean Salad*; sliced tomatoes and onions; ¼ melon*

Dinner: *1 serving Orange Prawns with Couscous*; 125g (5oz) steamed green beans; 1 Carob Nut Brownie**

Supplements: *Sinatra Foundation Programme*

Day 6

Breakfast: *50g (1¾oz) whole-grain cold cereal; 125ml (4fl oz) skimmed or soya milk; ½ sliced banana; 240ml (8fl oz) calcium-fortified orange juice; 1 cup coffee or tea*

Lunch: *Chef salad with 25g (¾oz) shredded soya cheese; 1 hard-boiled egg; 60g (2oz) turkey breast; green leaf lettuce, tomatoes, celery, and cucumbers and 2 Tbsp. Flaxseed Dressing*; 1 small wholemeal roll with 1 tsp. light margarine*

Snack: *1 apple*

Dinner: *1 serving Low-Fat Exceptional Hamburgers* on a wholemeal roll with lettuce, tomato, and 2 tsp. low-fat mayonnaise; 1 serving Veggie Coleslaw*; 120g (4oz) fresh sweet cherries*

Supplements: *Sinatra Foundation Programme*

Day 7

Breakfast: *1 Blueberry Bran Muffin*; 120g (4oz) low-fat low-sodium cottage cheese with ½ cup melon; 240ml (8fl oz) calcium-fortified orange juice; 1 cup coffee or tea*

Lunch: *1 serving Veggie Miso Soup*; 2 crisp crackers; 75g (2½oz) steamed kale; 1 small pear*

Snack: *1 Carob Nut Brownie*; 1 cup plain soya or skimmed milk*

Dinner: *1 serving Tofu with Sesame Seeds*; 1 serving Fresh Tomato Salsa*; 1 serving Three-Bean Salad*; 75g (2½oz) red grapes*

Supplements: *Sinatra Foundation Programme*

DAILY PLAN: WEEK 3

Day 1
Breakfast: Fruit Smoothie*
Lunch: 1 serving Salmon Salad*; sliced tomatoes; 1 apple
Dinner: 1 serving Tempeh Chilli*; large bowl tossed salad with 2 Tbsp. Flaxseed Dressing*; 100g (3½oz) strawberries
Supplements: Sinatra Foundation Programme plus the following:
  • 2g fish oil
  • 2 Tbsp. crushed flaxseed (preferred) or 1 Tbsp. flaxseed oil
Exercise: 20–30-minute walk

Day 2
Breakfast: 225ml (8fl oz) fat-free plain yogurt with 1 tsp. honey and 2 tsp. chopped walnuts; 80g (2¾oz) melon; 1 Blueberry Bran Muffin*; 1 cup coffee or tea
Lunch: 1 serving Salad Niçoise, Sinatra Style*; 1 apple
Dinner: 1 serving Scallop Kebab*; 1 serving Dr. Sinatra's Favourite Shiitake Recipe*; 1 serving Haricot Beans, Garlic, and Rosemary*; 180g (6oz) watermelon
Supplements: Sinatra Foundation Programme plus added fish oil and flaxseed
Exercise: 20–30-minute walk

Day 3
Breakfast: 2 scrambled eggs prepared with 2 Tbsp. skimmed milk; 2 slices wholemeal toast with 2 tsp. light margarine; 240g (8fl oz) calcium-fortified orange juice; 150g (5oz) blueberries; 1 cup coffee or tea
Lunch: Grilled soya cheese and tomato sandwich on wholemeal bread with 2 tsp. light margarine; 75g (2½oz) cup baby carrots; 1 apple
Dinner: 1 serving Roast Salmon*; 150g (5oz) steamed spinach; 100g (3½oz) black beans; 1 serving Israeli Chopped Salad*; 1 piece Spice Cake*
Supplements: Sinatra Foundation Programme plus added fish oil and flaxseed
Exercise: 20–30-minute walk

Day 4
Breakfast: 225ml (8oz) cooked oatmeal with 1 Tbsp. raisins; 125ml (4fl oz) skimmed or plain soya milk; 1 cup coffee or tea
Snack: 1 banana; 125ml (4fl oz) low-sodium low-fat cottage cheese
Lunch: 50g (1¾oz) fresh chopped spinach, 90g (3oz) navy beans, and 1 hard-boiled egg with Ginger Flaxseed Dressing*; 90g (3oz) honeydew melon
Snack: 180g (6oz) strawberries with Lemon Poppy Seed Dip*
Dinner: 1 serving Roast Vegetables*; 1 serving Grilled Tofu*; 1 serving Lentils with Garlic and Tomatoes*; ¼ melon
Supplements: Sinatra Foundation Programme plus added fish oil and flaxseed
Exercise: 20–30-minute walk

Day 5

Breakfast: *225g (8oz) low-sodium low-fat cottage cheese topped with 1 tsp. ground flaxseed, 2 tsp. wheat germ, and 125g (4½oz) cup crushed pineapple; 180g (6oz) mixed strawberries and melon; 1 cup coffee or tea*

Lunch: *1 serving Veggie Miso Soup*; 75g (2½oz) cooked brown rice; 125g (4½oz) steamed broccoli; 1 small pear*

Snack: *75g (2½oz) baby carrots*

Dinner: *1 serving Grilled Mediterranean Halibut*; 100g (3½oz) lima butter beans; large bowl tossed salad with Flaxseed Dressing*; 1 piece Spice Cake**

Supplements: *Sinatra Foundation Programme plus added fish oil and flaxseed*

Exercise: *20–30-minute walk*

Day 6

Breakfast: *2 eggs scrambled with 25g (¾oz) mushrooms, sliced tomato, and chopped onion in 1 tsp. olive oil; 1 slice wholemeal toast with 1 tsp. light margarine; 240ml (8fl oz) calcium-fortified orange juice; 1 cup coffee or tea*

Lunch: *1 serving TVP Chilli*; 180g (6oz) strawberries*

Dinner: *1 serving Stir-Fried Broccoli with Chicken*; 170g (5½oz) melon cubes; 1 piece Spice Cake**

Supplements: *Sinatra Foundation Programme plus added fish oil and flaxseed*

Exercise: *20–30-minute walk*

Day 7

Breakfast: *40g (1½oz) shredded wheat cereal with 125ml (4fl oz) plain soya or skimmed milk and 2 Tbsp. raisins; 1 cup coffee or tea*

Lunch: *Soya burger on a wholemeal roll with lettuce and tomato; 100g (3½oz) Bean Salad*; sliced tomatoes and cucumbers; 1 apple*

Dinner: *1 serving Grilled Red Snapper*; 100g (3oz) steamed cauliflower; large bowl tossed salad with diced celery and mushrooms and 2 Tbsp. Flaxseed Dressing*; 175g (5½oz) watermelon*

Supplements: *Sinatra Foundation Programme plus added fish oil and flaxseed*

Exercise: *20–30-minute walk*

DAILY PLAN: WEEK 4

Day 1

Breakfast: *225g (8oz) oatmeal with 1 Tbsp. diced figs or raisins; 125ml (4fl oz) skimmed or plain soya milk; 240g (8fl oz) calcium-fortified orange juice; 1 cup coffee or tea*

Lunch: *1 serving Tofu, Tomato, and Black Olive Salad*; 1 wholemeal pitta; 125g (4½oz) steamed broccoli; 1 apple*

Dinner: *1 serving Easy Broiled Chicken Breast*; Steamed Vegetables*; 75g (2½oz) cooked brown rice; 75g (2½oz) grapes and 80g (2¾oz) watermelon*

Supplements: *Sinatra Foundation Programme plus the following:*
- *2g fish oil*
- *2 Tbsp. crushed flaxseed (preferred) or 1 Tbsp. flaxseed oil*
- *2g L-Arginine*

Exercise: *Three flexibility exercises followed by a 20-minute walk*
Mind/Body: *Meditation or qi gong exercises*

Day 2

Breakfast: *225g (8oz) low-sodium low-fat cottage cheese; 170g (5½oz) diced melon; 150g (5oz) crushed pineapple; 1 cup coffee or tea*
Lunch: *60g (2oz) canned salmon on large bowl tossed salad and 1 medium tomato, sliced; 2 Tbsp. Flaxseed Dressing*; 1 apple*
Snack: *1 rye crisp cracker with 1 Tbsp. soya nut butter*
Dinner: *1 serving Stir-Fried Tofu and Vegetables*; 1 frozen banana*
Supplements: *Sinatra Foundation Programme plus added fish oil, flaxseed, and L-arginine*
Exercise: *Flexibility exercises followed by a 20-minute walk*
Mind/Body: *Meditation or qigong exercises*

Day 3

Breakfast: *2-egg spinach omelette made with 30g (1oz) feta cheese and 15g (1½oz) fresh chopped spinach; 1 slice wholemeal toast with 1 tsp. light margarine; 240ml (8fl oz) calcium-fortified orange juice; 1 cup coffee or tea*
Lunch: *1 serving Veggie Miso Soup*; 75g (2½oz) cooked brown rice with 2 Tbsp. dried figs; large bowl tossed salad with 2 Tbsp. Flaxseed Dressing*; 1 peach*
Dinner: *120g (4oz) grilled chicken breast; large bowl tossed salad with Ginger Flaxseed Dressing*; 1 serving Black Bean Salad*; 180g (6oz) strawberries*
Supplements: *Sinatra Foundation Programme plus added fish oil, flaxseed, L-arginine*
Exercise: *Flexibility exercises, followed by a 20-minute walk*
Mind/Body: *Meditation or qigong exercises*

Day 4

Breakfast: *225g (8oz) oatmeal with 1 Tbsp. soya powder; 125ml (4fl oz) plain soya or skimmed milk; 1 tsp. chopped nuts and cinnamon; ½ medium grapefruit; 1 cup coffee or tea*
Lunch: *120g (4oz) turkey burger on wholemeal roll with 2 tsp. light mayonnaise and sliced tomato and lettuce; 1 serving Three-Bean Salad*; 75g (2½oz) grapes*
Dinner: *1 serving Poached Salmon with Dill Sauce*; sliced cucumbers with dill; 1 serving Spinach with Pine Nuts and Garlic*; 1 frozen banana*
Supplements: *Sinatra Foundation Programme plus added fish oil, flaxseed, L-arginine*
Exercise: *Flexibility exercises, followed by a 20-minute walk*
Mind/Body: *Meditation or qigong exercises*

Day 5

Breakfast: *Blueberry or Apple-Cinnamon Bran Muffin*; 2 slices soya cheese; 180g (6oz) strawberries with 60ml (2fl oz) fat-free plain yogurt and 1 tsp. honey; 1 cup coffee or tea*

Snack: *1 orange*

Lunch: *1 serving Vegetable Soup*; large bowl tossed salad with 2 Tbsp. Flaxseed Dressing* and 1 hard-boiled egg*

Dinner: *1 serving Stir-Fried Chicken and Broccoli*; 170g (5½oz) blueberries*

Supplements: *Sinatra Foundation Programme plus added fish oil, flaxseed, L-arginine*

Exercise: *Flexibility exercises followed by a 20-minute walk*

Mind/Body: *Meditation or qigong exercises*

Day 6

Breakfast: *Fruit Smoothie*; 1 cup coffee or tea*

Snack: *125g (4½oz) low-sodium low-fat cottage cheese; 1 Tbsp. raisins*

Lunch: *Mushroom omelette made with 2 eggs and 2 Tbsp. skimmed milk and cooked in 1 tsp. olive oil; large bowl tossed salad with Ginger Flaxseed Dressing*; ¼ melon*

Dinner: *1 serving Prawns with Peppers, Tomatoes, and Garlic*; 1 serving Chickpea Salad with Rosemary*; 1 peach*

Supplements: *Sinatra Foundation Programme plus added fish oil, flaxseed, L-arginine*

Exercise: *Flexibility exercises followed by a 20-minute walk*

Mind/Body: *Meditation or qigong exercises*

Day 7

Breakfast: *50g (1¾oz) cold wholemeal cereal; 2 Tbsp. raisins; 125ml (4fl oz) plain soya or skimmed milk; 240ml (8fl oz) calcium-fortified orange juice; 1 cup coffee or tea*

Lunch: *15g (1½oz) feta cheese and 3 medium fresh figs in a wholemeal pitta; large bowl tossed salad with 2 Tbsp. Flaxseed Dressing**

Snack: *120g (4oz) low-sodium low-fat cottage cheese with 60g (2oz) crushed pineapple*

Dinner: *1 serving Roast Pork Tenderloin with Mustard*; 25g (1oz) onions and 170g (5½oz) sliced courgette sautéed in 1 tsp. olive oil; large bowl tossed salad with Ginger Flaxseed Dressing*; 180g (6oz) strawberries*

Supplements: *Sinatra Foundation Programme plus added fish oil, flaxseed, L-arginine*

Exercise: *Flexibility exercises followed by 20-minute walk*

Mind/Body: *Meditation or qigong exercises*

DAILY PLAN: WEEK 5

Day 1

Breakfast: *240ml (8fl oz) fat-free plain yogurt with 1 tsp. honey and 1 chopped banana; 2 tsp. chopped walnuts; 1 cup coffee or tea*

Lunch: *1 serving Tempeh and Stir-Fried Vegetables*; 180g (6oz) watermelon*

Dinner:	120g (4oz) grilled salmon; 120g (4oz) spinach sautéed in 1 tsp. olive oil; 75g (2½oz) brown rice with 1 Tbsp. raisins; 1 Oatmeal Date Biscuit*; 180g (6oz) honeydew melon
Supplements:	Sinatra Foundation Programme plus the following:

- 2g fish oil
- 2 Tbsp. crushed flaxseed (preferred) or 1 Tbsp. flaxseed oil
- 2g L-arginine
- 150–300mg grapeseed extract

Exercise:	Strength-training exercises
Mind/Body:	Anger management or emotional release exercises

Day 2

Breakfast:	2-egg omelette made with 50g (1¾oz) asparagus; 240ml (8fl oz) calcium-fortified orange juice; 1 slice wholemeal toast with 1 tsp. light margarine; 180g (6oz) strawberries; 1 cup coffee or tea
Lunch:	90g (3oz) turkey breast and ½ medium avocado in wholemeal pitta; 1 apple
Dinner:	1 serving Veggie Miso Soup*; 1 serving Grilled Tofu*; 1 serving Stir-Fry Mangetout and Sesame Seeds*; 90g (3oz) brown rice and lentils; 90g (3oz) grapes and 60g (2oz) blueberries
Supplements:	Sinatra Foundation Programme plus added fish oil, flaxseed, L-arginine, and grapeseed extract
Exercise:	20–30-minute walk
Mind/Body:	Anger management exercises

Day 3

Breakfast:	225g (8oz) cooked oatmeal with 25g (¾oz) chopped dried figs; 125ml (4fl oz) skimmed or plain soya milk; 240ml (8fl oz) calcium-fortified orange juice; 1 cup coffee or tea
Lunch:	60g (2oz) Hummus* with sliced cucumbers, tomatoes, endive, and black olives in wholemeal pitta; 180g (6oz) mixed berries
Dinner:	1 serving Grilled Mediterranean Halibut*; large bowl tossed salad with ½ medium avocado and Ginger Flaxseed Dressing*; ¼ melon
Supplements:	Sinatra Foundation Programme plus added fish oil, flaxseed, L-arginine, and grapeseed extract
Exercise:	Strength training
Mind/Body:	Anger management exercises

Day 4

Breakfast:	1 cup whole-grain cereal with 30g (1oz) blueberries, 1 Tbsp. ground flaxseed, and 240ml (8fl oz) skimmed or plain soya milk; 1 cup coffee or tea
Lunch:	1 serving Minestrone Soup*; large salad green lettuce with tomatoes, red peppers, and black olives with Ginger Flaxseed Dressing*; 180g (6oz) strawberries

Dinner: *1 serving Low-Fat Exceptional Hamburgers* with Fresh Tomato Salsa* on a wholemeal roll; 1 serving of Pinto Bean Salad*; 1 medium grilled yellow squash; 1 pear*
Supplements: *Sinatra Foundation Programme plus added fish oil, flaxseed, L-arginine, and grapeseed*
Exercise: *20–30-minute walk*
Mind/Body: *Anger management exercises*

Day 5
Breakfast: *2 slices wholemeal French toast made with 1 egg and 2 Tbsp. skimmed milk; 120ml (4fl oz) unsweetened stewed apples; 1 cup coffee or tea*
Lunch: *Grilled soya burger in a wholemeal pitta with lettuce, tomato and 2 tsp. light mayonnaise; 1 serving Bean Salad*; sliced cucumber salad with 1 tsp. olive oil and 1 tsp. cidar vinegar*
Dinner: *120g (4oz) chicken breast, grilled; 1 serving Black Bean Salad* with ½ medium avocado and 1 medium chopped tomato with Ginger Flaxseed Dressing*; 1 frozen banana*
Supplements: *Sinatra Foundation Programme plus added fish oil, flaxseed, L-arginine, and grapeseed extract*
Exercise: *Strength training*
Mind/Body: *Anger management exercises*

Day 6
Breakfast: *120g (4oz) low-sodium low-fat cottage cheese with 1 Tbsp. ground flaxseed; ¼ melon; 240ml (8fl oz) calcium-fortified orange juice; 1 cup coffee or tea*
Lunch: *120g (4oz) grilled tempeh; 1 serving Grilled Courgettes*; 90g (3oz) spinach with 1 hard-boiled egg, 1 Tbsp. olive oil, 1 Tbsp. vinegar, and crushed garlic*
Snack: *1 Oatmeal Date Biscuit**
Dinner: *1 serving Stir-Fried Chicken and Broccoli* with 50g (1¾oz) asparagus and 2 Tbsp. diced figs mixed into the rice; 180g (6oz) strawberries*
Supplements: *Sinatra Foundation Programme plus added fish oil, flaxseed, L-arginine, and grapeseed extract*
Exercise: *20–30-minute walk*
Mind/Body: *Anger management exercises*

Day 7
Breakfast: *Fruit Smoothie*; ½ grapefruit*
Lunch: *1 serving Asparagus with Tomatoes and Olive Oil*; grilled soya cheese sandwich on wholemeal bread with 2 tsp. light margarine*
Dinner: *1 serving Mussels Provençal*; large bowl tossed salad with 60g (2oz) firm cubed tofu, tomato, black olives, and Ginger Flaxseed Dressing*; 170g (5½oz) blueberries*

Supplements: *Sinatra Foundation Programme plus added fish oil, flaxseed,*
        L-arginine, and grapeseed extract
Exercise: *Strength training*
Mind/Body: *Anger management exercises*

DAILY PLAN: WEEK 6

Day 1
Breakfast: *120ml (4fl oz) cup fat-free plain yogurt, 2 tsp. chopped nuts, 1 Tbsp.*
        ground flaxseed; 90g (3oz) fresh berries; 1 Dried Fruit Spelt Muffin*;
        1 cup coffee or tea
Lunch: *90g (3oz) canned salmon; shredded raw vegetable salad of courgettes,*
        red peppers, and celery with 2 Tbsp. Flaxseed Dressing*; 125g (4½oz)
        raspberries
Dinner: *1 serving Spelt Pasta with Tomatoes, Basil, and Shiitake or Maitake*
        Mushrooms*; 1 serving of Dr. Sinatra's Favorite Shiitake Recipe*; large
        bowl tossed green salad with Ginger Flaxseed Dressing*
Supplements: *Sinatra Foundation Programme plus the following:*
        • *2g fish oil*
        • *2 Tbsp. crushed flaxseed (preferred) or 1 Tbsp. flaxseed oil*
        • *2g L-arginine*
        • *150–300mg grapeseed extract*
        • *500–1,000mg organic garlic capsules*
        • *10–15 drops Maitake D-Fraction Liquid three times daily (optional)*
Exercise: *20–30-minute walk and strength training*
Mind/Body: *Yogic breathing exercises*

Day 2
Breakfast: *50g (1¾oz) spelt (or wholegrain) cereal with 2 Tbsp. chopped figs and*
        120ml (4fl oz) plain soya or skimmed milk; 240ml (8fl oz) calcium-
        fortified orange juice; 1 cup coffee or tea
Lunch: *Soya burger on spelt (or wholemeal) toast with lettuce and tomato and*
        2 tsp. light mayonnaise; 1 apple
Dinner: *1 serving Turkey Meatloaf*; 1 serving Three-Bean Salad*;*
        120g (4oz) steamed broccoli; 1 piece Carrot Cake*
Supplements: *Sinatra Foundation Programme plus added fish oil, flaxseed,*
        L-arginine, grapeseed extract, and garlic
Exercise: *20–30-minute walk and strength training*
Mind/Body: *Yoga meditation exercises*

Day 3
Breakfast: *Fruit Smoothie*; 180g (6oz) strawberries*
Lunch: *1 serving Salmon Salad*; 170g (5½oz) watermelon*
Snack: *1 Carob Nut Brownie**
Dinner: *1 serving Grilled Tofu*; 1 serving Steamed Vegetables*;*
        75g (2½oz) brown rice; 150g (5oz) blueberries

Supplements: *Sinatra Foundation Programme plus added fish oil, flaxseed, L-arginine, grapeseed extract, and garlic*
Exercise: *Yoga asanas*
Mind/Body: *Yogic breathing exercises*

Day 4

Breakfast: *Tomato and asparagus omelette made with 2 eggs, 2 Tbsp. skimmed milk, ½ medium tomato, and 50g (1¾oz) asparagus; ¼ melon; 240ml (8fl oz) calcium-fortified orange juice; 1 cup coffee or tea*

Lunch: *1 serving Stir-Fried Tofu with Vegetables* and 25g (¾oz) fresh shiitake mushrooms; 180g (6oz) strawberries*

Dinner: *1 serving Roast Salmon*; 150g (5oz) steamed asparagus; 1 serving Lentils and Red Pepper Salad**

Supplements: *Sinatra Foundation Programme plus added fish oil, flaxseed, L-arginine, grapeseed extract, and garlic*

Exercise: *20–30-minute walk*

Mind/Body: *Yoga meditation exercises*

Day 5

Breakfast: *1 slice spelt (or wholemeal) toast with 1 tsp. light margarine; 1 scrambled egg; 180g (6oz) strawberries; 240ml (8fl oz) calcium-fortified juice; 1 cup coffee or tea*

Lunch: *120g (4oz) turkey burger on 2 slices spelt (or wholemeal) bread with lettuce, tomato, and 2 tsp. light mayonnaise; large bowl tossed salad with Ginger Flaxseed Dressing*; ¼ melon*

Dinner: *1 serving Grilled Prawns*; 1 serving Spelt Pilaf with Shiitake or Maitake Mushrooms*; ½ medium avocado and 1 medium tomato, sliced and seasoned with lemon juice*

Supplements: *Sinatra Foundation Programme plus added fish oil, flaxseed, L-arginine, grapeseed extract, and garlic*

Exercise: *Yoga asanas*

Mind/Body: *Yogic breathing exercises*

Day 6

Breakfast: *Fruit smoothie; ½ medium grapefruit*

Lunch: *1 serving Minestrone Soup*; large bowl tossed salad with 2 Tbsp. Flaxseed Dressing*; 1 apple*

Dinner: *1 serving Chicken and Red Pepper Kebab*; 1 serving Lentils and Courgettes Sauté*; 90g (3oz) fresh spinach with Ginger Flaxseed Dressing*; 125g (4½oz) raspberries*

Supplements: *Sinatra Foundation Programme plus added fish oil, flaxseed, L-arginine, grapeseed extract, and garlic*

Exercise: *20–30-minute walk and strength training*

Mind/Body: *Yoga meditation*

Day 7

Breakfast: *225g (8oz) cooked oatmeal with 2 tsp. walnuts and 1 tsp. honey; 120ml (4fl oz) plain soya or skimmed milk; 240ml (8fl oz) calcium-fortified orange juice; 1 cup coffee or tea*

Lunch: *½ 180g (6oz) can low-sodium tuna seasoned with 1 Tbsp. light mayonnaise on bed of lettuce, tomatoes, and cucumbers; 1 piece spelt (or wholemeal) bread with 1 tsp. light margarine; ¼ melon*

Dinner: *1 serving Tempeh Chilli*; 75g (2½oz) cooked brown rice; large bowl tossed salad with 2 Tbsp. Flaxseed Dressing*; 175g (5¾oz) frozen grapes*

Supplements: *Sinatra Foundation Programme plus added fish oil, flaxseed, L-arginine, grapeseed extract, and garlic*

Exercise: *Yoga asanas*

Mind/Body: *Yogic breathing exercises*

DAILY PLAN: WEEK 7

Day 1

Breakfast: *225g (8oz) cooked oatmeal with 2 tsp. wheat germ drizzled with 1 tsp. honey; 120ml (4fl oz) skimmed or plain soya milk; 175g (5¾oz) melon cubes; 1 cup green tea*

Lunch: *1 serving Vegetable Soup*; large bowl tossed salad with 60g (2oz) cooked chicken breast and 1 medium diced tomato, seasoned with garlic, 2 tsp. olive oil, and lemon juice*

Snack: *1 Peanut Butter Biscuit*; 240ml (8fl oz) soya milk*

Dinner: *1 serving Poached Salmon with Dill Sauce*; 120g (4oz) steamed spinach; 175g (5¾oz) frozen grapes*

Supplements: *Sinatra Foundation Programme plus the following:*
- *2g fish oil*
- *2 Tbsp. crushed flaxseed (preferred) or 1 Tbsp. flaxseed oil*
- *2g L-arginine*
- *150–300mg grapeseed extract*
- *500–1,000mg organic garlic capsules*
- *500mg hawthorn two or three times daily*
- *10–15 drops Maitake D-Fraction Liquid three times daily (optional)*

Exercise: *Upper-body workout*

Mind/Body: *Biofeedback exercises, qigong, or yoga*

Day 2

Breakfast: *1 serving Blueberry Buckwheat Pancakes with Wheat Germ*; 1 cup coffee or green tea*

Lunch: *1 serving Stir-Fried Tofu and Vegetables*; 1 apple*

Dinner: *1 serving Spelt (or wholemeal) Pasta with Asparagus and Tomatoes*; large bowl tossed salad with Ginger Flaxseed Dressing*; ¼ melon*

Supplements: *Sinatra Foundation Programme plus added fish oil, flaxseed, L-arginine, grapeseed extract, garlic, and hawthorn*

Exercise: *20–30-minute walk*
Mind/Body: *Biofeedback exercises, qigong, or yoga*

Day 3

Breakfast: *Tomato omelette made with 2 eggs, 2 Tbsp. skimmed milk, and
½ medium tomato; 1 slice spelt (or wholemeal) toast with 1 tsp. light
margarine; 240ml (8fl oz) calcium-fortified orange juice; 1 cup coffee or
green tea*

Lunch: *1 serving Grilled Chicken Teriyaki*; 1 serving Stir-Fry Mangetout and
Sesame Seeds*; 90g (3oz) pineapple*

Snack: *1 frozen banana*

Dinner: *1 serving Sandy's Crab Cakes*; 1 serving Lentils with Garlic and
Tomatoes*; 180g (6oz) strawberries with 120ml (4fl oz) fat-free plain
yogurt and 1 tsp. honey*

Supplements: *Sinatra Foundation Programme plus added fish oil, flaxseed,
L-arginine, grapeseed extract, garlic, and hawthorn*

Exercise: *Upper-body exercises*

Mind/Body: *Biofeedback exercises, qigong, or yoga*

Day 4

Breakfast: *1 Blueberry or Apple-Cinnamon Bran Muffin*; 120g (4oz) low-
sodium low-fat cottage cheese; 175g (5½oz) melon; 240ml (8fl oz)
calcium-fortified orange juice; 1 cup coffee or green tea*

Lunch: *1 serving Tofu, Tomato, and Black Olive Salad*; 75g (2½oz) brown
rice; 75g (2½oz) grapes*

Dinner: *120g (4oz) grilled chicken breast; 1 serving Roast Vegetables*;
1 serving Black Bean Salad*; 1 baked apple*

Supplements: *Sinatra Foundation Programme plus added fish oil, flaxseed,
L-arginine, grapeseed extract, garlic, and hawthorn*

Exercise: *20–30-minute walk*

Mind/Body: *Biofeedback exercises, qigong, or yoga*

Day 5

Breakfast: *Fruit Smoothie*; ½ grapefruit*

Lunch: *2 slices soya cheese in a wholemeal pitta with 25g (¾oz) fresh
maitake/shiitake mushrooms; large bowl tossed salad with
1 medium tomato and ½ small jar marinated artichoke hearts;
1 apple*

Dinner: *1 serving Tempeh Chilli*; large bowl tossed salad with ½ medium
chopped avocado and 25g (¾oz) chopped red onion and seasoned with
lemon juice; 90g (3oz) fresh pineapple*

Supplements: *Sinatra Foundation Programme plus added fish oil, flaxseed,
L-arginine, grapeseed extract, garlic, and hawthorn*

Exercise: *Upper-body exercise*

Mind/Body: *Biofeedback exercises, qigong, or yoga*

Day 6

Breakfast: 1 hard-boiled egg; 1 slice spelt (or wholemeal) toast with 1 tsp. light margarine; 175g (5¼oz) melon cubes; 1 cup coffee or green tea
Lunch: 1 serving Lentil Soup*; large bowl tossed salad with 2 Tbsp. Flaxseed Dressing*; 1 baked apple
Dinner: 1 serving Grilled Mediterranean Halibut*; asparagus, tomato, and red onion salad with Ginger Flaxseed Dressing*; 1 serving Haricot Beans, Garlic, and Rosemary Salad*; 180g (6oz) strawberries
Supplements: Sinatra Foundation Programme plus added fish oil, flaxseed, L-arginine, grapeseed extract, garlic, and hawthorn
Exercise: 20–30-minute walk
Mind/Body: Biofeedback exercises, qigong, or yoga

Day 7

Breakfast: 1 cup low-sodium low-fat cottage cheese mixed with 175g (5¼oz) melon cubes and ½ banana and topped with 1 Tbsp. ground flaxseed; 1 cup coffee or green tea
Lunch: 1 serving Salad Niçoise, Sinatra Style*; 240ml (8fl oz) calcium-fortified orange juice; 1 piece spelt (or wholemeal) bread with 1 tsp. light margarine; 1 apple
Dinner: 1 serving Wholemeal Pasta with Broccoli and Feta*; 180g (6oz) pineapple
Supplements: Sinatra Foundation Programme plus added fish oil, flaxseed, L-arginine, grapeseed extract, garlic, and hawthorn
Exercise: Upper-body workout
Mind/Body: Biofeedback exercises, qigong, or yoga

DAILY PLAN: WEEK 8

Day 1

Breakfast: 225g (8oz) cooked oatmeal enriched with 1 Tbsp. soya powder and 1 Tbsp. ground flaxseed and drizzled with 1 tsp. honey; 240ml (8fl oz) calcium-fortified orange juice; 1 cup coffee or green tea
Lunch: 1 serving Veggie Miso Soup*; 1 serving Steamed Vegetables*; 1 apple
Snack: 1 Peanut Butter Biscuit*; 240ml (8fl oz) plain soya or skimmed milk
Dinner: 1 serving Roast Salmon*; large bowl tossed salad with Ginger Flaxseed Dressing*; 1 medium baked potato with 2 Tbsp. fat-free plain yogurt; 180g (6oz) pineapple
Supplements: Sinatra Foundation Programme plus the following:
- 2g fish oil
- 2 Tbsp. crushed flaxseed (preferred) or 1 Tbsp. flaxseed oil
- 2g L-arginine
- 150–300mg grapeseed extract
- 500–1,000mg organic garlic capsules
- 500mg hawthorn two or three times daily

- 10–15 drops Maitake D-Fraction Liquid three times daily (optional)
- DHEA supplement (optional)

Exercise: Lower-body exercises
Mind/Body: Music therapy

Day 2
Breakfast: 1 Blueberry or Apple-Cinnamon Bran Muffin*; 120g (4oz) low-sodium low-fat cottage cheese; ¼ melon; 240ml (8fl oz) calcium-fortified orange juice; 1 cup coffee or green tea
Lunch: 1 serving Antiguan Black Bean Soup*; 50g (1¾oz) grilled maitake/shiitake mushrooms with ½ medium avocado, diced and topped with 2 Tbsp. Flaxseed Dressing*
Dinner: 1 serving Roast Pork Tenderloin with Rosemary and Garlic*; 1 serving Roast Vegetables; 1 baked apple
Supplements: Sinatra Foundation Programme plus added fish oil, flaxseed, L-arginine, grapeseed extract, garlic, and hawthorn
Exercise: 20–30-minute walk
Mind/Body: Music therapy

Day 3
Breakfast: 240ml (8fl oz) fat-free plain yogurt mixed with 1 tsp. honey, 180g (6oz) fresh strawberries, and 1 Tbsp. wheat germ; 1 cup coffee or green tea
Lunch: 1 serving Salmon Salad* with sliced cucumbers and tomatoes; 1 slice spelt (or wholemeal) bread with 1 tsp. light margarine
Dinner: 1 serving Stir-Fried Tempeh and Maitake/Shiitake Mushrooms and Mangetout*; 170g (5½oz) red grapes
Supplements: Sinatra Foundation Programme plus added fish oil, flaxseed, L-arginine, grapeseed extract, garlic, and hawthorn
Exercise: Lower-body exercises
Mind/Body: Music therapy

Day 4
Breakfast: 2 Tbsp. feta cheese and 25g (¾oz) chopped figs on 2 slices spelt (or wholemeal) toast; 240ml (8fl oz) calcium-fortified orange juice; 1 cup coffee or green tea
Lunch: Soya burger on a wholemeal roll with lettuce, tomato, and 2 tsp. light mayonnaise; 1 serving Veggie Coleslaw*; 1 apple
Dinner: 1 serving of Chinese Chicken Salad*; ¼ melon
Supplements: Sinatra Foundation Programme plus added fish oil, flaxseed, L-arginine, grapeseed extract, garlic, and hawthorn
Exercise: 20–30-minute walk
Mind/Body: Music therapy

Day 5

Breakfast: 2 slices wholemeal French toast made with 1 egg, 2 Tbsp. skimmed milk, and cinnamon, topped with 60g (2oz) stewed apple; 240ml (8fl oz) calcium-fortified orange juice; 1 cup coffee or green tea

Lunch: 1 serving Chicken Vegetable Soup*; large bowl tossed salad with Ginger Flaxseed Dressing*; 1 apple

Dinner: 120g (4oz) tenderloin of beef; 1 serving Grilled Courgettes*; 1 serving Spinach and Tomato Salad*; 1 frozen banana

Supplements: Sinatra Foundation Programme plus added fish oil, flaxseed, L-arginine, grapeseed extract, garlic, and hawthorn

Exercise: Lower-body exercises

Mind/Body: Music therapy

Day 6

Breakfast: 50g (1¾oz) cold wholemeal cereal; 2 Tbsp. raisins; 120ml (4fl oz) plain soya or skimmed milk; 240ml (8fl oz) calcium-fortified orange juice; 1 cup coffee or green tea

Lunch: 1 serving Pasta à la Sinatra*; 1 apple

Dinner: 1 serving Grilled Prawns*; large bowl tossed salad with crushed dried nori seaweed and 2 Tbsp. Flaxseed Dressing*

Supplements: Sinatra Foundation Programme plus added fish oil, flaxseed, L-arginine, grapeseed extract, garlic, and hawthorn

Exercise: 20–30-minute walk

Mind/Body: Music therapy

Day 7

Breakfast: Fruit Smoothie*; ½ grapefruit

Lunch: 65g (2oz) Hummus* with black olives, diced red onions, lettuce, and tomato in a wholemeal pitta; 1 apple

Dinner: 1 serving Chicken Breasts Stuffed with Spinach*; 1 medium baked potato with 2 Tbsp. fat-free plain yogurt; large bowl tossed salad with 1 Tbsp. sunflower seeds, grated red cabbage, and 2 Tbsp. Flaxseed Dressing*

Supplements: Sinatra Foundation Programme plus added fish oil, flaxseed, L-arginine, grapeseed extract, garlic, and hawthorn

Exercise: Lower-body exercises

Mind/Body: Music therapy

1,800-Calorie Meal Plan (Men)

WEEK ONE

Day One
Calories: 1,770
Calories from Fat: 430
Total Fat: 48g
Saturated Fat: 9g
Cholesterol: 375mg
Sodium: 1,440mg
Total Carbohydrate: 252g
Dietary Fibre: 33g
Sugars: 104g
Protein: 95g
% of Calories from Carbohydrate/Protein/Fat: 55/21/23

WEEK ONE

Day Two
Calories: 1,790
Calories from Fat: 700
Total Fat: 78g
Saturated Fat: 12g
Cholesterol: 105mg
Sodium: 1,140mg
Total Carbohydrate: 217g
Dietary Fibre: 37g
Sugars: 66g
Protein: 79g
% of Calories from Carbohydrate/Protein/Fat: 46/17/37

WEEK ONE

Day Three
Calories: 1,810
Calories from Fat: 520
Total Fat: 58g
Saturated Fat: 9g
Cholesterol: 120mg
Sodium: 770mg
Total Carbohydrate: 261g
Dietary Fibre: 45g
Sugars: 111g
Protein: 83g
% of Calories from Carbohydrate/Protein/Fat: 55/18/27

WEEK ONE

Day Four
Calories: 1,810
Calories from Fat: 580
Total Fat: 65g
Sodium: 1,080mg
Total Carbohydrate: 233g
Dietary Fibre: 52g

Saturated Fat: 11g   Sugars: 88g
Cholesterol: 520mg   Protein: 95g
% of Calories from Carbohydrate/Protein/Fat: 49/20/31

WEEK ONE

Day Five
Calories: 1,810   Sodium: 1,160mg
Calories from Fat: 500   Total Carbohydrate: 261g
Total Fat: 56g   Dietary Fibre: 41g
Saturated Fat: 8g   Sugars: 122g
Cholesterol: 150mg   Protein: 90g
% of Calories from Carbohydrate/Protein/Fat: 55/19/26

WEEK ONE

Day Six
Calories: 1,810   Sodium: 1,310mg
Calories from Fat: 590   Total Carbohydrate: 231g
Total Fat: 65g   Dietary Fibre: 29g
Saturated Fat: 11g   Sugars: 113g
Cholesterol: 585mg   Protein: 92g
% of Calories from Carbohydrate/Protein/Fat: 49/19/31

WEEK ONE

Day Seven
Calories: 1,790   Sodium: 1,210mg
Calories from Fat: 450   Total Carbohydrate: 262g
Total Fat: 50g   Dietary Fibre: 49g
Saturated Fat: 9g   Sugars: 110g
Cholesterol: 325mg   Protein: 93g
% of Calories from Carbohydrate/Protein/Fat: 56/20/24

WEEK TWO

Day One
Calories: 1,810   Sodium: 1,650mg
Calories from Fat: 510   Total Carbohydrate: 259g
Total Fat: 56g   Dietary Fibre: 30g
Saturated Fat: 8g   Sugars: 106g
Cholesterol: 140mg   Protein: 92g
% of Calories from Carbohydrate/Protein/Fat: 54/19/26

WEEK TWO

Day Two

Calories: 1,830	Sodium: 1,460mg
Calories from Fat: 550	Total Carbohydrate: 267g
Total Fat: 61g	Dietary Fibre: 30g
Saturated Fat: 9g	Sugars: 102g
Cholesterol: 5mg	Protein: 69g

% of Calories from Carbohydrate/Protein/Fat: 56/15/29

WEEK TWO

Day Three

Calories: 1,800	Sodium: 1,150mg
Calories from Fat: 620	Total Carbohydrate: 241g
Total Fat: 68g	Dietary Fibre: 44g
Saturated Fat: 9g	Sugars: 111g
Cholesterol: 95mg	Protein: 81g

% of Calories from Carbohydrate/Protein/Fat: 57/17/32

WEEK TWO

Day Four

Calories: 1,790	Sodium: 940mg
Calories from Fat: 420	Total Carbohydrate: 248g
Total Fat: 47g	Dietary Fibre: 47g
Saturated Fat: 8g	Sugars: 110g
Cholesterol: 150mg	Protein: 116g

% of Calories from Carbohydrate/Protein/Fat: 53/25/23

WEEK TWO

Day Five

Calories: 1,800	Sodium: 1,490mg
Calories from Fat: 540	Total Carbohydrate: 234g
Total Fat: 60g	Dietary Fibre: 40g
Saturated Fat: 11g	Sugars: 86g
Cholesterol: 670mg	Protein: 95g

% of Calories from Carbohydrate/Protein/Fat: 51/20/29

WEEK TWO

Day Six

Calories: 1,780	Sodium: 1,270mg
Calories from Fat: 590	Total Carbohydrate: 218g

Total Fat: 65g   Dietary Fibre: 32g
Saturated Fat: 12g   Sugars: 102g
Cholesterol: 370mg   Protein: 98g
% of Calories from Carbohydrate/Protein/Fat: 47/21/32

WEEK TWO

Day Seven
Calories: 1,810   Sodium: 1,870mg
Calories from Fat: 320   Total Carbohydrate: 314g
Total Fat: 36g   Dietary Fibre: 42g
Saturated Fat: 6g   Sugars: 166g
Cholesterol: 55mg   Protein: 82g
% of Calories from Carbohydrate/Protein/Fat: 65/17/17

WEEK THREE

Day One
Calories: 1,820   Sodium: 870mg
Calories from Fat: 610   Total Carbohydrate: 255g
Total Fat: 68g   Dietary Fibre: 49g
Saturated Fat: 9g   Sugars: 110g
Cholesterol: 80mg   Protein: 71g
% of Calories from Carbohydrate/Protein/Fat: 53/15/32

WEEK THREE

Day Two
Calories: 1,800   Sodium: 1,190mg
Calories from Fat: 530   Total Carbohydrate: 241g
Total Fat: 59g   Dietary Fibre: 42g
Saturated Fat: 8g   Sugars: 107g
Cholesterol: 205mg   Protein: 101g
% of Calories from Carbohydrate/Protein/Fat: 51/21/28

WEEK THREE

Day Three
Calories: 1,810   Sodium: 1,380mg
Calories from Fat: 540   Total Carbohydrate: 261g
Total Fat: 60g   Dietary Fibre: 42g
Saturated Fat: 10g   Sugars: 113g
Cholesterol: 515mg   Protein: 84g
% of Calories from Carbohydrate/Protein/Fat: 55/17/28

WEEK THREE

Day Four

Calories: 1,830
Calories from Fat: 350
Total Fat: 39g
Saturated Fat: 8g
Cholesterol: 435mg

Sodium: 1,120mg
Total Carbohydrate: 287g
Dietary Fibre: 45g
Sugars: 149g
Protein: 105g

% of Calories from Carbohydrate/Protein/Fat: 60/22/18

WEEK THREE

Day Five

Calories: 1,770
Calories from Fat: 460
Total Fat: 51g
Saturated Fat: 8g
Cholesterol: 85mg

Sodium: 870mg
Total Carbohydrate: 244g
Dietary Fibre: 44g
Sugars: 122g
Protein: 99g

% of Calories from Carbohydrate/Protein/Fat: 53/22/25

WEEK THREE

Day Six

Calories: 1,820
Calories from Fat: 530
Total Fat: 59g
Saturated Fat: 11g
Cholesterol: 525mg

Sodium: 1,670mg
Total Carbohydrate: 245g
Dietary Fibre: 41g
Sugars: 96g
Protein: 99g

% of Calories from Carbohydrate/Protein/Fat: 51/21/28

WEEK THREE

Day Seven

Calories: 1,820
Calories from Fat: 410
Total Fat: 45g
Saturated Fat: 9g
Cholesterol: 65mg

Sodium: 1,190mg
Total Carbohydrate: 275g
Dietary Fibre: 49g
Sugars: 92g
Protein: 94g

% of Calories from Carbohydrate/Protein/Fat: 58/20/22

WEEK FOUR

Day One

Calories: 1,800
Calories from Fat: 480

Sodium: 900mg
Total Carbohydrate: 277g

Total Fat: 53g   Dietary Fibre: 38g
Saturated Fat: 8g   Sugars: 132g
Cholesterol: 95mg   Protein: 80g
% of Calories from Carbohydrate/Protein/Fat: 58/17/25

WEEK FOUR

Day Two
Calories: 1,800   Sodium: 1,230mg
Calories from Fat: 580   Total Carbohydrate: 238g
Total Fat: 64g   Dietary Fibre: 31g
Saturated Fat: 11g   Sugars: 126g
Cholesterol: 95mg   Protein: 84g
% of Calories from Carbohydrate/Protein/Fat: 51/18/31

WEEK FOUR

Day Three
Calories: 1,780   Sodium: 1,480mg
Calories from Fat: 610   Total Carbohydrate: 207g
Total Fat: 68g   Dietary Fibre: 44g
Saturated Fat: 15g   Sugars: 89g
Cholesterol: 550mg   Protein: 102g
% of Calories from Carbohydrate/Protein/Fat: 45/22/23

WEEK FOUR

Day Four
Calories: 1,810   Sodium: 1,090mg
Calories from Fat: 530   Total Carbohydrate: 232g
Total Fat: 59g   Dietary Fibre: 54g
Saturated Fat: 10g   Sugars: 83g
Cholesterol: 170mg   Protein: 110g
% of Calories from Carbohydrate/Protein/Fat: 49/23/28

WEEK FOUR

Day Five
Calories: 1,800   Sodium: 1,220mg
Calories from Fat: 570   Total Carbohydrate: 247g
Total Fat: 64g   Dietary Fibre: 35g
Saturated Fat: 10g   Sugars: 118g
Cholesterol: 325mg   Protein: 81g
% of Calories from Carbohydrate/Protein/Fat: 52/17/30

WEEK FOUR

Day Six

Calories: 1,780
Calories from Fat: 520
Total Fat: 58g
Saturated Fat: 10g
Cholesterol: 670mg

Sodium: 730mg
Total Carbohydrate: 235g
Dietary Fibre: 39g
Sugars: 94g
Protein: 93g

% of Calories from Carbohydrate/Protein/Fat: 51/20/28

WEEK FOUR

Day Seven

Calories: 1,780
Calories from Fat: 460
Total Fat: 51g
Saturated Fat: 12g
Cholesterol: 110mg

Sodium: 1,520mg
Total Carbohydrate: 264g
Dietary Fibre: 38g
Sugars: 118g
Protein: 88g

% of Calories from Carbohydrate/Protein/Fat: 57/19/24

WEEK FIVE

Day One

Calories: 1,790
Calories from Fat: 410
Total Fat: 46g
Saturated Fat: 8g
Cholesterol: 110mg

Sodium: 1,240mg
Total Carbohydrate: 267g
Dietary Fibre: 29g
Sugars: 127g
Protein: 100g

% of Calories from Carbohydrate/Protein/Fat: 57/21/22

WEEK FIVE

Day Two

Calories: 1,740
Calories from Fat: 580
Total Fat: 65g
Saturated Fat: 12g
Cholesterol: 495mg

Sodium: 1,920mg
Total Carbohydrate: 223g
Dietary Fibre: 43g
Sugars: 95g
Protein: 92g

% of Calories from Carbohydrate/Protein/Fat: 48/20/31

WEEK FIVE

Day Three

Calories: 1,770
Calories from Fat: 550

Sodium: 800mg
Total Carbohydrate: 251g

Total Fat: 61g   Dietary Fibre: 36g
Saturated Fat: 9g   Sugars: 113g
Cholesterol: 70mg   Protein: 71g
% of Calories from Carbohydrate/Protein/Fat: 54/16/30

WEEK FIVE

Day Four
Calories: 1,800   Sodium: 1,400mg
Calories from Fat: 480   Total Carbohydrate: 268g
Total Fat: 53g   Dietary Fibre: 62g
Saturated Fat: 9g   Sugars: 96g
Cholesterol: 75mg   Protein: 86g
% of Calories from Carbohydrate/Protein/Fat: 57/18/25

WEEK FIVE

Day Five
Calories: 1,810   Sodium: 1,380mg
Calories from Fat: 550   Total Carbohydrate: 238g
Total Fat: 61g   Dietary Fibre: 58g
Saturated Fat: 11g   Sugars: 87g
Cholesterol: 280mg   Protein: 98g
% of Calories from Carbohydrate/Protein/Fat: 50/21/29

WEEK FIVE

Day Six
Calories: 1,860   Sodium: 990mg
Calories from Fat: 550   Total Carbohydrate: 239g
Total Fat: 61g   Dietary Fibre: 33g
Saturated Fat: 11g   Sugars: 117g
Cholesterol: 315mg   Protein: 105g
% of Calories from Carbohydrate/Protein/Fat: 50/22/28

WEEK FIVE

Day Seven
Calories: 1,780   Sodium: 1,710mg
Calories from Fat: 540   Total Carbohydrate: 268g
Total Fat: 60g   Dietary Fibre: 41g
Saturated Fat: 8g   Sugars: 130g
Cholesterol: 115mg   Protein: 75g
% of Calories from Carbohydrate/Protein/Fat: 56/16/28

WEEK SIX

Day One

Calories: 1,800
Calories from Fat: 590
Total Fat: 66g
Saturated Fat: 10g
Cholesterol: 290mg

Sodium: 1,120mg
Total Carbohydrate: 245g
Dietary Fibre: 46g
Sugars: 89g
Protein: 77g

% of Calories from Carbohydrate/Protein/Fat: 52/16/32

WEEK SIX

Day Two

Calories: 1,730
Calories from Fat: 350
Total Fat: 38g
Saturated Fat: 6g
Cholesterol: 125mg

Sodium: 1,420mg
Total Carbohydrate: 285g
Dietary Fibre: 47g
Sugars: 116g
Protein: 86g

% of Calories from Carbohydrate/Protein/Fat: 62/19/19

WEEK SIX

Day Three

Calories: 1,800
Calories from Fat: 510
Total Fat: 56g
Saturated Fat: 8g
Cholesterol: 130mg

Sodium: 1,360mg
Total Carbohydrate: 273g
Dietary Fibre: 33g
Sugars: 122g
Protein: 75g

% of Calories from Carbohydrate/Protein/Fat: 57/16/27

WEEK SIX

Day Four

Calories: 1,790
Calories from Fat: 540
Total Fat: 60g
Saturated Fat: 11g
Cholesterol: 490mg

Sodium: 1,350mg
Total Carbohydrate: 240g
Dietary Fibre: 39g
Sugars: 102g
Protein: 92g

% of Calories from Carbohydrate/Protein/Fat: 51/20/29

WEEK SIX

Day Five

Calories: 1,820
Calories from Fat: 500

Sodium: 1,290mg
Total Carbohydrate: 247g

Total Fat: 55g   Dietary Fibre: 45g
Saturated Fat: 11g   Sugars: 64g
Cholesterol: 575mg   Protein: 104g
% of Calories from Carbohydrate/Protein/Fat: 52/22/26

WEEK SIX

Day Six
Calories: 1,750   Sodium: 760mg
Calories from Fat: 510   Total Carbohydrate: 256g
Total Fat: 57g   Dietary Fibre: 60g
Saturated Fat: 8g   Sugars: 119g
Cholesterol: 110mg   Protein: 79g
% of Calories from Carbohydrate/Protein/Fat: 55/17/28

WEEK SIX

Day Seven
Calories: 1,740   Sodium: 750mg
Calories from Fat: 450   Total Carbohydrate: 266g
Total Fat: 50g   Dietary Fibre: 37g
Saturated Fat: 7g   Sugars: 130g
Cholesterol: 65mg   Protein: 76g
% of Calories from Carbohydrate/Protein/Fat: 59/17/25

WEEK SEVEN

Day One
Calories: 1,810   Sodium: 990mg
Calories from Fat: 460   Total Carbohydrate: 270g
Total Fat: 51g   Dietary Fibre: 32g
Saturated Fat: 9g   Sugars: 134g
Cholesterol: 135mg   Protein: 89g
% of Calories from Carbohydrate/Protein/Fat: 57/19/24

WEEK SEVEN

Day Two
Calories: 1,750   Sodium: 1,090mg
Calories from Fat: 390   Total Carbohydrate: 282g
Total Fat: 43g   Dietary Fibre: 31g
Saturated Fat: 9g   Sugars: 134g
Cholesterol: 125mg   Protein: 83g
% of Calories from Carbohydrate/Protein/Fat: 61/18/21

WEEK SEVEN

Day Three

Calories: 1,720
Calories from Fat: 360
Total Fat: 40g
Saturated Fat: 8g
Cholesterol: 660mg

Sodium: 1,550mg
Total Carbohydrate: 248g
Dietary Fibre: 38g
Sugars: 119g
Protein: 103g

% of Calories from Carbohydrate/Protein/Fat: 56/23/20

WEEK SEVEN

Day Four

Calories: 1,780
Calories from Fat: 440
Total Fat: 48g
Saturated Fat: 9g
Cholesterol: 140mg

Sodium: 420mg
Total Carbohydrate: 246g
Dietary Fibre: 36g
Sugars: 135g
Protein: 106g

% of Calories from Carbohydrate/Protein/Fat: 53/23/24

WEEK SEVEN

Day Five

Calories: 1,760
Calories from Fat: 390
Total Fat: 43g
Saturated Fat: 5g
Cholesterol: 85mg

Sodium: 1,070mg
Total Carbohydrate: 301g
Dietary Fibre: 59g
Sugars: 130g
Protein: 81g

% of Calories from Carbohydrate/Protein/Fat: 63/17/20

WEEK SEVEN

Day Six

Calories: 1,770
Calories from Fat: 540
Total Fat: 61g
Saturated Fat: 10g
Cholesterol: 475mg

Sodium: 940mg
Total Carbohydrate: 223g
Dietary Fibre: 45g
Sugars: 97g
Protein: 95g

% of Calories from Carbohydrate/Protein/Fat: 49/21/30

WEEK SEVEN

Day Seven

Calories: 1,770
Calories from Fat: 440

Sodium: 850mg
Total Carbohydrate: 264g

Total Fat: 49g   Dietary Fibre: 38g
Saturated Fat: 10g   Sugars: 128g
Cholesterol: 200mg   Protein: 90g
% of Calories from Carbohydrate/Protein/Fat: 57/19/24

WEEK EIGHT

Day One
Calories: 1,770   Sodium: 940mg
Calories from Fat: 400   Total Carbohydrate: 290g
Total Fat: 45g   Dietary Fibre: 39g
Saturated Fat: 6g   Sugars: 145g
Cholesterol: 120mg   Protein: 81g
% of Calories from Carbohydrate/Protein/Fat: 61/17/21

WEEK EIGHT

Day Two
Calories: 1,750   Sodium: 420mg
Calories from Fat: 550   Total Carbohydrate: 234g
Total Fat: 61g   Dietary Fibre: 37g
Saturated Fat: 12g   Sugars: 126g
Cholesterol: 105mg   Protein: 85g
% of Calories from Carbohydrate/Protein/Fat: 51/19/30

WEEK EIGHT

Day Three
Calories: 1,750   Sodium: 1,330mg
Calories from Fat: 400   Total Carbohydrate: 278g
Total Fat: 44g   Dietary Fibre: 32g
Saturated Fat: 8g   Sugars: 117g
Cholesterol: 90mg   Protein: 78g
% of Calories from Carbohydrate/Protein/Fat: 61/17/22

WEEK EIGHT

Day Four
Calories: 1,810   Sodium: 2,000mg
Calories from Fat: 490   Total Carbohydrate: 257g
Total Fat: 55g   Dietary Fibre: 47g
Saturated Fat: 11g   Sugars: 126g
Cholesterol: 115mg   Protein: 90g
% of Calories from Carbohydrate/Protein/Fat: 55/19/26

WEEK EIGHT

Day Five

Calories: 1,760

Calories from Fat: 690

Total Fat: 77g

Saturated Fat: 15g

Cholesterol: 405mg

Sodium: 1,190mg

Total Carbohydrate: 186g

Dietary Fibre: 32g

Sugars: 97g

Protein: 101g

% of Calories from Carbohydrate/Protein/Fat: 40/22/38

WEEK EIGHT

Day Six

Calories: 1,820

Calories from Fat: 460

Total Fat: 52g

Saturated Fat: 7g

Cholesterol: 280mg

Sodium: 1,170mg

Total Carbohydrate: 281g

Dietary Fibre: 52g

Sugars: 122g

Protein: 79g

% of Calories from Carbohydrate/Protein/Fat: 59/17/24

WEEK EIGHT

Day Seven

Calories: 1,770

Calories from Fat: 510

Total Fat: 57g

Saturated Fat: 8g

Cholesterol: 105mg

Sodium: 900mg

Total Carbohydrate: 270g

Dietary Fibre: 42g

Sugars: 122g

Protein: 66g

% of Calories from Carbohydrate/Protein/Fat: 58/14/27

1,800-CALORIE DAILY PLAN: WEEK 1

Day 1

Breakfast: *225ml (8fl oz) cooked oatmeal (not instant packages) with 1 Tbsp. raisins; 120ml (4fl oz) skimmed or plain soya milk; 1 hard-boiled egg; 1 cup tea or coffee*

Lunch: *60g (2oz) canned low-sodium or fresh cooked salmon in a wholemeal pitta with lettuce, tomato, and onion, seasoned with lemon juice and 2 tsp. olive oil; 1 apple*

Snack: *1 Apricot Oatmeal Bar*; 240ml (8fl oz) soya milk*

Dinner: *1 serving Steamed Mussels*; 125g (4½oz) steamed broccoli; 1 medium baked potato with 2 Tbsp. fat-free plain yogurt; ¼ melon*

Day 2

Breakfast: *2 slices wholemeal toast; 2 Tbsp. soya nut butter; ¼ melon; 1 cup coffee or tea*

Lunch: *1 serving Grilled Rosemary Chicken Breast*; large bowl tossed salad with 2 Tbsp. Flaxseed Dressing*; 180g (6oz) strawberries*

Dinner: *1 serving Wholemeal Pasta with Aubergine Tomato Sauce*; 1 serving Spinach and Tomato Salad*; 1 serving Carrot Cake*; 240ml (8fl oz) soya milk*

Day 3

Breakfast: *40g (1½oz) unsweetened shredded wheat, 2 tsp. walnuts, 3 Tbsp. raisins, 240ml (8fl oz) skimmed or soya milk; 1 cup coffee or tea*

Snack: *1 orange*

Lunch: *1 serving Vegetable Soup*; large bowl tossed salad with 2 Tbsp. Flaxseed Dressing*; 1 small wholemeal roll with 2 tsp. light margarine; 1 Apricot Oatmeal Bar**

Dinner: *1 serving Roast Pork Tenderloin with Rosemary and Garlic*; large bowl tossed salad with Ginger Flaxseed Dressing*; 1 serving Lentils with Garlic and Tomatoes*; 60g (2oz) raspberries with 120ml (4fl oz) fat-free plain yogurt and 2 tsp. honey*

Day 4

Breakfast: *2 scrambled eggs prepared with 2 Tbsp. skimmed milk; 2 slices wholemeal toast with 2 tsp. light margarine; ¼ melon; 1 cup coffee or tea*

Lunch: *1 serving Tempeh Chilli*; 3 wholemeal crackers; large bowl tossed salad with Ginger Flaxseed Dressing*; 1 apple*

Snack: *1 Apricot Oatmeal Bar**

Dinner: *1 serving Roast Salmon*; 1 serving Spinach with Pine Nuts and Garlic*; 1 serving Chickpea Salad with Rosemary*; 1 peach*

Day 5

Breakfast: *2 slices wholemeal toast with 2 Tbsp. unsalted natural peanut butter and 1 Tbsp. all-fruit preserves; 240ml (8fl oz) calcium-fortified orange juice; 1 cup coffee or tea*

Snack: *1 pear*

Lunch: *1 serving Chickpea and Chicory Soup*; 4 wholemeal crackers; 125g (4½oz) steamed broccoli; 180g (6oz) strawberries; 25g (¾oz) walnuts*

Snack: *1 banana*

Dinner: *150g (5oz) sliced roast turkey breast with rocket and 25g (¾oz) sun-dried oil-packed tomatoes (drained) stuffed in a wholemeal pitta; 1 piece Carrot Cake**

Day 6

Breakfast: *2-egg omelette made with 2 Tbsp. skimmed milk, 25g (¾oz) mushrooms, and 1 slice soya cheese; 2 pieces wholemeal toast with 2 tsp. light margarine; 240ml (8fl oz) calcium-fortified orange juice; 1 cup coffee or tea*

Lunch: *½ of a 180g (6oz) can low-sodium water-packed tuna, drained and seasoned with lemon juice; large bowl tossed salad with 2 Tbsp. Flaxseed Dressing*; 2 rye crisp crackers; 1 apple*

Snack: *1 banana*

Dinner: *1 serving Turkey Meatloaf*; 1 medium baked potato with 2 Tbsp. fat-free plain yogurt; 1 serving Grilled Courgettes*; large bowl tossed salad with Ginger Flaxseed Dressing*; 1 piece Carrot Cake**

Day 7

Breakfast: *2 slices wholemeal French toast made with 1 egg and 2 Tbsp. skimmed milk and seasoned with cinnamon; 60g (2oz) unsweetened stewed apples; 240ml (8fl oz) calcium-fortified orange juice; 1 cup coffee or tea*

Lunch: *1 serving Chicken Vegetable Soup*; 4 wholemeal crackers; 1 Apricot Oatmeal Bar**

Snack: *75g (2½oz) unsalted soya nuts and 6 dried apricots*

Dinner: *1 serving Pasta à la Sinatra*; large bowl tossed salad with 2 Tbsp. Ginger Flaxseed Dressing*; 1 small wholemeal roll with 1 tsp. margarine; 75g (2½oz) red grapes and 100g (3½oz) strawberries*

DAILY PLAN: WEEK 2

Day 1

Breakfast: *Fruit Smoothie**

Lunch: *1 serving Stir-Fried Tofu and Vegetables*; 1 orange*

Snack: *1 Carob Nut Brownie*; 240ml (8fl oz) plain soya milk*

Dinner: *1 serving Breaded Sole or Flounder*; 1 serving Spinach and Tomato Salad; 1 small baked sweet potato; 60g (2oz) blueberries with 120g (4oz) fat-free plain yogurt and 1 tsp. honey*

Supplements: *A good multivitamin/mineral supplement containing all the essential vitamins and minerals recommended with the suggested doses below. The supplements should contain natural carotenoids, flavonoids, vitamin E with gamma tocopherol, as well as some grapeseed, lutein, alpha lipoic acid, lycopene in combination with full vitamin B support, and minerals such as magnesium, selenium and chromium, to mention a few. Suggested doses for the Sinatra Foundation Programme include the following:*

- *10,000 units (6,000µg) of mixed carotenoids with beta carotene, or 2,500 units (750µg retinol)/(4,500µg) of vitamin A with 7,500 units of mixed carotenoids with beta carotene*

- Vitamin C in divided doses of 200–400mg/day
- Vitamin E 200–400 IU with some gamma tocopherol
- Magnesium 400–800 mg/day
- Calcium 250–1,000 mg/day
- CoQ10 15–30 mg 4 times daily
- L-carnitine fumarate 250–500mg 4 times daily

Each week we will build on this programme. Remember to take supplements with meals in divided dosages.

Day 2

Breakfast: 225g (8oz) cooked oatmeal enriched with 1 Tbsp. soya powder; 120ml (4fl oz) plain soya or skimmed milk; 240ml (8fl oz) calcium-fortified orange juice; 1 cup coffee or tea

Lunch: 1 serving Tofu, Tomato, and Black Olive Salad*; 1 small wholemeal roll with 1 tsp. light margarine; 1 apple

Snack: 4 wholemeal crackers with 2 Tbsp. unsalted natural peanut butter and 240ml (8fl oz) plain soya milk

Dinner: Tempeh and Stir-Fried Vegetables*; 90g (3oz) diced pineapple with 120g (4oz) fat-free plain yogurt and 1 tsp. honey

Supplements: Sinatra Foundation Programme

Day 3

Breakfast: ½ medium grapefruit; 2 slices soya cheese tucked into a wholemeal pitta and toasted in the grill/oven; 1 banana; 1 cup coffee or tea

Lunch: 1 serving Antiguan Black Bean Soup*; 4 wholemeal crackers; large salad tossed salad with 2 Tbsp. Ginger Flaxseed Dressing*; 175g (5¾oz) grapes

Snack: 75g (2½oz) baby carrots with 2 Tbsp. Hummus*

Dinner: 1 serving Grilled Rosemary Chicken Breast*; 1 serving Spinach with Pine Nuts and Garlic*; 1 medium tomato, sliced, and 4 black olives; 1 apple; 1 Peanut Butter Biscuit*

Supplements: Sinatra Foundation Programme

Day 4

Breakfast: 225g (8oz) low-sodium low-fat cottage cheese with 175g (5¾oz) melon cubes and 4 tsp. chopped walnuts; 1 banana; 1 cup coffee or tea

Lunch: 60g (2oz) sliced roast turkey breast on 2 slices wholemeal bread with lettuce, tomato, and 2 tsp. light soya-based mayonnaise; 1 serving Bean Salad*; 1 apple

Snack: 1 Peanut Butter Biscuit*; 240ml (8fl oz) plain soya or skimmed milk

Dinner: 1 serving Roast Pork Tenderloin with Mustard*; 1 small baked potato with 1 tsp. light margarine; 1 serving Grilled Courgettes*; 1 medium baked potato with 2 tsp. light margarine; 1 medium tomato, chopped and mixed with fresh basil; 180g (6oz) strawberries with 120ml (4fl oz) fat-free plain yogurt and 1 tsp. honey

Supplements: Sinatra Foundation Programme

Day 5

Breakfast: *2 poached eggs on 2 slices wholemeal toast; 180g (6oz) strawberries or organic blueberries; 240ml (8fl oz) calcium-fortified orange juice; 1 cup coffee or tea*

Lunch: *Soya burger on a wholemeal roll with sliced tomato and onion; 1 serving Pinto Bean Salad*; sliced tomatoes and onions; ¼ melon*

Snack: *1 stalk celery with 2 Tbsp. unsalted natural peanut butter*

Dinner: *1 serving Orange Prawns with Couscous*; 120g (4oz) steamed green beans; 1 Carob Nut Brownie**

Supplements: *Sinatra Foundation Programme*

Day 6

Breakfast: *50g (1½oz) cold wholemeal cereal; 120ml (4fl oz) skimmed or soya milk; ½ sliced banana; 240ml (8fl oz) calcium-fortified orange juice; 1 cup coffee or tea*

Lunch: *Chef salad with 30g (1oz) shredded soya cheese; 1 hard-boiled egg; 90g (3oz) turkey breast; green leaf lettuce, tomatoes, celery, and cucumbers with 2 Tbsp. Flaxseed Dressing*; 1 small wholemeal roll with 1 tsp. light margarine; 1 Peanut Butter Biscuit**

Snack: *1 apple*

Dinner: *1 serving Low-Fat Exceptional Hamburgers* on a wholemeal roll with lettuce, tomato, and 2 tsp. low-fat mayonnaise; 1 serving Veggie Coleslaw*; 80g (2¾oz) pinto beans; 100g (3½oz) fresh sweet cherries*

Supplements: *Sinatra Foundation Programme*

Day 7

Breakfast: *1 Blueberry Bran Muffin*; 225g (8oz) low-fat low-sodium cottage cheese with 175g (5¾oz) melon; 240ml (8fl oz) calcium-fortified orange juice; 1 cup coffee or tea*

Snack: *1 banana*

Lunch: *1 serving Veggie Miso Soup*; 2 rye crisp crackers; 80g (2¾oz) steamed kale; 75g (2½oz) cooked brown rice; 1 small pear*

Snack: *1 Carob Nut Brownie*; 240ml (8fl oz) plain soya or skim milk*

Dinner: *1 serving Tofu with Sesame Seeds*; 1 serving Fresh Tomato Salsa*; 1 serving Three-Bean Salad*; 75g (2½oz) red grapes and 175g (5¾oz) watermelon*

Supplements: *Sinatra Foundation Programme*

DAILY PLAN: WEEK 3

Day 1

Breakfast: *Fruit Smoothie*; ½ grapefruit*

Lunch: *1 serving Salmon Salad* with sliced tomatoes; 1 apple*

Snack: *2 Tbsp. Hummus* and 75g (2½oz) baby carrots*

Dinner: 1 serving Tempeh Chilli*; large bowl tossed salad with 2 Tbsp. Flaxseed
Dressing*; 1 small wholemeal roll with 2 tsp. light margarine; 75g
(2½oz) strawberries; 1 Peanut Butter Biscuit*
Supplements: Sinatra Foundation Programme plus the following:
  • 2g fish oil
  • 2 Tbsp. crushed flaxseed (preferred) or 1 Tbsp. flaxseed oil
Exercise: 20–30-minute walk

Day 2
Breakfast: 225ml (8fl oz) fat-free plain yogurt with 1 tsp. honey and 2 tsp.
chopped walnuts; 175g (5¾oz) melon; 1 Blueberry Bran Muffin*; 1
cup coffee or tea
Snack: 1 banana
Lunch: 1 serving Salad Niçoise, Sinatra Style*; 1 apple
Snack: 2 rye crisp crackers with 2 Tbsp. unsalted natural peanut butter
Dinner: 1 serving Scallop Kebab*; 1 serving Dr. Sinatra's Favourite Shiitake
Recipe*; 1 serving White Beans, Garlic, and Rosemary*; 175g (5¾oz)
watermelon
Supplements: Sinatra Foundation Programme plus added fish oil and flaxseed
Exercise: 20–30-minute walk

Day 3
Breakfast: 2 scrambled eggs prepared with 2 Tbsp. skimmed milk; 2 slices
wholemeal toast with 2 tsp. light margarine; 240ml (8fl oz) calcium-
fortified orange juice; 170g (5½oz) blueberries; 1 cup coffee or tea
Snack: 1 banana
Lunch: Grilled soya cheese and tomato sandwich on wholemeal bread with
2 tsp. light margarine; 75g (2½oz) baby carrots; 1 apple
Snack: 2 Tbsp. unsalted peanuts and 2 Tbsp. raisins
Dinner: 1 serving Roast Salmon*; 120g (5oz) steamed spinach;
100g (3½oz) black beans; 1 serving Israeli Chopped Salad*;
1 piece Spice Cake*
Supplements: Sinatra Foundation Programme plus added fish oil and flaxseed
Exercise: 20–30-minute walk

Day 4
Breakfast: 225g (8oz) cooked oatmeal with 1 Tbsp. raisins; 120ml (4fl oz)
skimmed or plain soya milk; 1 slice wholemeal toast with 1 tsp. light
margarine; 1 cup coffee or tea
Snack: 1 banana; 225g (8oz) low-sodium low-fat cottage cheese; 4 Tbsp.
raisins
Lunch: 50g (1¾oz) fresh chopped spinach, 90g (3oz) navy beans, and
2 hard-boiled eggs with Ginger Flaxseed Dressing*; 90g (3oz)
honeydew melon
Snack: 180g (6oz) strawberries with Lemon Poppy Seed Dip*

Dinner: *1 serving Roast Vegetables*; 1 serving Grilled Tofu*;*
                1 serving Lentils with Garlic and Tomatoes; ¼ melon*
Supplements: *Sinatra Foundation Programme plus added fish oil and flaxseed*
Exercise: *20–30-minute walk*

Day 5

Breakfast: *225g (8oz) low-sodium low-fat cottage cheese topped with 3 tsp. ground*
                flaxseed, 3 tsp. wheat germ, and 60g (2oz) crushed pineapple;
                200g (6½oz) mixed strawberries and melon; 1 cup coffee or tea
Snack: *1 banana*
Lunch: *1 serving Veggie Miso Soup*; 75g (2½oz) brown rice; 1 small*
                wholemeal roll with 1 tsp. margarine; 125g (4½oz) steamed broccoli;
                1 small pear
Snack: *75g (2½oz) baby carrots with 2 Tbsp. Hummus**
Dinner: *1 serving Grilled Mediterranean Halibut*; 100g (3½oz) lima butter*
                beans; large bowl tossed salad with Flaxseed Dressing; 1 piece Spice*
                *Cake**
Supplements: *Sinatra Foundation Programme plus added fish oil and flaxseed*
Exercise: *20–30-minute walk*

Day 6

Breakfast: *2 eggs scrambled with 25g (¾oz) mushrooms, sliced tomato, and*
                chopped onion in 1 tsp. olive oil; 2 slices wholemeal toast with
                2 tsp. light margarine; 240ml (8fl oz) calcium-fortified orange juice;
                1 cup coffee or tea
Lunch: *1 serving TVP Chilli*; 180g (6oz) strawberries*
Snack: *2 rye crisp cracker; 2 Tbsp. soya nut butter*
Dinner: *1 serving Stir-Fried Chicken and Broccoli*; 175g (5¾oz) melon cubes;*
                *1 piece Spice Cake**
Supplements: *Sinatra Foundation Programme plus added fish oil and flaxseed*
Exercise: *20–30-minute walk*

Day 7

Breakfast: *Med. bowl shredded wheat cereal with 120ml (4fl oz) plain soya or*
                skimmed milk and 2 Tbsp. raisins; 1 cup coffee or tea
Snack: *1 banana; 120g (4oz) cottage cheese*
Lunch: *Soya burger on a wholemeal roll with lettuce and tomato;*
                100g (3½oz) Bean Salad; sliced tomatoes and cucumbers; 1 apple*
Dinner: *1 serving Grilled Red Snapper*; 75g (2½oz) steamed cauliflower;*
                1 medium baked potato with 1 tsp. light margarine; 2 cups tossed salad
                with diced celery and mushrooms and 2 Tbsp. Flaxseed Dressing;*
                175g (5¾oz) watermelon
Supplements: *Sinatra Foundation Programme plus added fish oil and flaxseed*
Exercise: *20–30-minute walk*

DAILY PLAN: WEEK 4

Day 1

Breakfast: 225g (8oz) cooked oatmeal with 2 Tbsp. diced figs or raisins; 120ml (2fl oz) skimmed or plain soya milk; 240ml (8fl oz) calcium-fortified orange juice; 1 cup coffee or tea

Snack: 1 banana

Lunch: 1 serving Tofu, Tomato, and Black Olive Salad*; 1 wholemeal pitta; 125g (4½oz) steamed broccoli; 1 apple

Snack: 1 Oatmeal Date Biscuit*; 240ml (8fl oz) plain soya milk

Dinner: 1 serving Easy Grilled Chicken Breast*; Steamed Vegetables*; 75g (2½oz) brown rice; 75g (2½oz) grapes and 125g (4½oz) watermelon

Supplements: Sinatra Foundation Programme plus the following:
- 2g fish oil
- 2 Tbsp. crushed flaxseed (preferred) or 1 Tbsp. flaxseed oil
- 2g L-arginine

Exercise: Three flexibility exercises followed by a 20-minute walk

Mind/Body: Meditation or qigong exercises

Day 2

Breakfast: 225g (8oz) low-sodium low-fat cottage cheese; 175g (5¾oz) diced melon; 125g (4½oz) crushed pineapple; 1 cup coffee or tea

Lunch: 60g (2oz) canned low-sodium salmon on large bowl tossed salad and 1 medium tomato, sliced; 2 Tbsp. Flaxseed Dressing*; 1 apple; 1 piece Apple Raisin Bread

Snack: 2 rye crisp crackers with 2 Tbsp. soya nut butter

Dinner: 1 serving Stir-Fried Tofu and Vegetables*; 1 frozen banana

Supplements: Sinatra Foundation Programme plus added fish oil, flaxseed, and L-arginine

Exercise: Flexibility exercises followed by a 20-minute walk

Mind/Body: Meditation or qigong exercises

Day 3

Breakfast: 2-egg spinach omelette made with 30g (1oz) feta cheese and 25g (¾oz) fresh chopped spinach; 2 slices wholemeal toast with 2 tsp. light margarine; 240ml (8fl oz) calcium-fortified orange juice; 1 cup coffee or tea

Lunch: 1 serving Veggie Miso Soup*; 75g (2½oz) brown rice with 2 Tbsp. dried figs; large bowl tossed salad with 2 Tbsp. Flaxseed Dressing*; 1 peach

Snack: 2 celery sticks with 2 Tbsp. unsalted natural peanut butter

Dinner: 180g (6oz) grilled chicken breast; large bowl tossed salad with Ginger Flaxseed Dressing*; 1 serving Black Bean Salad*; 180g (6oz) strawberries

Supplements: Sinatra Foundation Programme plus added fish oil, flaxseed, L-arginine

Exercise: Flexibility exercises, followed by a 20-minute walk

Mind/Body: Meditation or qigong exercises

Day 4

Breakfast: *225g (8oz) oatmeal with 1 Tbsp. soya powder; 120ml (4fl oz) plain soya or skimmed milk; 1 tsp. chopped nuts and cinnamon; ½ medium grapefruit; 1 cup coffee or tea*

Lunch: *120g (4oz) turkey burger on wholemeal roll with 2 tsp. light mayonnaise and sliced tomato and lettuce; 1 serving Three-Bean Salad*; 75g (2½oz) grapes*

Snack: *1 Oatmeal Date Biscuit**

Dinner: *1 serving Poached Salmon with Dill Sauce*; sliced cucumbers with dill; 1 serving Spinach with Pine Nuts and Garlic*; 1 serving of Lentils and Red Pepper Salad*; 1 frozen banana*

Supplements: *Sinatra Foundation Programme plus added fish oil, flaxseed, L-arginine*

Exercise: *Flexibility exercises, followed by a 20-minute walk*

Mind/Body: *Meditation or qigong exercises*

Day 5

Breakfast: *1 Blueberry or Apple-Cinnamon Bran Muffin*; 2 slices soya cheese; 180g (6oz) strawberries with 60ml (2fl oz) fat-free plain yogurt and 1 tsp. honey; 1 cup coffee or tea*

Snack: *1 orange*

Lunch: *1 serving Vegetable Soup*; large bowl tossed salad with 2 Tbsp. Flaxseed Dressing* and 1 hard-boiled egg; 1 Oatmeal Date Biscuit*; 240ml (8fl oz) plain soya or skimmed milk*

Snack: *2 dried figs and 2 dried apricots*

Dinner: *1 serving Stir-Fried Chicken and Broccoli*; 170g (5½oz) blueberries*

Supplements: *Sinatra Foundation Programme plus added fish oil, flaxseed, L-arginine*

Exercise: *Flexibility exercises followed by a 20-minute walk*

Mind/Body: *Meditation or qigong exercises*

Day 6

Breakfast: *Fruit Smoothie*; 1 cup coffee or tea*

Snack: *120g (4oz) low-sodium low-fat cottage cheese; 1 Tbsp. raisins*

Lunch: *Mushroom omelette made with 2 eggs and 2 Tbsp. skimmed milk and cooked in 1 tsp. olive oil; large bowl tossed salad with 2 Tbsp. Flaxseed Dressing*; ¼ melon*

Dinner: *1 serving Prawns with Peppers, Tomatoes, and Garlic*; 1 serving Chickpea Salad with Rosemary*; 1 peach; 1 Oatmeal Date Biscuit**

Supplements: *Sinatra Foundation Programme plus added fish oil, flaxseed, L-arginine*

Exercise: *Flexibility exercises followed by a 20-minute walk*

Mind/Body: *Meditation or qigong exercises*

Day 7

Breakfast: *40g (1½oz) whole-grain cereal; 2 Tbsp. raisins; 1 cup plain soya or skimmed milk; 240ml (8fl oz) calcium-fortified orange juice; 1 cup coffee or tea*

Snack: *225g (8oz) low-sodium low-fat cottage cheese; 125g (4½oz) crushed pineapple*

Lunch: *15g (½oz) feta cheese and 3 medium fresh figs in a wholemeal pitta; large bowl tossed salad with 2 Tbsp. Flaxseed Dressing**

Dinner: *1 serving Roast Pork Tenderloin with Mustard*; 25g (¾oz) onions and 120g (4oz) sliced courgette sautéed in 1 tsp. olive oil; 1 medium baked potato with 1 tsp. light margarine; large bowl tossed salad with Ginger Flaxseed Dressing*; 180g (6oz) strawberries*

Supplements: *Sinatra Foundation Programme plus added fish oil, flaxseed, L-arginine*

Exercises: *Flexibility exercises followed by 20-minute walk*

Mind/Body: *Meditation or qigong exercises*

DAILY PLAN: WEEK 5

Day 1

Breakfast: *225g (8oz) fat-free plain yogurt with 1 tsp. honey and 1 chopped banana; 2 tsp. chopped walnuts; 1 cup coffee or tea*

Snack: *25g (¾oz) unsalted soya nuts*

Lunch: *1 serving Tempeh and Stir-Fried Vegetables*; 175g (5¾oz) watermelon*

Snack: *1 Oatmeal Date Biscuit**

Dinner: *120g (4oz) grilled salmon; 120g (4oz) spinach sautéed in 1 tsp. olive oil; 75g (2½oz) brown rice with 1 Tbsp. raisins; 1 Oatmeal Date Biscuit*; 175g (5¾oz) honeydew melon*

Supplements: *Sinatra Foundation Programme plus the following:*
- *2g fish oil*
- *2 Tbsp. crushed flaxseed (preferred) or 1 Tbsp. flaxseed oil*
- *2g L-arginine*
- *150–300mg grapeseed extract*

Exercise: *Strength-training exercises*

Mind/Body: *Anger management or emotional release exercises*

Day 2

Breakfast: *2-egg omelette made with 50g (1¾oz) asparagus; 2 slices toast with 2 tsp. light margarine; 240ml (8fl oz) calcium-fortified orange juice; 180g (6oz) strawberries; 1 cup coffee or tea*

Lunch: *90g (3oz) turkey breast and ½ medium avocado in wholemeal pitta; 1 apple*

Snack: *2 stalks celery with 2 Tbsp. unsalted peanut butter*

Dinner: *1 serving Veggie Miso Soup*; 1 serving Grilled Tofu*; 1 serving Stir-Fry Mangetout and Sesame Seeds*; 75g (2½oz) brown rice and lentils; 75g (2½oz) grapes and 75g (2½oz) blueberries*

Supplements: *Sinatra Foundation Programme plus added fish oil, flaxseed, L-arginine, and grapeseed extract*

Exercise: *20–30-minute walk*

Mind/Body: *Anger management exercises*

Day 3

Breakfast: *Small bowl cooked oatmeal with 25g (¾oz) chopped dried figs; 120ml (4fl oz) skimmed or plain soya milk; 240ml (8fl oz) calcium-fortified orange juice; 1 cup coffee or tea*

Snack: *240ml (8fl oz) plain soya milk; 1 banana*

Lunch: *60ml (2fl oz) Hummus* with sliced cucumbers, tomatoes, endive, and black olives in a wholemeal pitta pocket; 170g (5½oz) mixed berries*

Dinner: *1 serving Mediterranean Halibut*; large bowl tossed salad with ½ medium avocado and 2 Tbsp. Flaxseed Dressing*; ¼ melon*

Supplements: *Sinatra Foundation Programme plus added fish oil, flaxseed, L-arginine, and grapeseed extract*

Exercise: *Strength training exercises*

Mind/Body: *Anger management exercises*

Day 4

Breakfast: *Medium to large bowl whole-grain cereal with 60g (2oz) blueberries, 1 Tbsp. ground flaxseed, and 240ml (8fl oz) skim or plain soya milk; 1 cup coffee or tea*

Lunch: *1 serving Minestrone Soup*; large bowl green lettuce with tomatoes, red peppers, and black olives with Ginger Flaxseed Dressing*; 180g (6oz) strawberries*

Snack: *¼ melon*

Dinner: *1 serving Exceptional Hamburgers* with Fresh Tomato Salsa* on a wholemeal roll; 1 serving of Pinto Bean Salad*; 1 medium grilled yellow squash; 1 pear*

Supplements: *Sinatra Foundation Programme plus added fish oil, flaxseed, L-arginine, and grapeseed extract*

Exercise: *20–30-minute walk*

Mind/Body: *Anger management exercises*

Day 5

Breakfast: *2 slices wholemeal French toast made with 1 egg and 2 Tbsp. skimmed milk; 125g (4½oz) unsweetened stewed apples; 1 cup coffee or tea*

Lunch: *Grilled soya burger in a wholemeal pitta with lettuce, tomato, and 2 tsp. light mayonnaise; 1 serving Bean Salad*; sliced cucumber salad with 1 tsp. olive oil and 1 tsp. cider vinegar*

Snack: *260g (9oz) honeydew melon with Lemon Poppy Seed Dip**

Dinner: *120g (4oz) chicken breast, grilled; 1 serving Black Bean Salad* with ½ medium avocado and 1 medium chopped tomato with 2 Tbsp. Flaxseed Dressing*; 1 frozen banana*

Supplements: *Sinatra Foundation Programme plus added fish oil, flaxseed, L-arginine, and grapeseed extract*

Exercise: *Strength training exercises*

Mind/Body: *Anger management exercises*

Day 6

Breakfast: 225g (8oz) low-sodium low-fat cottage cheese with 1 Tbsp. ground flaxseed; ¼ melon; 240ml (8fl oz) calcium-fortified orange juice; 1 cup coffee or tea

Snack: 1 banana

Lunch: 120g (4oz) grilled tempeh; 1 serving Grilled Courgettes*; 100g (3½oz) spinach with 1 hard-boiled egg, 1 Tbsp. olive oil, 1 Tbsp. vinegar, and crushed garlic

Snack: 1 Oatmeal Date Biscuit*; 240ml (8fl oz) plain soya milk

Dinner: 1 serving Stir-Fried Chicken and Broccoli* with added 50g (1¾oz) asparagus and 2 Tbsp. diced figs mixed into the rice; 180g (6oz) strawberries and 175g (5¼oz) watermelon

Supplements: Sinatra Foundation Programme plus added fish oil, flaxseed, L-arginine, and grapeseed extract

Exercise: 20–30-minute walk

Mind/Body: Anger management exercises

Day 7

Breakfast: Fruit Smoothie*; ½ grapefruit

Snack: 1 piece Apple Raisin Bread*

Lunch: 1 serving Asparagus with Tomatoes and Olive Oil*; grilled soya cheese sandwich on wholemeal bread with 2 tsp. light margarine

Dinner: 1 serving Mussels Provençal*; large bowl tossed salad with 60g (2oz) of firm cubed tofu, tomato, black olives, and Ginger Flaxseed Dressing*; 1 small wholemeal roll with 1 tsp. light margarine; 150g (5oz) blueberries

Supplements: Sinatra Foundation Programme plus added fish oil, flaxseed, L-arginine, and grapeseed extract

Exercise: Strength training exercises

Mind/Body: Anger management exercises

DAILY PLAN: WEEK 6

Day 1

Breakfast: 120g (4oz) fat-free plain yogurt with 2 tsp. chopped nuts and 1 Tbsp. ground flaxseed; 60g (2oz) fresh berries; 1 Dried Fruit Spelt Muffin*; 1 cup coffee or tea

Lunch: 90g (3oz) low-sodium canned salmon; 1 hard-boiled egg; shredded raw vegetable salad of courgettes, red peppers, and celery with 2 Tbsp. Flaxseed Dressing*; 125g (4½oz) raspberries

Snack: 1 rye crisp cracker with 1 Tbsp. soya nut butter

Dinner: 1 serving Spelt (or Wholemeal) Pasta with Tomato, Basil, and Shiitake or Maitake Mushrooms*; 1 serving of Dr. Sinatra's Favourite Shiitake Recipe*; large bowl tossed green salad with Ginger Flaxseed Dressing*; 1 frozen banana

Supplements: Sinatra Foundation Programme plus the following:
  • 2g fish oil

- *2 Tbsp. crushed flaxseed (preferred) or 1 Tbsp. flaxseed oil*
- *2g L-arginine*
- *150–300mg grapeseed extract*
- *500–1,000mg organic garlic capsules*
- *10–15 drops Maitake D-Fraction Liquid three times daily (optional)*

Exercise: *20–30-minute walk and strength training exercises*
Mind/Body: *Yogic breathing exercises*

Day 2

Breakfast: *40g (1½oz) spelt (or wholemeal) cereal with 2 Tbsp. chopped figs and 240ml (8fl oz) plain soya or skimmed milk; 240ml (8fl oz) calcium-fortified orange juice; 1 cup coffee or tea*
Snack: *1 banana*
Lunch: *Soya burger on spelt (or wholemeal) toast with lettuce and tomato and 2 tsp. light mayonnaise; 1 apple*
Dinner: *1 serving Turkey Meatloaf*; 1 serving Three-Bean Salad*; 120g (4oz) steamed broccoli; 1 small wholemeal roll with 1 tsp. light margarine; 1 piece Carrot Cake**
Supplements: *Sinatra Foundation Programme plus added fish oil, flaxseed, L-arginine, grapeseed extract, and garlic*
Exercise: *20–30-minute walk and strength exercises*
Mind/Body: *Yoga meditation exercises*

Day 3

Breakfast: *Fruit Smoothie*; 180g (6oz) strawberries; 1 Dried Fruit Spelt Muffin**
Lunch: *1 serving Salmon Salad*; 350g (14oz) watermelon*
Snack: *1 Carob Nut Brownie*, 240g (8fl oz) skimmed or plain soya milk*
Dinner: *1 serving Grilled Tofu*; 1 serving Steamed Vegetables*; 75g (2½oz) brown rice; 150g (5oz) blueberries*
Supplements: *Sinatra Foundation Programme plus added fish oil, flaxseed, L-arginine, grapeseed extract, and garlic*
Exercise: *Yoga asanas*
Mind/Body: *Yogic breathing exercises*

Day 4

Breakfast: *Tomato and asparagus omelette made with 2 eggs, 2 Tbsp. skimmed milk, ½ medium tomato, and 50g (1¾oz) asparagus; ¼ melon; 1 slice wholemeal toast with 1 tsp. light margarine; 240ml (8fl oz) calcium-fortified orange juice; 1 cup coffee or tea*
Lunch: *1 serving Stir-Fried Tofu and Vegetables* and 25g (¾oz) fresh shiitake mushrooms; 225g (8oz) strawberries*
Snack: *1 rye crisp cracker with 1 Tbsp. soya nut butter*
Dinner: *1 serving Roast Salmon*; 150g (5oz) steamed asparagus; 1 serving Lentils and Red Pepper Salad*; 1 frozen banana*

Supplements: *Sinatra Foundation Programme plus added fish oil, flaxseed,*
                  L-arginine, grapeseed extract, and garlic
Exercise: *20–30-minute walk*
Mind/Body: *Yoga meditation exercises*

Day 5

Breakfast: *2 slices spelt (or wholemeal) toast with 2 tsp. light margarine;*
                1 scrambled egg; 180g (6oz) strawberries; 240ml (8 fl oz) calcium-
                fortified juice; 1 cup coffee or tea
Lunch: *120g (4oz) turkey burger on 2 slices spelt (or wholemeal) bread with*
                lettuce, tomato, and 2 tsp. light mayonnaise; 1 serving of Black Bean
                Salad*; large bowl tossed salad with Ginger Flaxseed Dressing*; ¼ melon
Dinner: *1 serving Grilled Prawns*; 1 serving Spelt Pilaf with Shiitake or*
                Maitake Mushrooms*; ½ medium avocado and 1 medium tomato, sliced
                and seasoned with lemon juice
Supplements: *Sinatra Foundation Programme plus added fish oil, flaxseed,*
                  L-arginine, grapeseed extract, and garlic
Exercise: *Yoga asanas*
Mind/Body: *Yogic breathing exercises*

Day 6

Breakfast: *Fruit smoothie*; ½ medium grapefruit*
Snack: *1 Dried Fruit Spelt Muffin**
Lunch: *1 serving Minestrone Soup*; 4 wholemeal crackers; large bowl tossed*
                salad with 2 Tbsp. Ginger Flaxseed Dressing*; 1 apple
Dinner: *1 serving Chicken and Red Pepper Kebab*; 1 serving Lentils and*
                Courgettes Sauté*; 3 cups fresh spinach with Ginger Flaxseed
                Dressing*; 125g (4½oz) raspberries
Supplements: *Sinatra Foundation Programme plus added fish oil, flaxseed,*
                  L-arginine, grapeseed extract, and garlic
Exercise: *20–30-minute walk and strength training*
Mind/Body: *Yoga meditation*

Day 7

Breakfast: *225g (8oz) cooked oatmeal with 2 tsp. walnuts and 1 tsp. honey;*
                120ml (4fl oz) plain soya or skimmed milk; 240ml (8fl oz) calcium-
                fortified orange juice; 1 cup coffee or tea
Snack: *1 Dried Fruit Spelt Muffin**
Lunch: *180g (6oz) can low-sodium tuna seasoned with 1 Tbsp. light*
                mayonnaise on bed of lettuce, tomatoes, and cucumbers; 1 piece spelt
                (or wholemeal) bread with 1 tsp. light margarine; ¼ melon
Dinner: *1 serving Tempeh Chilli*; 75g (2½oz) brown rice; large bowl tossed*
                salad with 2 Tbsp. Flaxseed Dressing*; 175g (5¾oz) frozen grapes
Supplements: *Sinatra Foundation Programme plus added fish oil, flaxseed,*
                  L-arginine, grapeseed extract, and garlic
Exercise: *Yoga asanas*
Mind/Body: *Yogic breathing exercises*

DAILY PLAN: WEEK 7

Day 1

Breakfast: *225g (8oz) cooked oatmeal with 2 tsp. wheat germ drizzled with 1 tsp. honey; 120ml (4oz) skimmed or plain soya milk; 175g (5¾oz) melon cubes; 1 cup green tea*

Snack: *1 banana*

Lunch: *1 serving Vegetable Soup*; large bowl tossed salad with 60g (2oz) cooked chicken breast and 1 medium diced tomato, seasoned with garlic, 2 tsp. olive oil, and lemon juice; 1 small wholemeal roll with 1 tsp. light margarine*

Snack: *1 Peanut Butter Biscuit*; 240ml (8fl oz) soya milk*

Dinner: *1 serving Poached Salmon with Dill Sauce*; 120g (4oz) steamed spinach; 1 medium baked potato with 1 tsp. light margarine; 175g (5¾oz) frozen grapes*

Supplements: *Sinatra Foundation Programme plus the following:*
- *2g fish oil*
- *2 Tbsp. crushed flaxseed (preferred) or 1 Tbsp. flaxseed oil*
- *2g L-arginine*
- *150–300mg grapeseed extract*
- *500–1,000mg organic garlic capsules*
- *500mg hawthorn two or three times daily*
- *10–15 drops Maitake D-Fraction Liquid three times daily (optional)*

Exercise: *Upper-body workout*

Mind/Body: *Biofeedback exercises, qigong, or yoga*

Day 2

Breakfast: *1 serving Blueberry Buckwheat Pancakes with Wheat Germ*; 1 cup coffee or green tea*

Lunch: *1 serving Stir-Fried Tofu and Vegetables*; 1 apple*

Snack: *225g (8oz) low-sodium low-fat cottage cheese; 1 banana*

Dinner: *1 serving Spelt (or Wholemeal) Pasta with Asparagus and Tomatoes*; large bowl tossed salad with Ginger Flaxseed Dressing*; ¼ melon*

Supplements: *Sinatra Foundation Programme plus added fish oil, flaxseed, L-arginine, grapeseed extract, garlic, and hawthorn*

Exercise: *20–30-minute walk*

Mind/Body: *Biofeedback exercises, qigong, or yoga*

Day 3

Breakfast: *Tomato omelette made with 2 eggs, 2 Tbsp. skimmed milk, and ½ medium tomato; 2 slices spelt (or wholemeal) toast with 2 tsp. light margarine; 240ml (8fl oz) calcium-fortified orange juice; 1 cup coffee or green tea*

Lunch: *1 serving Grilled Chicken Teriyaki*; 1 serving Stir-Fry Mangetout and Sesame Seeds*; 75g (2½oz) brown rice; 180g (6oz) pineapple*

Snack: *1 frozen banana*

Dinner: *1 serving Sandy's Crab Cakes*; 1 serving Lentils with Garlic and Tomatoes*; 180g (6oz) strawberries with 125ml (4fl oz) fat-free plain yogurt and 1 tsp. honey*

Supplements: *Sinatra Foundation Programme plus added fish oil, flaxseed, L-arginine, grapeseed extract, garlic, and hawthorn*

Exercise: *Upper-body exercises*

Mind/Body: *Biofeedback exercises, qigong, or yoga*

Day 4

Breakfast: *1 Blueberry or Apple-Cinnamon Bran Muffin*; 225ml (8fl oz) low-sodium low-fat cottage cheese; 170g (5½oz) melon; 240ml (8fl oz) calcium-fortified orange juice; 1 cup coffee or green tea*

Snack: *1 banana*

Lunch: *1 serving Tofu, Tomato, and Black Olive Salad*; 75g (2½oz) brown rice; 75g (2½oz) grapes; 1 Peanut Butter Biscuit**

Dinner: *120g (4oz) grilled chicken breast; 1 serving Roast Vegetables*; 1 serving Black Bean Salad*; 1 baked apple*

Supplements: *Sinatra Foundation Programme plus added fish oil, flaxseed, L-arginine, grapeseed extract, garlic, and hawthorn*

Exercise: *20–30-minute walk*

Mind/Body: *Biofeedback exercises, qigong, or yoga*

Day 5

Breakfast: *Fruit Smoothie*; ½ grapefruit*

Snack: *1 Dried Fruit Spelt Muffin**

Lunch: *2 slices soya cheese and 60g (2oz) roasted turkey breast in a wholemeal pitta with 25g (¾oz) fresh maitake/shiitake mushrooms; large bowl tossed salad with 1 medium tomato and ½ small jar marinated artichoke hearts; 1 apple*

Dinner: *1 serving Tempeh Chilli*; large bowl tossed salad with ½ medium chopped avocado and 30g (1oz) chopped red onion and seasoned with lemon juice; 60g (2oz) fresh pineapple*

Supplements: *Sinatra Foundation Programme plus added fish oil, flaxseed, L-arginine, grapeseed extract, garlic, and hawthorn*

Exercise: *Upper-body exercise*

Mind/Body: *Biofeedback exercises, qigong, or yoga*

Day 6

Breakfast: *2 hard-boiled eggs; 2 slice spelt (or wholemeal) toast with 2 tsp. light margarine; 175g (5¾oz) melon cubes; 1 cup coffee or green tea*

Lunch: *1 serving Lentil Soup*; large bowl tossed salad with 2 Tbsp. Flaxseed Dressing*; 1 baked apple*

Dinner: *1 serving Grilled Mediterranean Halibut*; asparagus, tomato, and red onion salad with Ginger Flaxseed Dressing*; 1 serving Haricot Beans, Garlic, and Rosemary Salad*; 180g (6oz) strawberries with Poppy Seed Lemon Dip**

Supplements: *Sinatra Foundation Programme plus added fish oil, flaxseed,*
                   L-arginine, grapeseed extract, garlic, and hawthorn
Exercise: *20–30-minute walk*
Mind/Body: *Biofeedback exercises, qigong, or yoga*

Day 7

Breakfast: *225g (8oz) low-sodium low-fat cottage cheese mixed with 175g (5¼oz)*
                   melon cubes, ½ banana, and 1 Tbsp. ground flaxseed; 1 cup coffee or
                   green tea
Snack: *1 Dried Fruit Spelt Muffin**
Lunch: *1 serving Salad Niçoise, Sinatra Style*; 240ml (8fl oz) calcium-fortified*
                   orange juice; 1 piece spelt (or wholemeal) bread with 1 tsp. light
                   margarine; 1 apple
Snack: *1 rye crisp cracker with 1 Tbsp. soya nut butter*
Dinner: *1 serving Wholemeal Pasta with Broccoli and Feta*;*
                   170g (5½oz) pineapple
Supplements: *Sinatra Foundation Programme plus added fish oil, flaxseed,*
                   L-arginine, grapeseed extract, garlic, and hawthorn
Exercise: *Upper-body workout*
Mind/Body: *Biofeedback exercises, qigong, or yoga*

DAILY PLAN: WEEK 8

Day 1

Breakfast: *225g (8oz) oatmeal enriched with 1 Tbsp. soya powder and 1 Tbsp.*
                   ground flaxseed and drizzled with 1 tsp. honey; 240ml (8fl oz) calcium-
                   fortified orange juice; 1 cup coffee or green tea
Snack: *1 Dried Fruit Spelt Muffin*; 1 banana*
Lunch: *1 serving Veggie Miso Soup*; 1 serving Steamed Vegetables*; 1 apple*
Snack: *1 Peanut Butter Biscuit*; 240ml (8fl oz) plain soya or skimmed milk*
Dinner: *1 serving Roast Salmon*; large bowl tossed salad with Ginger Flaxseed*
                   Dressing*; 1 medium baked potato with 2 Tbsp. fat-free plain yogurt;
                   170g (5½oz) pineapple
Supplements: *Sinatra Foundation Programme plus the following:*
                   - *2g fish oil*
                   - *2 Tbsp. crushed flaxseed (preferred) or 1 Tbsp. flaxseed oil*
                   - *2g L-arginine*
                   - *150–300mg grapeseed extract*
                   - *500–1,000mg organic garlic capsules*
                   - *500mg hawthorn two or three times daily*
                   - *10–15 drops Maitake D-Fraction Liquid three times daily (optional)*
                   - *DHEA supplement (optional)*
Exercise: *Lower-body exercises*
Mind/Body: *Music therapy*

Day 2

Breakfast: 1 Blueberry or Apple/Cinnamon Bran Muffin*; 225g (8oz) low-sodium low-fat cottage cheese; ¼ melon; 240ml (8fl oz) calcium-fortified orange juice; 1 cup coffee or green tea

Lunch: 1 serving Antiguan Black Bean Soup*; 50g (1¾oz) grilled maitake/shiitake mushrooms with ½ medium avocado, diced, and topped with 2 Tbsp. Flaxseed Dressing*; 175g (5¾oz) grapes

Dinner: 1 serving Roast Pork Tenderloin with Rosemary and Garlic*; 1 serving Roast Vegetables; 1 medium sweet potato; 1 baked apple

Supplements: Sinatra Foundation Programme plus added fish oil, flaxseed, L-arginine, grapeseed extract, garlic, and hawthorn

Exercise: 20–30-minute walk

Mind/Body: Music therapy

Day 3

Breakfast: 225ml (8fl oz) fat-free plain yogurt mixed with 1 tsp. honey; ½ banana; 180g (6oz) fresh strawberries and 1 Tbsp. wheat germ; 1 cup coffee or green tea

Lunch: 1 serving Salmon Salad* with sliced cucumbers and tomatoes; 1 slice spelt (or wholemeal) bread with 1 tsp. light margarine

Snack: 1 Oatmeal Date Biscuit*; 240ml (8fl oz) skimmed or plain soya milk

Dinner: 1 serving Stir-Fried Tempeh and Maitake/Shiitake Mushrooms and Mangetout*; 175g (5¾oz) red grapes

Supplements: Sinatra Foundation Programme plus added fish oil, flaxseed, L-arginine, grapeseed extract, garlic, and hawthorn

Exercise: Lower-body exercises

Mind/Body: Music therapy

Day 4

Breakfast: 2 Tbsp. feta cheese and 25g (¾oz) chopped figs on 2 slices spelt (or wholemeal) toast; 240ml (8fl oz) calcium-fortified orange juice; 1 cup coffee or green tea

Snack: 1 banana

Lunch: Soya burger on a wholemeal roll with lettuce, tomato and 2 tsp. light mayonnaise; 1 serving Veggie Coleslaw*; 1 serving of Bean Salad*; 1 apple

Dinner: 1 serving of Chinese Chicken Salad*; ¼ melon

Supplements: Sinatra Foundation Programme plus added fish oil, flaxseed, L-arginine, grapeseed extract, garlic, and hawthorn

Exercise: 20–30-minute walk

Mind/Body: Music therapy

Day 5

Breakfast: 2 slices wholemeal French toast made with 1 egg, 2 Tbsp. skimmed milk, and cinnamon, topped with 120ml (4fl oz) unsweetened stewed apple; 240ml (8fl oz) calcium-fortified orange juice; 1 cup coffee or green tea

Lunch: 1 serving Chicken Vegetable Soup*; large bowl tossed salad with 2 Tbsp. Flaxseed Dressing*; 1 apple

Dinner: 120g (4oz) tenderloin of beef; 1 serving Grilled Courgettes*; 1 serving Spinach and Tomato Salad*; 1 piece Carrot Cake*

Supplements: Sinatra Foundation Programme plus added fish oil, flaxseed, L-arginine, grapeseed extract, garlic, and hawthorn

Exercise: Lower-body exercises

Mind/Body: Music therapy

Day 6

Breakfast: 40g (1½oz) whole-grain cereal; 2 Tbsp. raisins; 120g (4oz) low-sodium low-fat cottage cheese; 240ml (8fl oz) plain soya or skimmed milk; 240ml (8fl oz) calcium-fortified orange juice; 1 cup coffee or green tea

Lunch: 1 serving Pasta à la Sinatra*; 1 apple

Dinner: 1 serving Grilled Prawns*; 1 medium baked potato with 1 tsp. light margarine; large bowl tossed salad with crushed dried nori seaweed and 2 Tbsp. Ginger Flaxseed Dressing*

Supplements: Sinatra Foundation Programme plus added fish oil, flaxseed, L-arginine, grapeseed extract, garlic, and hawthorn

Exercise: 20–30-minute walk

Mind/Body: Music therapy

Day 7

Breakfast: Fruit Smoothie*; ½ grapefruit

Snack: 1 banana

Lunch: 120g (4oz) Hummus* with black olives, diced red onions, lettuce, and tomato in a wholemeal pitta; 1 apple

Dinner: 1 serving Chicken Breasts Stuffed with Spinach*; 1 medium baked potato with 2 Tbsp. fat-free plain yogurt; large bowl tossed salad with 1 Tbsp. sunflower seeds, grated red cabbage, and 2 Tbsp. Flaxseed Dressing*; 1 piece Carrot Cake*

Supplements: Sinatra Foundation Programme plus added fish oil, flaxseed, L-arginine, grapeseed extract, garlic, and hawthorn

Exercise: Lower-body exercises

Mind/Body: Music therapy

RECIPES

Salads
1. Bean Salad
2. Black Bean Salad
3. Chickpea Salad with Rosemary
4. Veggie Coleslaw
5. Chinese Chicken Salad
6. Israeli Chopped Salad
7. Lentils and Red Pepper Salad
8. Salad Niçoise, Sinatra Style
9. Salmon Salad
10. Spinach and Tomato Salad
11. Three-Bean Salad
12. Tofu, Tomato, and Black Olive Salad
13. Haricot Bean Salad
14. Pinto Bean Salad

Vegetables
15. Asparagus with Tomatoes and Olive Oil
16. Dr. Sinatra's Favourite Shiitake Recipe
17. Grilled Courgettes
18. Lentils with Garlic and Tomatoes
19. Lentils and Courgettes Sauté
20. Roast Vegetables
21. Spinach with Pine Nuts and Garlic
22. Spelt Pilaf with Shiitake or Maitake Mushrooms
23. Steamed Vegetables
24. Stir Fried Mangetout and Sesame Seeds
25. Haricot Beans, Garlic, and Rosemary

Soups
26. Antiguan Black Bean Soup
27. Chicken Vegetable Soup
28. Chickpea and Chicory Soup
29. Lentil Soup
30. Minestrone Soup

31. Vegetable Soup
32. Veggie Miso Soup

Tofu/Tempeh
33. Grilled Tofu
34. Stir-Fried Tempeh and Maitake/Shiitake Mushrooms and Mangetout
35. Stir-Fried Tofu and Vegetables
36. Tempeh and Stir-Fried Vegetables
37. TVP Chilli
38. Tempeh Chilli
39. Tofu with Sesame Seeds

Poultry, Beef, and Pork
40. Chicken Breasts Stuffed with Spinach
41. Chicken and Red Pepper Kebab
42. Easy Grilled Chicken Breast
43. Grilled Chicken Teriyaki
44. Grilled Rosemary Chicken Breast
45. Low-Fat Exceptional Hamburgers
46. Roast Pork Tenderloin with Mustard
47. Roast Pork Tenderloin with Rosemary and Garlic
48. Stir-Fried Chicken and Broccoli
49. Turkey Meatloaf

Seafood
50. Breaded Sole or Flounder
51. Grilled Mediterranean Halibut
52. Grilled Red Snapper
53. Grilled Prawns
54. Mussels Provençal
55. Poached Salmon with Dill Sauce
56. Roast Salmon
57. Sandy's Crab Cakes
58. Scallop Kebab
59. Orange Prawns with Couscous
60. Prawns with Peppers, Tomatoes, and Garlic
61. Steamed Mussels

Pasta
62. Pasta à la Sinatra
63. Spelt (or Wholemeal) Pasta with Asparagus and Tomatoes
64. Spelt (or Wholemeal) Pasta with Tomato, Basil, and Shiitake or Maitake Mushrooms
65. Wholemeal Pasta with Broccoli and Feta
66. Wholemeal Pasta with Aubergine Tomato Sauce

Condiments
67. Flaxseed Dressing
68. Ginger Flaxseed Dressing
69. Fresh Tomato Salsa
70. Hummus

Breakfast Foods
71. Apple Raisin Bread
72. Blueberry or Apple-Cinnamon Bran Muffins
73. Blueberry Buckwheat Pancakes with Wheat Germ
74. Fruit Smoothie
75. Dried Fruit Spelt Muffins

Desserts and Snacks
76. Carrot Cake
77. Apricot Oatmeal Bars
78. Peanut Butter Biscuits
79. Carob Nut Brownies
80. Spice Cake
81. Oatmeal Date Biscuits
82. Lemon Poppy Seed Dip

SALADS

1. BEAN SALAD

1 350g (14oz) can unsalted or low-sodium beans, drained and rinsed (choose from kidney, black, haricot, cannelli, or lentil)
2 Tbsp. chopped red onion
2 Tbsp. chopped parsley
2 Tbsp. chopped tomato
1 tsp. sherry vinegar

Combine all ingredients in a medium bowl and chill for several hours.

SERVES 2

Nutrition Facts per Serving

Calories: 170	Sodium: 30mg
Calories from Fat: 0	Total Carbohydrate: 31g
Total Fat: 0	Dietary Fibre: 17g
Saturated Fat: 0	Sugar: 1g
Cholesterol: 0	Protein: 13g

2. BLACK BEAN SALAD

2 350g (14oz) cans unsalted or low-sodium black beans, drained and rinsed
2 Tbsp. fresh lemon juice
1 tsp. cumin
¼ tsp. crushed dried red pepper
2 spring onions, chopped
2 Tbsp. chopped coriander
1 red pepper, diced

Combine all ingredients in a medium bowl and chill for several hours.

SERVES 4

Nutrition Facts per Serving

Calories: 190

Calories from Fat: 10

Total Fat: 1g

Saturated Fat: 0

Cholesterol: 0

Sodium: 0

Total Carbohydrate: 36g

Dietary Fibre: 13g

Sugar: 4g

Protein: 13g

3. CHICKPEA SALAD with ROSEMARY

1 350g (14oz) can unsalted or low-sodium chickpeas, drained and rinsed

2 Tbsp. chopped red onion

2 tsp. chopped fresh rosemary

1 tsp. olive oil

1 tsp. balsamic vinegar

1 Tbsp. chopped fresh parsley

1 small tomato, diced

¼ lemon wedge, squeezed

Combine all ingredients in a medium bowl and chill for several hours.

SERVES 2

Nutrition Facts per Serving

Calories: 290

Calories from Fat: 60

Total Fat: 7g

Saturated Fat: 1g

Cholesterol: 0

Sodium: 15mg

Total Carbohydrate: 47g

Dietary Fibre: 13g

Sugar: 4g

Protein: 14g

4. VEGGIE COLESLAW

2 Tbsp. red wine vinegar

2 tsp. celery seed

2 Tbsp. Dijon mustard

2 tsp. honey

3 Tbsp. light soya mayonnaise

2 Tbsp. olive oil

1 medium red onion, finely chopped

300g (10oz) shredded cabbage

1 medium orange pepper, chopped

1 medium green pepper, chopped

In a large bowl whisk together vinegar, celery seed, mustard, honey, mayonnaise, and oil. Mix in remaining ingredients and chill several hours.

SERVES 4

Nutrition Facts per Serving

Calories: 150	Sodium: 310mg
Calories from Fat: 80	Total Carbohydrate: 17g
Total Fat: 9g	Dietary Fibre: 3g
Saturated Fat: 1g	Sugar: 10g
Cholesterol: 0	Protein: 2g

5. CHINESE CHICKEN SALAD

DRESSING:

> 1½ tsp. olive oil
> 1½ tsp. honey
> 1½ tsp. sesame oil
> 2 Tbsp. natural unsalted peanut butter
> 2 Tbsp. unseasoned rice wine vinegar
> 2 Tbsp. lime juice
> 1 Tbsp. low-sodium soya sauce
> ⅛ tsp. garlic powder
> ⅛ tsp. ground ginger

SALAD:

> 225g (½lb) diced cooked chicken breast
> 2 spring onions, chopped
> 1 stalk of celery, chopped
> ½ red pepper, chopped
> 100g (3½oz) baby spinach
> 125g (4½oz) Chinese cabbage, shredded
> 2 tsp. toasted sesame seeds

In medium bowl whisk together dressing ingredients. Add chicken, spring onions, celery, and red pepper. Serve over spinach and cabbage, and garnish with sesame seeds.

SERVES 2

Nutrition Facts per Serving

Calories: 420	Sodium: 410mg
Calories from Fat: 190	Total Carbohydrate: 18g
Total Fat: 21g	Dietary Fibre: 5g
Saturated Fat: 3.5g	Sugar: 9g
Cholesterol: 95mg	Protein: 42g

6. ISRAELI CHOPPED SALAD

1 medium cucumber, peeled and diced
1 red pepper, diced
3 stalks celery, diced
200g (6½oz) cherry tomatoes, quartered
2 Tbsp. chopped red onion
2 Tbsp. finely chopped fresh parsley
1 Tbsp. lemon juice
6 black olives, pitted and diced

Combine all ingredients in a medium bowl and chill for several hours.

SERVES 2

Nutrition Facts per Serving

Calories: 90	Sodium: 200mg
Calories from Fat: 25	Total Carbohydrate: 16g
Total Fat: 2.5g	Dietary Fibre: 5g
Saturated Fat: 0	Sugar: 5g
Cholesterol: 0	Protein: 3g

7. LENTILS and RED PEPPER SALAD

1 350g (14oz) can unsalted or low-sodium lentils, drained and rinsed
1 Tbsp. olive oil
½ cup red pepper, finely chopped
2 spring onions, chopped
1 Tbsp. lemon juice
1 Tbsp. red wine vinegar
½ Tbsp. Dijon mustard
⅛ tsp. black pepper
½ tsp. dried parsley

Combine all ingredients in a medium bowl and chill for several hours.

SERVES 2

Nutrition Facts per Serving

Calories: 270	Sodium: 95mg
Calories from Fat: 70	Total Carbohydrate: 37g
Total Fat: 7g	Dietary Fibre: 14g
Saturated Fat: 1g	Sugar: 5g
Cholesterol: 0	Protein: 15g

8. SALAD NIÇOISE, SINATRA STYLE

125g (4½oz) canned unsalted or low-sodium haricot beans, drained and rinsed
1 180g (6oz) can low-sodium salmon or 180g (6oz) of cooked fresh salmon
1 large egg, boiled and sliced
90g (3oz) cherry tomatoes, cut in half
60g (2oz) cooked green beans, cut in 2-inch pieces
1 Tbsp. chopped black olives
½ green pepper, chopped
1 Tbsp. olive oil
2 tsp. lemon juice
120g (4oz) baby spinach or green leaf lettuce

Toss all ingredients except spinach in a medium bowl. Serve on top of the baby spinach or lettuce.

SERVES 2

Nutrition Facts per Serving

Calories: 340	Sodium: 190mg
Calories from Fat: 160	Total Carbohydrate: 21g
Total Fat: 17g	Dietary Fibre: 8g
Saturated Fat: 3.5g	Sugar: 3g
Cholesterol: 145mg	Protein: 28g

9. SALMON SALAD

DRESSING:

1 Tbsp. balsamic vinegar
1 Tbsp. Dijon mustard
2 Tbsp. olive oil
2 Tbsp. water
1 Tbsp. lemon juice
1 tsp. dried basil
1 tsp. honey

SALAD:

225g (8oz) cooked fresh salmon, chopped
2 unpeeled cooked red potatoes, quartered and cooled
120g (4oz) chopped spinach or green leaf lettuce

Whisk dressing ingredients together in large bowl. Add all salad ingredients and toss gently.

SERVES 2

Nutrition Facts per Serving

Calories: 460	Sodium: 300mg
Calories from Fat: 200	Total Carbohydrate: 39g
Total Fat: 22g	Dietary Fibre: 5g
Saturated Fat: 3g	Sugar: 6g
Cholesterol: 60mg	Protein: 28g

10. SPINACH and TOMATO SALAD

3 tsp. olive oil, divided
2 cloves garlic, slivered
1 slice wholemeal bread, cut into cubes
120g (4oz) mushrooms, thinly sliced
75g (3oz) cherry tomatoes, halved
225g (½lb) fresh spinach (preferably baby spinach)
1 tsp. lemon rind
1 tsp. rice wine vinegar

Heat 2 teaspoons olive oil in a small frying pan over medium-high heat. Cook garlic until lightly browned and then discard. Fry the bread cubes in the garlic-flavoured oil until crispy, stirring frequently. Drain on a paper towel. Combine mushrooms, tomatoes, spinach, and bread cubes in a large bowl. Toss with remaining teaspoon of olive oil, lemon rind, and vinegar.

SERVES I

Nutrition Facts per Serving

Calories: 290	Sodium: 340mg
Calories from Fat: 150	Total Carbohydrate: 31g
Total Fat: 16g	Dietary Fibre: 10g
Saturated Fat: 2.5g	Sugar: 4g
Cholesterol: 0	Protein: 12g

11. THREE-BEAN SALAD

1 350g (14oz) can unsalted or low-sodium chickpeas, drained and rinsed
1 350g (14oz) can unsalted or low-sodium black beans, drained and rinsed
1 350g (14oz) can unsalted or low-sodium kidney beans, drained and rinsed
2 stalks celery, chopped
2 Tbsp. olive oil
1 Tbsp. lemon juice
3 Tbsp. light soya mayonnaise
1½ tsp. honey
1 Tbsp. cider vinegar
1 medium cucumber, peeled and diced
½ medium onion, chopped

Combine all ingredients in a large bowl and chill for several hours.

SERVES 8

Nutrition Facts per Serving

Calories: 190	Sodium: 60mg
Calories from Fat: 60	Total Carbohydrate: 23g
Total Fat: 7g	Dietary Fibre: 9g
Saturated Fat: 1g	Sugar: 3g
Cholesterol: 0	Protein: 10g

12. TOFU, TOMATO, and BLACK OLIVE SALAD

6 leaves fresh basil, slivered
120g (4oz) block of firm tofu, cut into cubes
2 plum tomatoes, diced
2 Tbsp. diced black olives
1 Tbsp. chopped fresh parsley
1 tsp. red wine vinegar
1 Tbsp. olive oil
1 Tbsp. chopped red onion

Combine all ingredients in a medium bowl and chill for several hours.

SERVES I

Nutrition Facts per Serving

Calories: 260	Sodium: 115mg
Calories from Fat: 180	Total Carbohydrate: 11g
Total Fat: 20g	Dietary Fibre: 2g
Saturated Fat: 2.5g	Sugar: 5g
Cholesterol: 0	Protein: 10g

13. HARICOT SALAD

225g (½lb) dried white beans, washed and soaked overnight
875ml (28fl oz) water
1 medium onion, coarsely chopped
2 garlic cloves, chopped
1 medium red onion, finely chopped
1 medium yellow or red pepper, chopped
1 garlic clove, minced
½ tsp. dried mustard
1 Tbsp. flaxseed oil or olive oil
Lemon juice to taste
Balsamic vinegar to taste
1 bunch fresh parsley, stems removed and chopped

Drain the beans and place in a pot with water, coarsely chopped onion, and chopped garlic cloves. Bring to a boil; reduce heat and simmer for 1½ hours or until tender. Drain and reserve 60ml (2fl oz) of the cooking liquid.

Mix the red onion, pepper, minced garlic, mustard, flaxseed oil, lemon juice, and vinegar with the reserved liquid in a large bowl. Add the warm beans and toss with parsley. Chill several hours before serving.

SERVES 4

Nutrition Facts per Serving

Calories: 270	Sodium: 20mg
Calories from Fat: 40	Total Carbohydrate: 45g
Total Fat: 4g	Dietary Fibre: 11g
Saturated Fat: 0g	Sugar: 12g
Cholesterol: 0	Protein: 15g

14. PINTO BEAN SALAD

1 Tbsp. olive oil
1 350g (14oz) can unsalted or low-sodium pinto beans, drained and rinsed
1 medium tomato, chopped
25g (¾oz) diced red onion
1 tsp. dried basil
½ tsp. lemon rind
1½ tsp. lemon juice
1 Tbsp. balsamic vinegar
½ tsp. honey
⅛ tsp. black pepper

Combine all ingredients in a medium bowl and chill for several hours.

SERVES 2

Nutrition Facts per Serving

Calories: 260	Sodium: 35mg
Calories from Fat: 60g	Total Carbohydrate: 38g
Total Fat: 7g	Dietary Fibre: 11g
Saturated Fat: 1g	Sugar: 6g
Cholesterol: 0	Protein: 11g

VEGETABLES

15. ASPARAGUS with TOMATOES and OLIVE OIL

60g (2oz) finely chopped onion
1 clove garlic, chopped
60ml (2fl oz) extra virgin olive oil
700g (1½lb) fresh asparagus, ends removed and cut into 2-inch pieces
325g (12oz) chopped fresh tomatoes
Black pepper to taste
1 Tbsp. lemon juice

In a large saucepan, cook the onion and garlic in olive oil until the onion is golden and starting to brown. Rinse the asparagus and add to the onions. Mix well, cover, and cook on medium-low for about 5 minutes. Add tomatoes and pepper. Cover and cook about 40 minutes, until asparagus is soft and tomatoes have dissolved into a sauce. Stir in lemon juice.

SERVES 4

Nutrition Facts per Serving

Calories: 170	Sodium: 20mg
Calories from Fat: 130	Total Carbohydrate: 10g
Total Fat: 14g	Dietary Fibre: 3g
Saturated Fat: 2g	Sugar: 5g
Cholesterol: 0	Protein: 3g

16. DR. SINATRA'S FAVOURITE SHIITAKE RECIPE

225g (½lb) fresh shiitake mushroom, diced
12 garlic cloves, finely chopped
4 Tbsp. water
2 180g (6oz) jars of marinated artichoke hearts
Chopped fresh coriander
Chopped fresh parsley
Freshly ground black pepper

Lightly cook the shiitakes and garlic in the water in a frying pan. Cover the pan briefly while they cook. When heated through, add the artichoke hearts with their liquid. Sauté a few minutes longer until the artichoke hearts are heated through. Sprinkle with coriander and parsley. Add pepper to taste.

SERVES 2

Nutrition Facts per Serving

Calories: 160	Sodium: 390mg
Calories from Fat: 50	Total Carbohydrate: 23g
Total Fat: 5g	Dietary Fibre: 5g
Saturated Fat: 0	Sugar: 2g
Cholesterol: 0	Protein: 7g

17. GRILLED COURGETTES

3 medium courgettes (approximately 2 lb), sliced lengthways
2 Tbsp. olive oil, divided
2 cloves garlic, minced
4 leaves of fresh basil, chopped

Heat a grill pan. Brush courgettes with 1 Tbsp. olive oil. Grill on each side for 2 minutes or until lightly browned. Remove to a platter. Sprinkle on garlic, basil, and remaining 1 Tbsp. olive oil. Cover with plastic wrap and allow flavours to mellow for 2 hours at room temperature.

SERVES 3

Nutrition Facts per Serving

Calories: 130	Sodium: 10mg
Calories from Fat: 80	Total Carbohydrate: 9g
Total Fat: 9g	Dietary Fibre: 4g
Saturated Fat: 1.5g	Sugar: 3g
Cholesterol: 0	Protein: 4g

18. LENTILS with GARLIC and TOMATOES

1 350g (14oz) can unsalted or low-sodium lentils, drained and rinsed
1 clove garlic, crushed
1 medium tomato, diced
2 tsp. red wine vinegar
1 Tbsp. chopped fresh parsley
1 tsp. extra virgin olive oil

Combine all ingredients in a medium bowl. Allow to sit at room temperature for 30 minutes to blend flavours.

SERVES 2

Nutrition Facts per Serving

Calories: 220

Calories from Fat: 30

Total Fat: 3g

Saturated Fat: 0g

Cholesterol: 0

Sodium: 10mg

Total Carbohydrate: 36g

Dietary Fibre: 14g

Sugar: 5g

Protein: 15g

19. LENTILS and COURGETTES SAUTÉ

1 Tbsp. olive oil

1 shallot, finely chopped

225g (8oz) thinly sliced courgettes

125g (4½oz) unsalted or low-sodium canned lentils, drained and rinsed,
or 125g (4½oz) cooked lentils

1 tsp. sherry vinegar

Chopped fresh parsley

Heat oil in a frying pan over medium heat. Sauté shallots until softened and lightly brown. Add courgettes and cook for 2 minutes. Stir in lentils and heat through. Season with sherry vinegar and parsley.

SERVES 2

Nutrition Facts per Serving

Calories: 140

Calories from Fat: 60

Total Fat: 7g

Saturated Fat: 1g

Cholesterol: 0

Sodium: 5mg

Total Carbohydrate: 16g

Dietary Fibre: 6g

Sugar: 4g

Protein: 6g

20. ROAST VEGETABLES

120g (4oz) cubed courgettes

100g (3½oz) cubed aubergine

6 medium mushrooms, stems removed

2 small onions, peeled

4 plum tomatoes, quartered

150g (5oz) cubed yellow squash

1 Tbsp. olive oil

2 cloves of garlic, minced

3 sprigs fresh thyme or oregano

Mix all vegetables with olive oil and minced garlic. Place on a shallow baking sheet and top with herbs. Roast at 220°C/425°F/Gas mark 6 for 30 minutes.

SERVES 2

Nutrition Facts per Serving

Calories: 160

Calories from Fat: 70

Total Fat: 8g

Saturated Fat: 1g

Cholesterol: 0

Sodium: 20mg

Total Carbohydrate: 22g

Dietary Fibre: 5g

Sugar: 11g

Protein: 5g

21. SPINACH with PINE NUTS and GARLIC

1 Tbsp. olive oil

2 cloves garlic, minced

500g (1lb) spinach

1 Tbsp. pine nuts

Heat olive oil with garlic in large frying pan over medium heat until garlic is golden. Toss in spinach and cook several minutes or until wilted. Top with pine nuts and serve.

SERVES 2

Nutrition Facts per Serving

Calories: 140

Calories from Fat: 90

Total Fat: 10g

Saturated Fat: 1g

Cholesterol: 0

Sodium: 180mg

Total Carbohydrate: 10g

Dietary Fibre: 2g

Sugar: 0

Protein: 8g

22. SPELT PILAF with SHIITAKE or MAITAKE MUSHROOMS

1 Tbsp. olive oil

1 medium onion, chopped

375g (¾lb) of fresh shiitake or maitake mushrooms, stems removed and chopped

140g (4¾oz) spelt grain or brown rice, cooked according to package directions using low-sodium chicken stock in place of water

½ tsp. dried thyme

2 tsp. Worcestershire sauce

¼ tsp. black pepper

2 Tbsp. fresh parsley, chopped

Heat oil in a frying pan over medium heat. Sauté onions and mushrooms till lightly browned. Add spelt grain and seasonings; heat through. Fold in parsley and serve.

SERVES 4

Nutrition Facts per Serving

Calories: 260

Calories from Fat: 50

Total Fat: 6g

Saturated Fat: 1g

Cholesterol: 0

Sodium: 85mg

Total Carbohydrate: 49g

Dietary Fibre: 2g

Sugar: 3g

Protein: 10g

23. STEAMED VEGETABLES

4–6 Tbsp. water

125g (4½oz) sliced carrots

240g (8½oz) diced courgettes

240g (8½oz) chopped fresh broccoli

240g (8½oz) diced summer squash

50g (1¾oz) chopped mushrooms

75g (2½oz) chopped cauliflower

3 cloves garlic, minced

2 tsp. dried basil

1 Tbsp. olive oil

Freshly ground black pepper

2 Tbsp. grated Parmesan cheese

1 Tbsp. chopped fresh parsley

Place the water in a wok or frying pan. Use a steaming rack or tray if available. Place the chopped vegetables in the wok. Sprinkle garlic and basil on top and cover. Steam for several minutes until the vegetables are tender, stirring frequently if not using a rack. When tender, sprinkle olive oil over the mixture and add pepper to taste. Sprinkle cheese and parsley over the steamed vegetables.

SERVES 4

Nutrition Facts per Serving

Calories: 110

Calories from Fat: 45

Total Fat: 5g

Saturated Fat: 1g

Cholesterol: 0

Sodium: 105mg

Total Carbohydrate: 14g

Dietary Fibre: 6g

Sugar: 5g

Protein: 6g

24. STIR-FRIED MANGETOUT and SESAME SEEDS

1 tsp. olive oil
225g (8oz) mangetout
2 tsp. toasted sesame seeds

Heat olive oil in a frying pan over medium heat. Toss in mangetout and cook, stirring frequently for 1 minute. Remove to plate, sprinkle with sesame seeds, and serve.

SERVES 2

Nutrition Facts per Serving

Calories: 90	Sodium: 5mg
Calories from Fat: 40	Total Carbohydrate: 9g
Total Fat: 4g	Dietary Fibre: 3g
Saturated Fat: 0.5g	Sugar: 5g
Cholesterol: 0	Protein: 4g

25. HARICOT BEANS, GARLIC, and ROSEMARY

2 tsp. olive oil
2 cloves garlic, crushed
½ tsp. rosemary
1 350g (14oz) can unsalted or low-sodium haricot beans, drained and rinsed

Heat oil in a frying pan over medium heat. Cook garlic until golden. Add rosemary and beans. Stir frequently until heated through.

SERVES 2

Nutrition Facts per Serving

Calories: 210	Sodium: 10mg
Calories from Fat: 45	Total Carbohydrate: 31g
Total Fat: 5g	Dietary Fibre: 8g
Saturated Fat: 0.5g	Sugar: 6g
Cholesterol: 0	Protein: 12g

SOUPS

26. ANTIGUAN BLACK BEAN SOUP

1 Tbsp. olive oil
1 medium green pepper, chopped
1 medium onion, chopped
2 cloves garlic, minced
1 450g (15oz) can unsalted or low-sodium black beans, drained and rinsed
¼ tsp. black pepper
2 tsp. honey
240ml (8fl oz) low-sodium vegetable juice
950ml (32fl oz) low-sodium or reduced-sodium chicken stock
140g (4¾oz) cooked brown rice
Fresh parsley, chopped

In a large pot, heat oil over medium heat. Sauté green pepper, onion, and garlic until tender. Add rest of ingredients except rice and parsley, and simmer uncovered for 30–40 minutes. Stir in rice and garnish with fresh parsley.

SERVES 4

Nutrition Facts per Serving

Calories: 240	Sodium: 150mg
Calories from Fat: 60	Total Carbohydrate: 32g
Total Fat: 7g	Dietary Fibre: 7g
Saturated Fat: 1.5g	Sugar: 10g
Cholesterol: 5mg	Protein: 13g

27. CHICKEN VEGETABLE SOUP

1 medium onion, chopped
2 cloves garlic, minced
2 celery stalks, chopped
1 medium turnip, diced
50g (1¾oz) sliced mushrooms

2 tsp. each of dried thyme, tarragon, and parsley
½ tsp. black pepper
2 tsp. honey
1 Tbsp. Worcestershire sauce
1,125ml (140fl oz) low-sodium or reduced-sodium chicken stock, divided
500g (1lb) chicken breast, cooked and chopped
1 medium courgette, quartered and sliced
1 medium yellow summer squash, quartered and sliced

Place all vegetables except courgette and summer squash and 2 Tbsp. of the chicken stock in a large pot. Cook covered over medium heat till vegetables are tender, about 30–40 minutes. Stir frequently to prevent sticking. Uncover and add rest of ingredients. Bring to boil, reduce heat to low, and simmer uncovered for 15 minutes.

SERVES 4

Nutrition Facts per Serving

Calories: 230	Sodium: 290mg
Calories from Fat: 35	Total Carbohydrate: 16g
Total Fat: 3.5g	Dietary Fibre: 3g
Saturated Fat: 1.5g	Sugar: 9g
Cholesterol: 70mg	Protein: 32g

28. CHICKPEA and CHICORY SOUP

1 Tbsp olive oil
1 medium onion, chopped
4 cloves garlic, chopped
2 carrots, diced
1 350g (14oz) can unsalted or low-sodium chickpeas, drained and rinsed
150g (5oz) loosely packed chopped broad leafed chicory (or spinach) leaves
225g (8oz) low-sodium vegetable juice
1 Tbsp. brown sugar or honey
1 Tbsp. Worcestershire sauce
1 tsp. black pepper
900ml (32fl oz) of low-sodium or reduced-sodium chicken stock

Heat oil in large pot over medium heat. Cook vegetables until tender. Stir in rest of ingredients and bring to boil. Reduce heat to low, cover and simmer for 2 hours.

SERVES 4

Nutrition Facts per Serving

Calories: 250
Calories from Fat: 60
Total Fat: 7g
Saturated Fat: 1.5g
Cholesterol: 5mg

Sodium: 260mg
Total Carbohydrate: 38g
Dietary Fibre: 10g
Sugar: 13g
Protein: 12g

29. LENTIL SOUP

1 Tbsp. olive oil
1 medium onion, chopped
2 shallots, chopped
2 cloves of garlic, chopped
3 carrots, chopped
3 stalks of celery, chopped
1 450ml (14½fl oz) can low-sodium or reduced-sodium vegetable stock
1 420ml (14fl oz) can unsalted or low-sodium lentils, drained and rinsed
2 bay leaves
1 tsp. dried thyme
2 tsp. honey
1½ tsp. Worcestershire sauce
900ml (32fl oz) low-sodium vegetable juice
¼ tsp. black pepper

Heat oil in large pot over medium heat and sauté onion, shallots, garlic, carrots, and celery until softened. Add rest of ingredients and bring to a boil. Reduce heat to low and simmer covered for 30 minutes. Remove bay leaves before serving.

SERVES 4

Nutrition Facts per Serving

Calories: 270
Calories from Fat: 40
Total Fat: 4.5g
Saturated Fat: 1g
Cholesterol: 0

Sodium: 260mg
Total Carbohydrate: 45g
Dietary Fibre: 12g
Sugar: 20g
Protein: 13g

30. MINESTRONE SOUP

1 Tbsp. olive oil
1 medium onion, chopped
2 cloves of garlic, minced
2 stalks celery, chopped
180g (6oz) shredded cabbage

400ml (32fl oz) low-sodium or reduced-sodium beef stock
1 450g (15oz) can no-salt-added diced tomatoes, undrained
1 tsp. dried oregano
2 bay leaves
2 Tbsp. Worcestershire sauce
1 Tbsp. brown sugar or honey
1 350g (14oz) can unsalted or low-sodium kidney beans, drained and rinsed
2 medium courgettes, chopped
¾ cup macaroni pasta (whole wheat or spelt)
Black pepper to taste
Grated Parmesan cheese

In large pot heat oil over medium heat. Cook onion, garlic, and celery until tender. Add cabbage, beef broth, tomatoes and their juice, seasonings, and the beans. Bring to a boil, add courgettes and macaroni pasta, simmer 15 minutes. Remove bay leaves, and add pepper to taste. Sprinkle each serving with Parmesan cheese.

SERVES 4

Nutrition Facts per Serving

Calories: 270	Sodium: 230mg
Calories from Fat: 45	Total Carbohydrate: 42g
Total Fat: 5g	Dietary Fibre: 14g
Saturated Fat: 1g	Sugar: 12g
Cholesterol: 0	Protein: 18g

31. VEGETABLE SOUP

2 Tbsp. olive oil
1 medium onion, chopped
125g (4½oz) shredded cabbage
2 stalks celery, chopped
300g (10oz) package sliced fresh mushrooms
3 cloves garlic, chopped
1 tsp. dried thyme
1 bay leaf
½ tsp. dried rosemary
½ tsp. dried parsley
1 tsp. honey
¼ tsp. pepper
1 Tbsp. Worcestershire sauce
175g (5¾oz) fresh or frozen sweetcorn
900ml (32fl oz) low-sodium or reduced-sodium chicken stock
1 450g (15oz) can unsalted stewed tomatoes, undrained

In a large pot, heat oil over medium heat and lightly sauté all vegetables except corn till tender. Add seasonings, corn, stock, and tomatoes. Bring to a boil. Reduce heat to low and simmer 1 hour uncovered. Discard bay leaf before serving.

SERVES 4

Nutrition Facts per Serving

Calories: 210

Calories from Fat: 80

Total Fat: 9g

Saturated Fat: 2g

Cholesterol: 5mg

Sodium: 190mg

Total Carbohydrate: 28g

Dietary Fibre: 5g

Sugar: 11g

Protein: 8g

32. VEGGIE MISO SOUP

1,400ml (48fl oz) water

4 cloves garlic, minced

4 carrots, chopped

1 medium onion, chopped

2 stalks celery, chopped

300g (10oz) shredded cabbage

225g (8oz) broccoli florets, chopped

4 shiitake mushrooms, quartered

2 Tbsp. miso (found in health food shops)

120g (4oz) firm tofu, cut into cubes

In a large covered pot, bring water, garlic, carrots, onion, celery, and cabbage to a boil. Uncover, reduce heat to low, and simmer for 30 minutes. Add broccoli, mushrooms, and miso. Simmer another 15 minutes. Add tofu just before serving.

SERVES 4

Nutrition Facts per Serving

Calories: 120

Calories from Fat: 20

Total Fat: 2g

Saturated Fat: 0g

Cholesterol: 0

Sodium: 370mg

Total Carbohydrate: 21g

Dietary Fibre: 6g

Sugar: 9g

Protein: 7g

TOFU/TEMPEH

33. GRILLED TOFU

2 Tbsp. low-sodium soya sauce
2 spring onions, slivered
1 tsp. grated fresh ginger
225g (8oz) block of firm tofu, cut into ½-inch slices
Olive oil for greasing the pan

Combine soya sauce, spring onions, and ginger. Lay slices of tofu in soya mixture to marinate for 10 minutes. Place tofu on a grill rack greased with olive oil and grill 2 minutes each side.

SERVES 2

Nutrition Facts per Serving

Calories: 100	Sodium: 540mg
Calories from Fat: 45	Total Carbohydrate: 6g
Total Fat: 5g	Dietary Fibre: <1g
Saturated Fat: 0.5g	Sugar: 1g
Cholesterol: 0	Protein: 10g

34. STIR-FRIED TEMPEH and MAITAKE/SHIITAKE MUSHROOMS and MANGETOUT

225g (8oz) salt-free tempeh, cut into slices
3 tsp. low-sodium soy sauce
1 Tbsp. toasted sesame oil
50g (1¾oz) fresh maitake or shiitake mushrooms, stems removed and sliced
2 cloves of garlic, minced
1 yellow pepper, chopped
1 tsp. grated fresh ginger
4 spring onions, chopped
120g (4oz) fresh mangetout
½ tsp. cornflour
120ml (4fl oz) unsweetened stewed apples
1 Tbsp. treacle
75g (2½oz) cooked brown rice

Soak tempeh in soy sauce for 10 minutes. Heat 1 tsp. sesame oil in a large frying pan over medium heat. Remove tempeh from soy sauce and reserve any remaining soy sauce. Lightly sauté tempeh strips on both sides and remove to a plate. Heat remaining 2 tsp. of sesame oil in the pan and sauté mushrooms and garlic for 2–3 minutes until lightly brown. Add yellow pepper, ginger, and spring onions and sauté until pepper is tender. Add mangetout and cook for 1 minute, stirring almost constantly. Remove all vegetables from the pan. Mix together cornflour, apple juice, treacle, and any remaining soy sauce in a small bowl. Add this mixture to the frying pan and cook till bubbly. Add vegetables and tempeh and heat through. Serve over rice.

SERVES 2

Nutrition Facts per Serving

Calories: 580	Sodium: 570mg
Calories from Fat: 110	Total Carbohydrate: 99g
Total Fat: 13g	Dietary Fibre: 12g
Saturated Fat: 3g	Sugar: 20g
Cholesterol: 0	Protein: 20g

35. STIR-FRIED TOFU and VEGETABLES

325g (12oz) package of firm tofu
2 Tbsp. low-sodium soy sauce
3 tsp. toasted sesame oil, divided
240g (8½oz) broccoli florets
1 orange pepper, chopped
1 medium courgette, sliced
90g (3oz) mangetout
2 tsp. cornflour
120g (4oz) unsweetened stewed apples
1 Tbsp. honey
⅛ tsp. ground ginger
60ml (2fl oz) water
1 tsp. low-sodium or less-sodium instant chicken stock (in health food shops)
75g (2½oz) cooked brown rice, cooked according to package directions

Marinate tofu in soy sauce for 10 minutes. Heat 1 tsp. sesame oil in a large frying pan over medium heat. Remove tofu from soy sauce and reserve any remaining soy sauce. Lightly sauté tofu on both sides and remove to a plate. Heat remaining 2 tsp. of sesame oil in the pan and sauté broccoli, covered, for 5 minutes until lightly brown. Remove cover, add orange pepper, and sauté until pepper is tender. Add courgette and cook for 3–5 minutes, or until courgette is tender. Add mangetout and cook 1 minute. Remove all vegetables from the pan.

Mix together cornflour, apple juice, honey, ginger, water, instant stock, and any remaining soy sauce in a small bowl. Add this mixture to the frying pan and cook till bubbly. Add vegetables and tofu and heat through. Serve over rice.

SERVES 2

Nutrition Facts per Serving

Calories: 510	Sodium: 680mg
Calories from Fat: 150	Total Carbohydrate: 73g
Total Fat: 17g	Dietary Fibre: 7g
Saturated Fat: 2.5g	Sugar: 22g
Cholesterol: 0	Protein: 22g

36. TEMPEH and STIR-FRIED VEGETABLES

225g (8oz) salt-free tempeh, cut into slices
2 tsp. honey
2 tsp. balsamic vinegar
1 Tbsp. grated fresh ginger
2 Tbsp. low-sodium soy sauce
3 tsp. toasted sesame oil
2 cloves of garlic, minced
2 carrots, thinly sliced
1 celery stalk, chopped
2 spring onions, chopped
1 medium courgette, sliced
2 tsp. cornflour
125g (4oz) unsweetened stewed apples
60ml (2fl oz) water
¼ tsp. black pepper
1 tsp. instant low-sodium or less-sodium chicken stock
75g brown rice, cooked according to package directions

Mix tempeh with honey, balsamic vinegar, ginger, and soy sauce and let soak for 10 minutes. Heat 1 tsp. sesame oil in a large frying pan over medium heat. Remove tempeh from marinade and reserve any remaining liquid. Lightly sauté tempeh strips on both sides and remove to a plate. Heat remaining 2 tsp. of sesame oil in the pan and sauté garlic, carrots, and celery for 5 minutes or until lightly brown, stirring frequently. Add spring onions and courgette and cook for 3–5 minutes, or until courgette is tender. Remove all vegetables from the pan. Mix together cornflour, apple juice, water, black pepper, instant stock, and any remaining marinade in a small bowl. Add this mixture to the frying pan and cook till bubbly. Add vegetables and tempeh and heat through. Serve over rice.

SERVES 2

Nutrition Facts per Serving

Calories: 560

Calories from Fat: 120

Total Fat: 13g

Saturated Fat: 3g

Cholesterol: 0

Sodium: 720mg

Total Carbohydrate: 93g

Dietary Fibre: 12g

Sugar: 23g

Protein: 20g

37. TVP CHILLI

1 Tbsp extra virgin olive oil

2 cloves garlic, diced

1 medium onion, diced

1 medium green pepper, diced

1 medium yellow pepper, diced

2 Tbsp. salt-free chilli powder (available in health food shops)

1 tsp. ground cumin

¼ tsp. black pepper

¼ tsp. cayenne pepper, optional

350ml (12fl oz) salt-free tomato puree

120g (4oz) of dehydrated TVP, rehydrated according to package directions

1 820g (28oz) can unsalted whole peeled tomatoes, undrained

2 450g (15oz) cans unsalted or low-sodium kidney beans, rinsed and drained

175g (5¾oz) fresh or frozen sweetcorn

2 tsp. honey

2 tsp. salt free tomato paste

125g (4½oz) shredded soya cheese

Heat oil in large pot over medium heat. Add garlic, onions, and peppers; cover pot and cook about 10 minutes or until vegetables are tender. Remove cover and add spices. Sauté 2 minutes. Lower heat and add remaining ingredients except soya cheese. Break up whole tomatoes with kitchen scissors or your fingers. Simmer uncovered 1–1½ hours. Sprinkle each serving with cheese.

Nutrition Facts per Serving

Calories: 330

Calories from Fat: 45

Total Fat: 5g

Saturated Fat: 0g

Cholesterol: 0

Sodium: 140mg

Total Carbohydrate: 54g

Dietary Fibre: 19g

Sugar: 15g

Protein: 27g

38. TEMPEH CHILLI

1 Tbsp. olive oil
3 cloves garlic, chopped
1 medium onion, chopped
1 green pepper, chopped
4 carrots, sliced
2 Tbsp. salt-free chilli powder (available in health food shops)
¼ tsp. cayenne pepper, or more to taste
1 tsp. cumin
1 450g (15oz) can unsalted or low-sodium pinto beans, drained and rinsed*
1 450g (15oz) can unsalted or low-sodium black beans, drained and rinsed*
4 tsp. honey
225g (8oz) salt-free tempeh, cut into slices
810g (28oz) can unsalted whole tomatoes in tomato puree, undrained
350ml (12fl oz) unsalted tomato puree
125g (4½oz) shredded soya cheddar cheese

Heat oil in large pot over medium heat. Add garlic, onions, peppers, and carrots; cover pot and cook about 10 minutes or until vegetables are tender. Remove cover and add spices. Sauté 2 minutes. Lower heat and add remaining ingredients except soya cheese. Break up whole tomatoes with kitchen scissors or your fingers. Simmer uncovered 1–1½ hours. Sprinkle each serving with cheese.

SERVES 4

Nutrition Facts per Serving

Calories: 340	Sodium: 150mg
Calories from Fat: 60	Total Carbohydrate: 51g
Total Fat: 7g	Dietary Fibre: 13g
Saturated Fat: 1g	Sugar: 17g
Cholesterol: 0	Protein: 21g

* If desired, you can substitute any type of low-salt canned or cooked beans

39. TOFU with SESAME SEEDS

225g (8oz) firm tofu
2 Tbsp. toasted sesame seeds
1 clove garlic, minced
8 spring onions, chopped
2 Tbsp. low-sodium soy sauce
60ml (2fl oz) rice wine

Chop tofu into 1-inch cubes. Sprinkle sesame seeds into tofu. Add garlic, spring onions, soy sauce, and rice wine and mix well. Chill several hours before serving.

SERVES 2

Nutrition Facts per Serving

Calories: 210

Calories from Fat: 90

Total Fat: 10g

Saturated Fat: 1.5g

Cholesterol: 0

Sodium: 550mg

Total Carbohydrate: 11g

Dietary Fibre: 3g

Sugar: 2g

Protein: 14g

POULTRY, BEEF, and PORK

40. CHICKEN BREASTS STUFFED with SPINACH

2 120–150g (4–5oz) boneless, skinless chicken breasts
1 Tbsp. extra virgin olive oil
50g (1¾oz) grated carrot
25g (¾oz) chopped fresh spinach
1 tsp. dried basil
4 Tbsp. grated Parmesan or Romano cheese
Black pepper to taste

Preheat oven to 400°F/200°C/Gas mark 5. Slice the chicken breasts halfway through the centre lengthways, forming a pocket. Heat 2 tsp. of the oil in a frying-pan over medium-low heat. Stir in the carrots and heat until softened, about 5 minutes. Add the spinach and basil. Cook about 3 minutes or until wilted. Remove from heat. Add the cheese and stir to combine. Stuff the mixture into the chicken pockets. Soak toothpicks in water and use them to secure the chicken pockets. Lightly brush with remaining oil and sprinkle with pepper. Bake for 30 minutes or until the chicken juices run clear.

SERVES 2

Nutrition Facts per Serving

Calories: 230	Sodium: 160mg
Calories from Fat: 80	Total Carbohydrate: 4g
Total Fat: 9g	Dietary Fibre: 2g
Saturated Fat: 2g	Sugar: 2g
Cholesterol: 75	Protein: 32g

41. CHICKEN and RED PEPPER KEBAB

1 Tbsp. olive oil
2 tsp. lime juice
1 tsp. cumin
1 225–300g (8–10oz) boneless, skinless chicken breast, cut into 3cm (1½-in)
cubes
1 medium red pepper, cut into 2cm (1-in) squares
1 medium onion, separated and cut into 2cm (1-in) pieces
1 Tbsp. chopped fresh coriander

Combine olive oil, lime juice, and cumin. Pour over chicken breast and marinate in refrigerator for 2 hours. Thread on skewers alternating with red pepper and onion. Grill 5–7 minutes, turning over once or twice. Sprinkle with coriander and serve.

SERVES 2

Nutrition Facts per Serving

Calories: 250	Sodium: 90mg
Calories from Fat: 80	Total Carbohydrate: 12g
Total Fat: 9g	Dietary Fibre: 3g
Saturated Fat: 1.5g	Sugar: 6g
Cholesterol: 75mg	Protein: 31g

42. EASY GRILLED CHICKEN BREAST

1 225–300g (8–10oz) boneless, skinless chicken breast
170ml (6fl oz) extra virgin olive oil
Black pepper to taste

Marinate the chicken in olive oil for at least 2 hours. (Marinating overnight provides a more flavourful chicken.) Remove from the marinade and discard the remaining marinade. Sprinkle the chicken with pepper, place on a grill pan, and grill 4–5 minutes on each side until cooked through.

SERVES 2

Nutrition Facts per Serving

Calories: 260	Sodium: 85mg
Calories from Fat: 140	Total Carbohydrate: 0
Total Fat: 15g	Dietary Fibre: 0
Saturated Fat: 2g	Sugar: 0
Cholesterol: 75mg	Protein: 29g

43. GRILLED CHICKEN TERIYAKI

1 225–300g (8–10oz) boneless, skinless chicken breast, split and pounded thin
2 Tbsp. low-sodium soy sauce
1 tsp. honey
1 Tbsp. dry sherry
120ml (4fl oz) unsweetened canned pineapple juice
1 tsp. grated ginger
2 slices canned pineapple
1 spring onion, slivered

Place chicken breast in a shallow glass or ceramic pan. Combine soy sauce, honey, sherry, pineapple juice, and ginger and pour over chicken breast. Cover with cling film and marinate in refrigerator for 2–4 hours. Heat up grill pan and cook chicken for 4–5 minutes on each side or until cooked through. Discard any remaining marinade. Grill pineapple briefly if desired. Garnish with spring onions and sliced pineapple.

SERVES 2

Nutrition Facts per Serving

Calories: 220	Sodium: 360mg
Calories from Fat: 15	Total Carbohydrate: 19g
Total Fat: 1.5g	Dietary Fibre: >1g
Saturated Fat: 0	Sugar: 16g
Cholesterol: 75mg	Protein: 30g

44. GRILLED ROSEMARY CHICKEN BREAST

1 Tbsp. olive oil
¼ tsp. black pepper
1 tsp. dried rosemary
½ tsp. paprika
½ tsp. onion powder
1 225–300g (8–10oz) boneless, skinless chicken breast, cut in half

Combine olive oil, pepper, rosemary, paprika and onion powder. Rub on chicken breast and refrigerate for 2 hours. Grill chicken approximately 4–5 minutes on each side, or until cooked through.

SERVES 2

Nutrition Facts per Serving

Calories: 210	Sodium: 85mg
Calories from Fat: 80	Total Carbohydrate: 1g
Total Fat: 9g	Dietary Fibre: 0
Saturated Fat: 1.5g	Sugar: 0
Cholesterol: 75mg	Protein: 30g

45. LOW-FAT EXCEPTIONAL HAMBURGERS

500g (1lb) extra lean mince
2 cloves garlic, minced
1 tsp. onion powder
¼ tsp. black pepper
1 Tbsp. Worcestershire sauce

Mix mince with seasoning. Form meat into 125g (4½oz) burgers. Fry burgers in a non-stick frying pan over medium heat until cooked to the desired degree.

SERVES 4

Nutrition Facts per Serving

Calories: 150	Sodium: 100mg
Calories from Fat: 40	Total Carbohydrate: 2g
Total Fat: 4.5g	Dietary Fibre: 0
Saturated Fat: 1g	Sugar: 0
Cholesterol: 55mg	Protein: 25g

46. ROAST PORK TENDERLOIN with MUSTARD

500g (1lb) boneless pork tenderloin
¼ tsp. black pepper
1 Tbsp. olive oil
1 tsp. crushed thyme
1 Tbsp. Dijon mustard

Season meat with black pepper. Heat oil in a pan and brown meat on all sides. Sprinkle with thyme and spread with Dijon mustard. Roast 45 minutes to 1 hour at 375°F/190°C/Gas mark 4.

SERVES 4

Nutrition Facts per Serving

Calories: 170	Sodium: 150mg
Calories from Fat: 70	Total Carbohydrate: 1g
Total Fat: 8g	Dietary Fibre: 0
Saturated Fat: 2g	Sugar: 0
Cholesterol: 75mg	Protein: 24g

47. ROAST PORK TENDERLOIN
with ROSEMARY and GARLIC

500g (1lb) boneless pork tenderloin
1 tsp. dried rosemary
1 Tbsp. olive oil
⅛ tsp. black pepper
2 cloves garlic, crushed

Season the meat with rosemary, oil, pepper, and garlic. Roast for 1 hour at 375°/190°/Gas mark 4.

SERVES 4

Nutrition Facts per Serving

Calories: 170	Sodium: 55mg
Calories from Fat: 70	Total Carbohydrate: 1g
Total Fat: 7g	Dietary Fibre: 0
Saturated Fat: 2g	Sugar: 0
Cholesterol: 75mg	Protein: 24g

48. STIR-FRIED CHICKEN and BROCCOLI

1 225–300g (8–10oz) boneless, skinless chicken breast, cut into cubes
2 Tbsp. low-sodium soy sauce
1 tsp. honey
1 tsp. cornflour
2 tsp. toasted sesame oil
3 tsp. olive oil
2 tsp. chopped fresh ginger
240g (8½oz) broccoli florets
2 spring onions, slivered
75g (2½oz) cooked brown rice, cooked according to package directions

Marinate chicken in soy sauce, honey, cornflour, and sesame oil. Heat 2 tsp. olive oil in pan. Add chicken and stir for 5 minutes, turning frequently. Remove chicken and set aside. Lower heat and add remaining 1 tsp. oil and ginger; cook for 30 seconds. Add broccoli and spring onions and cook for 2 minutes more. Add back chicken and mix into vegetables. Serve over rice.

SERVES 2

Nutrition Facts per Serving

Calories: 460	Sodium: 640mg
Calories from Fat: 130	Total Carbohydrate: 46g
Total Fat: 15g	Dietary Fibre: 4g
Saturated Fat: 2.5g	Sugar: 5g
Cholesterol: 75mg	Protein: 36g

49. TURKEY MEATLOAF

1 Tbsp. olive oil
1 medium onion, chopped
2 carrots, finely grated
650g (1⅓lb) ground turkey breast
150g (5oz) oatmeal
1 150g (5½fl oz) can of low-sodium V-8 juice
1 Tbsp. dried parsley
¼ tsp. black pepper
½ tsp. garlic powder
1 large egg, beaten
1 tsp. honey
2 tsp. Worcestershire sauce
1 Tbsp. Dijon mustard
½ tsp. dried marjoram

Topping:
120ml (14fl oz) unsalted tomato passata
1 tsp honey

Preheat oven to 350°F/180°C/Gas mark 3. Spray a 22cm × 12cm (9 × 5-in) loaf pan with non-stick spray. Heat oil in a medium frying pan over medium heat and sauté onion and carrots till tender. In a large bowl, combine all ingredients except topping. Pat turkey mixture into 22cm × 12cm (9 × 5-in) loaf pan. Mix topping ingredients and spread on turkey mixture. Bake 45 minutes.

SERVES 4

Nutrition Facts per Serving

Calories: 220	Sodium: 170mg
Calories from Fat: 40	Total Carbohydrate: 15g
Total Fat: 4.5g	Dietary Fibre: 3g
Saturated Fat: 1g	Sugar: 6g
Cholesterol: 100mg	Protein: 26g

SEAFOOD

50. BREADED SOLE or FLOUNDER

1 large egg
1 large egg white
70g (2¼oz) wholemeal bread crumbs
1 tsp. paprika
¼ tsp. black pepper
2 tsp. dried parsley
500g (1lb) sole or flounder, cut in 4 pieces
2 Tbsp. olive oil
Lemon slices

Beat together egg and egg white. Mix together the bread crumbs and seasoning. Dip fish in beaten eggs then roll in bread crumbs. Heat olive oil in a large frying pan over medium high heat and fry fish several minutes on each side or until fish flakes easily. Serve with lemon slices.

SERVES 4

Nutrition Facts per Serving

Calories: 220	Sodium: 210mg
Calories from Fat: 90	Total Carbohydrate: 7g
Total Fat: 10g	Dietary Fibre: 1g
Saturated Fat: 2g	Sugar: 1g
Cholesterol: 105mg	Protein: 25g

51. GRILLED MEDITERRANEAN HALIBUT

Juice of 1 lemon
2 Tbsp. olive oil
3 cloves garlic, crushed
½ tsp. grated lemon peel
3 Tbsp. fresh basil or 1 Tbsp dried
2 tsp. drained capers
4 150–180g (5–6oz) halibut steaks
Freshly ground black pepper to taste

Preheat grill. Combine lemon juice, olive oil, garlic, and lemon peel in a small bowl. Stir in 2 tablespoons basil and capers. Season halibut with pepper and brush with 1 tablespoon of lemon vinaigrette. Grill until cooked through, about 4 minutes on each side. Transfer to a plate. Rewhisk remaining vinaigrette and pour over fish. Garnish with remaining tablespoon of basil.

SERVES 4

Nutrition Facts per Serving

Calories: 240	Sodium: 125mg
Calories from Fat: 90	Total Carbohydrate: 2g
Total Fat: 10g	Dietary Fibre: 0
Saturated Fat: 1.5g	Sugar: 0
Cholesterol: 50mg	Protein: 33g

52. GRILLED RED SNAPPER

1 Tbsp. olive oil
1 Tbsp. lemon juice
500g (1lb) snapper fillet
Black pepper

Preheat grill. Combine olive oil and lemon juice and brush on fillet. Dust with black pepper. Grill 12cm (5 in) from grill for 5 minutes or until fish flakes easily.

SERVES 4

Nutrition Facts per Serving

Calories: 140	Sodium: 75mg
Calories from Fat: 45	Total Carbohydrate: 0
Total Fat: 5g	Dietary Fibre: 0
Saturated Fat: 1g	Sugar: 0
Cholesterol: 40mg	Protein: 23g

53. GRILLED PRAWNS

3 cloves garlic, crushed
1 Tbsp. olive oil
1 Tbsp. lemon juice
1 tsp. paprika
Pinch red pepper
500g (1lb) fresh prawns, peeled

Combine garlic, olive oil, lemon juice, paprika, and red pepper and pour over prawns. Mix well and marinate in refrigerator for several hours, stirring several

times. Heat a large frying pan over medium heat and cook prawns in their marinade 3 minutes on each side or until prawns are opaque.

SERVES 2

Nutrition Facts per Serving

Calories: 210
Calories from Fat: 80
Total Fat: 8g
Saturated Fat: 1.5g
Cholesterol: 270mg

Sodium: 310mg
Total Carbohydrate: 3g
Dietary Fibre: 0
Sugar: 0
Protein: 29g

54. MUSSELS PROVENÇAL

2 tsp. olive oil
3 Tbsp. chopped shallots
4 cloves garlic, minced
½ medium red pepper, chopped
240ml (8fl oz) no-salt-added whole tomatoes with juice
½ tsp. ground tumeric
¼ tsp. black pepper
1 tsp. thyme
1 tsp. sherry vinegar
2 tsp. dried parsley
Red pepper flakes, to taste
500g (1lb) mussels, washed in cold water
2 Tbsp. chopped fresh basil

Heat oil in a large frying pan over medium heat and cook shallots, garlic, and
red pepper till tender, stirring often. Add tomatoes and seasonings; bring to a
boil, reduce heat, and simmer for 2 minutes. Add mussels and fresh basil; cover
and cook until mussels open, 5–6 minutes. Discard any shells that do not open.

SERVES 2

Nutrition Facts per Serving

Calories: 290
Calories from Fat: 90
Total Fat: 10g
Saturated Fat: 1.5g
Cholesterol: 65mg

Sodium: 670mg
Total Carbohydrate: 21g
Dietary Fibre: 3g
Sugar: 9g
Protein: 29g

55. POACHED SALMON with DILL SAUCE

3 lemon slices
2 peppercorns
2 slices white onion
1 parsley sprig
450ml (16fl oz) water
225g (8oz) salmon fillet, cut into two servings

Yogurt Sauce:
1 Tbsp. light soya mayonnaise
3 Tbsp. fat-free plain yogurt
2 tsp. fresh dill
1–2 Tbsp. skimmed milk

Place all ingredients, except salmon, into a large pan and simmer, covered, for 10 minutes. Add salmon fillet and cook for 10 minutes over medium heat until flesh is cooked through. Remove fish from poaching liquid and chill in refrigerator for 1–2 hours. Meanwhile make yogurt sauce. In a small bowl mix the mayonnaise, yogurt, and dill and thin with milk until desired consistency. Serve sauce with salmon.

SERVES 2

Nutrition Facts per Serving

Calories: 200	Sodium: 130mg
Calories from Fat: 90	Total Carbohydrate: 3g
Total Fat: 10g	Dietary Fibre: 0
Saturated Fat: 1.5g	Sugar: 2g
Cholesterol: 65mg	Protein: 24g

56. ROAST SALMON

225g (8oz) salmon fillet
1 Tbsp. olive oil
1 clove garlic, crushed
1 Tbsp. chopped fresh dill
Black pepper to taste
1 Tbsp. chopped fresh parsley
1 lemon

Preheat oven to 425°F/220°C/Gas mark 6. Cut salmon in half to form two pieces. Rub with olive oil, garlic, dill, and pepper. Roast 6–8 minutes, depending on thickness. Garnish with parsley and fresh lemon.

SERVES 2

Nutrition Facts per Serving

Calories: 230

Calories from Fat: 130

Total Fat: 14g

Saturated Fat: 2g

Cholesterol: 60mg

Sodium: 50mg

Total Carbohydrate: 2g

Dietary Fibre: 0

Sugar: 1g

Protein: 23g

57. SANDY'S CRAB CAKES

2 180g (6oz) cans lump crab meat, drained

2 eggs

30g (1oz) instant potato flakes

30g (1oz) amaranth flour

30g (1oz) minced onion

2 tsp. dried basil

2 tsp. dried parsley

Dash of hot sauce

1 tsp. paprika

1 stalk celery, finely chopped

2 tsp. skimmed milk

Pepper to taste

1 Tbsp. extra virgin olive oil for sautéing

Easy Remoulade Sauce (recipe follows)

Using your hands, thoroughly mix together all the ingredients for the crab cakes, except the oil, in a large bowl. Hand form mixture into patties and sauté them in a skillet in hot olive oil. After a minute or so, flip the cakes so they are browned on both sides. Remove from the oil and drain on paper towels. Serve hot with Remoulade sauce.

EASY REMOULADE SAUCE

In a small bowl, mix together equal amounts of salsa and light soya mayonnaise. Add horseradish if desired.

SERVES 4

Nutrition Facts per Serving

Calories: 250

Calories from Fat: 110

Total Fat: 12g

Saturated Fat: 2.5g

Cholesterol: 160mg

Sodium: 600mg

Total Carbohydrate: 15g

Dietary Fibre: 2g

Sugar: 3g

Protein: 19g

58. SCALLOP KEBAB

1 Tbsp. olive oil
6 basil leaves, sliced
2 cloves garlic, slivered
225g (8oz) sea scallops
1 lemon, thinly sliced

Combine olive oil, basil, and garlic and pour over scallops to marinate. Keep scallops refrigerated for 3 hours. Thread scallops on skewers, separated by slices of lemon. Grill 3–5 minutes or until lightly browned on all sides.

SERVES 2

Nutrition Facts per Serving

Calories: 160

Calories from Fat: 70

Total Fat: 8g

Saturated Fat: 1g

Cholesterol: 35mg

Sodium: 180mg

Total Carbohydrate: 4g

Dietary Fibre: 0

Sugar: 0

Protein: 19g

59. ORANGE PRAWNS with COUSCOUS

½ Tbsp. olive oil
1 medium red onion, chopped
½ Tbsp. fresh ginger, finely grated
1 green pepper, chopped
2 tsp. cornflour
160ml (5½fl oz) orange juice
¼ tsp. black pepper
1 Tbsp. all-fruit orange marmalade
½ Tbsp. lime juice
500g (1lb) cooked large prawns
300g (10oz) can mandarin orange segments, drained
125g (4½oz) couscous, cooked according to package directions

Heat oil in a large frying pan over medium heat and sauté onion, ginger, and green pepper until tender. Dissolve cornflour in orange juice and add to pan along with black pepper, orange marmalade, lime juice, and prawns. Bring to a boil; remove from heat and gently stir in orange segments. Serve over couscous.

SERVES 4

Nutrition Facts per Serving

Calories: 320

Calories from Fat: 30

Total Fat: 3g

Saturated Fat: 0.5g

Cholesterol: 220mg

Sodium: 260mg

Total Carbohydrate: 42g

Dietary Fibre: 3g

Sugar: 14g

Protein: 29g

60. PRAWNS with PEPPERS, TOMATOES, and GARLIC

1 Tbsp. olive oil

2 cloves garlic, minced

1 green pepper, chopped

1 red pepper, chopped

1 medium onion, chopped

60ml (2fl oz) cooking sherry

1 tsp. ground coriander seed

250ml (8fl oz) no-salt-added crushed tomatoes

240ml (8fl oz) no-salt-added tomato sauce

¼ tsp. black pepper

½ tsp. brown sugar or honey

500g (1lb) cooked large prawns

225g (8oz) wholemeal pasta, cooked according to package directions

Heat oil in a large frying pan over medium heat and sauté garlic, peppers, and onion until tender. Add sherry and bring to a boil. Add rest of ingredients, bring to a boil again, and then serve over pasta.

SERVES 4

Nutrition Facts per Serving

Calories: 430

Calories from Fat: 50

Total Fat: 6g

Saturated Fat: 1g

Cholesterol: 220mg

Sodium: 370mg

Total Carbohydrate: 59g

Dietary Fibre: 11g

Sugar: 9g

Protein: 35g

61. STEAMED MUSSELS

1 Tbsp. olive oil
1 small onion, chopped
2 cloves garlic, minced
500g (1lb) mussels, washed
500g (1lb) fresh tomatoes, chopped
2 Tbsp. white wine
Chopped fresh parsley for garnish

Heat olive oil in a large pan. Cook onion until soft. Add garlic. Stir in mussels, tomatoes, and wine. Cover and cook until mussels open, about 3–4 minutes. Discard shells that do not open. Serve in soup bowls. Garnish with parsley.

SERVES 2

Nutrition Facts per Serving

Calories: 340	Sodium: 640mg
Calories from Fat: 110	Total Carbohydrate: 24g
Total Fat: 13g	Dietary Fibre: 2g
Saturated Fat: 2g	Sugar: 12g
Cholesterol: 65mg	Protein: 29g

PASTA

62. PASTA à la SINATRA

½ Tbsp. olive oil
4 cloves garlic, minced
3 small onions, chopped
1 225g (8oz) jar sun-dried tomatoes in olive oil, puréed in food processor
225g (8oz) chopped courgettes
Fresh chopped basil
Freshly ground black pepper to taste
225g (8oz) wholemeal pasta, cooked according to package directions
Grated Parmesan cheese
Chopped fresh parsley

Heat olive oil over medium heat in a saucepan. Add garlic and onions and sauté for a few minutes. Add tomatoes and cook a few minutes more. Add courgettes and continue to cook a few minutes longer. Add fresh basil and pepper. Pour sauce over pasta. Garnish with Parmesan cheese and parsley.

SERVES 4

Nutrition Facts per Serving

Calories: 460	Sodium: 180mg
Calories from Fat: 130	Total Carbohydrate: 69g
Total Fat: 15g	Dietary Fibre: 23g
Saturated Fat: 1.5g	Sugar: 10g
Cholesterol: 5mg	Protein: 17g

63. SPELT (OR WHOLEMEAL) PASTA with ASPARAGUS and TOMATOES

1 Tbsp. olive oil
3 cloves garlic, chopped
120g (4oz) asparagus, cleaned and cut into 1cm (½-in) pieces
100g (3½oz) cherry tomatoes
120g (4oz) spelt (or wholemeal) pasta, cooked according to package directions
6 basil leaves, slivered
Parmesan cheese

Heat olive oil over medium heat in a medium frying pan. Add garlic and asparagus and stir-fry until asparagus is tender. Add tomatoes and cook for 2 minutes longer. Spoon mixture over pasta and garnish with basil and Parmesan.

SERVES 2

Nutrition Facts per Serving

Calories: 320	Sodium: 125mg
Calories from Fat: 90	Total Carbohydrate: 49g
Total Fat: 10g	Dietary Fibre: 7g
Saturated Fat: 2.5g	Sugar: 4g
Cholesterol: 5mg	Protein: 13g

64. SPELT (OR WHOLEMEAL) PASTA with TOMATO, BASIL, and SHIITAKE or MAITAKE MUSHROOMS

1 Tbsp. olive oil
2 cloves garlic, chopped
2 shallots, chopped
6 fresh shiitake or maitake mushrooms, stems removed and sliced
420g (14½oz) can unsalted chopped tomatoes, undrained
225g (8oz) can unsalted tomato sauce
1 Tbsp. unsalted tomato paste
½ tsp. honey
1 tsp. red wine vinegar
¼ tsp. black pepper
6 basil leaves, slivered
120g (4oz) spelt (or wholemeal) pasta, cooked according to package directions
Parmesan cheese

Heat oil over medium heat in a large frying pan. Cook garlic, shallots, and mushrooms until lightly browned. Add chopped tomatoes, tomato sauce, tomato paste, honey, vinegar, black pepper, and basil. Bring to a boil. Reduce heat to low and simmer for 5 minutes. Serve over pasta and sprinkle with Parmesan cheese.

SERVES 2

Nutrition Facts per Serving

Calories: 440	Sodium: 170mg
Calories from Fat: 90	Total Carbohydrate: 78g
Total Fat: 10g	Dietary Fibre: 14g
Saturated Fat: 2.5g	Sugar: 12g
Cholesterol: 5mg	Protein: 16g

65. WHOLEMEAL PASTA with BROCCOLI and FETA

1 Tbsp. olive oil
3 cloves garlic, crushed
450g (15oz) can unsalted chopped tomatoes, undrained
180g (6oz) fresh broccoli florets
½ cup low-sodium or reduced-sodium chicken stock
1 tsp. honey
½ tsp. dried basil
2 Tbsp. crumbled feta cheese
3 Tbsp. tomato paste
120g (4oz) wholemeal pasta, cooked according to package directions

Heat olive oil over medium heat in a large frying pan. Cook garlic until lightly browned. Add chopped tomatoes, broccoli, chicken broth, honey, and basil. Bring to a boil. Reduce heat to low and simmer for 5 minutes or until broccoli is tender. Stir in feta cheese and tomato paste; heat through. Serve over pasta.

SERVES 2

Nutrition Facts per Serving

Calories: 370	Sodium: 180mg
Calories from Fat: 90	Total Carbohydrate: 62g
Total Fat: 10g	Dietary Fibre: 9g
Saturated Fat: 2.5g	Sugar: 12g
Cholesterol: 10mg	Protein: 15g

66. WHOLEMEAL PASTA with AUBERGINE TOMATO SAUCE

2 Tbsp. olive oil
200g (6½oz) cubed black aubergine
1 medium onion, chopped
3 cloves garlic, chopped
1 tsp. sherry or red wine vinegar
2 225g (8oz) cans unsalted tomato sauce
½ tsp. dried basil
½ tsp. dried parsley
½ tsp. honey
2 Tbsp. dried currants
Red pepper flakes to taste
225g (8oz) wholemeal pasta, cooked according to package directions
Parmesan cheese

Preheat oven to 400°F/200°C/Gas mark 5. Mix 1 Tbsp. olive oil with the aubergine. Place on baking sheet and roast for 20 minutes or until golden brown.

In a large frying pan, heat the remaining tablespoon of olive oil over medium heat and sauté onions and garlic until golden. Add sherry vinegar, aubergine, tomato sauce, basil, parsley, honey, currants, and red pepper flakes and bring to a boil. Reduce heat to low and simmer, uncovered, for 20 minutes. Serve over pasta and sprinkle with Parmesan cheese.

SERVES 4

Nutrition Facts per Serving

Calories: 370	Sodium: 140mg
Calories from Fat: 90	Total Carbohydrate: 62g
Total Fat: 10g	Dietary Fibre: 9g
Saturated Fat: 2.5g	Sugar: 10g
Cholesterol: 5mg	Protein: 14g

CONDIMENTS

67. FLAXSEED DRESSING

8 cloves garlic, minced
1 bunch fresh parsley, chopped
2 Tbsp. chopped fresh coriander
3 Tbsp. toasted organic sesame seeds (toast in frying pan then grind
in a coffee mill)
¼ tsp. black pepper
½ tsp. crushed oregano
2 stalks fresh rosemary, chopped
Juice of 1 lemon
450ml (16fl oz) extra virgin olive oil
120ml (4fl oz) flaxseed oil
60ml (2fl oz) extra virgin sesame seed oil
3 Tbsp. dark sesame oil
60ml (2fl oz) walnut oil

Whisk all ingredients together in a large bowl. Store in the refrigerator in tightly sealed containers.

YIELD: 900ML (32FL OZ), 36 SERVINGS

1 SERVING = 2 TBSP.

Nutrition Facts per Serving

Calories: 180	Sodium: 0
Calories from Fat: 170	Total Carbohydrate: 0
Total Fat: 19g	Dietary Fibre: 0
Saturated Fat: 2.5g	Sugar: 0
Cholesterol: 0	Protein: 0

68. GINGER FLAXSEED DRESSING

1 tsp. fresh grated ginger
2 tsp. lime juice
1 tsp. whole flaxseed, ground in a coffee mill
1 Tbsp. low sodium tomato juice

Mix all ingredients together in a small bowl and toss with salad.

SERVES I

Nutrition Facts per Serving

Calories: 20	Sodium: 0
Calories from Fat: 10	Total Carbohydrate: 3g
Total Fat: 1g	Dietary Fibre: 0
Saturated Fat: 0	Sugar: 1g
Cholesterol: 0	Protein: 1g

69. FRESH TOMATO SALSA

2 large tomatoes, diced
2 Tbsp. chopped red onion
1 clove garlic, minced
1 medium green pepper, chopped
30g (1oz) chopped fresh coriander
1 Tbsp. fresh lime juice
1 small jalapeno pepper, seeded and finely chopped

Combine all ingredients in a medium bowl and chill several hours before serving.

SERVES 2

Nutrition Facts per Serving

Calories: 70	Sodium: 20mg
Calories from Fat: 10	Total Carbohydrate: 16g
Total Fat: 1g	Dietary Fibre: 3g
Saturated Fat: 0	Sugar: 8g
Cholesterol: 0	Protein: 3g

70. HUMMUS

1 450g (15oz) can unsalted or low-sodium chickpeas, drained and rinsed
1 clove garlic, minced
1 Tbsp. tahini (sesame seed paste)
Juice of ½ lemon
Black pepper to taste
1 Tbsp. olive oil
2 Tbsp. finely chopped fresh parsley
Paprika

In a food processor, combine chickpeas, garlic, tahini, lemon juice, pepper, and olive oil until smooth. Garnish with parsley and paprika if desired. Store covered in the refrigerator for up to 2 weeks.

YIELD: 270G (9½OZ)

1 SERVING = 2 TBSP.

Nutrition Facts per Serving

Calories: 60
Calories from Fat: 25
Total Fat: 3g
Saturated Fat: 0
Cholesterol: 0

Sodium: 0
Total Carbohydrate: 7g
Dietary Fibre: 2g
Sugar: 0
Protein: 2g

BREAKFAST FOODS

71. APPLE RAISIN BREAD

120ml (4fl oz) light-tasting olive oil
120ml (4fl oz) honey
240ml (8fl oz) treacle
4 eggs
180g (6oz) seedless raisins
2 tsp. vanilla extract
325g (12oz) wholemeal flour
125g (½oz) wheat germ
4 tsp. baking powder
1 tsp. cinnamon
1 tsp. lemon rind
1 tsp. nutmeg
2 medium apples, peeled and grated

Preheat oven to 350°F/180°C/Gas mark 3. Spray a 22cm × 12cm (9 × 5-in) loaf pan with non-stick cooking spray. Combine all ingredients in a large bowl and mix until well combined. Pour in pan and bake 1 hour or until a toothpick inserted in the centre of the bread comes out clean.

SERVES 16

Nutrition Facts per Serving

Calories: 260
Calories from Fat: 80
Total Fat: 9g
Saturated Fat: 1.5g
Cholesterol: 55mg

Sodium: 120mg
Total Carbohydrate: 41g
Dietary Fibre: 4g
Sugar: 24g
Protein: 6g

72. BLUEBERRY or APPLE-CINNAMON BRAN MUFFINS

90g (3oz) bran flakes cereal
240ml (8fl oz) skimmed milk or plain soya milk
2 Tbsp. grapeseed oil
1 egg
1 Tbsp. honey
80ml (2½fl oz) treacle
1 tsp. vanilla extract
200g (6½oz) wholemeal flour
1 tsp. baking powder
300g (10oz) blueberries; or 2 apples, grated and 1 tsp. cinnamon

Preheat oven to 350°F/180°C/Gas mark 3. Spray twelve 5–6-cm (2½-in) muffin cups with non-stick cooking spray. Mix bran cereal and milk in a medium bowl and let stand 5 minutes. In a large bowl mix oil, egg, honey, treacle, vanilla extract, and cereal. Add flour and baking powder. Fold in blueberries or apple-cinnamon mixture. Divide batter into 12 muffin cups. Bake 25 minutes. Freeze individual muffins in freezer bags.

YIELD: 12 MUFFINS

Nutrition Facts per Muffin

Calories: 150
Calories from Fat: 30
Total Fat: 3.5g
Saturated Fat: 0
Cholesterol: 20mg

Sodium: 110g
Total Carbohydrate: 28g
Dietary Fibre: 4g
Sugar: 12g
Protein: 4g

73. BLUEBERRY BUCKWHEAT PANCAKES with WHEAT GERM

160g (5½oz) buckwheat flour
125g (4½oz) wholemeal flour
2 Tbsp. wheat germ
1 tsp. baking powder
350ml (12fl oz) skimmed milk or plain soya milk
2 eggs, beaten
1 Tbsp. honey
2 Tbsp. olive oil
150g (5oz) blueberries (in frozen section of supermarket)
Real maple syrup

Stir together dry ingredients. Add milk, eggs, honey, and oil. Mix briefly. Fold in blueberries. Cook on a hot frying pan sprayed with nonstick spray.

YIELD: 12 PANCAKES (3 PANCAKES AND 2½ TBSP. MAPLE SYRUP PER SERVING)

SERVES 4

Nutrition Facts per Serving

Calories: 460

Calories from Fat: 100

Total Fat: 11g

Saturated Fat: 2g

Cholesterol: 110mg

Sodium: 210mg

Total Carbohydrate: 81g

Dietary Fibre: 6g

Sugar: 46g

Protein: 13g

74. FRUIT SMOOTHIE

2 tsp. whole flaxseed, ground in a coffee mill

300ml (10fl oz) plain soya milk

½ medium banana

4 strawberries, sliced

2 Tbsp. blueberries

1 tsp. honey

4 ice cubes

Whip all ingredients in a blender.

SERVES I

Nutrition Facts per Serving

Calories: 310

Calories from Fat: 45

Total Fat: 5g

Saturated Fat: 0

Cholesterol: 0

Sodium: 120mg

Total Carbohydrate: 63g

Dietary Fibre: 6g

Sugar: 33g

Protein: 8g

75. DRIED FRUIT SPELT MUFFINS

150g (5oz) spelt flour

125g (4½oz) wholemeal flour

25g (¾oz) soya flour

2 tsp. baking powder

2 tsp. cinnamon

240ml (8fl oz) plain fat-free yogurt

1 tsp. vanilla extract

2 eggs

60ml (2fl oz) olive oil

240ml (8fl oz) honey

60g (2oz) seedless raisins

75g (2½oz) dried apricots, chopped

80g (2¾oz) chopped dried dates

Preheat oven to 350°F/180°C/Gas mark 3. Spray twelve 5–6cm (2½-in) muffin cups with non-stick cooking spray. Mix dry ingredients in a medium bowl.

In a large bowl mix the remaining ingredients except dried fruits. Mix in the flour mixture until just moistened. Fold in the dried fruits. Divide into muffin cups, filling almost full. Bake 25–30 minutes or until toothpick inserted in centre of muffin comes out clean.

YIELD: 12 MUFFINS

Nutrition Facts per Muffin

Calories: 240

Calories from Fat: 60

Total Fat: 6g

Saturated Fat: 1g

Cholesterol: 35mg

Sodium: 110mg

Total Carbohydrate: 44g

Dietary Fibre: 5g

Sugar: 25g

Protein: 7g

DESSERTS and SNACKS

76. CARROT CAKE

120ml (4fl oz) olive oil
240ml (8fl oz) honey
2 eggs
225g (8oz) grated carrots
80g (2¾oz) seedless raisins
1 225g (8oz) can crushed pineapple in juice, undrained
2 tsp. vanilla extract
260g (9oz) wholemeal flour
1 Tbsp. baking powder
2 tsp. cinnamon
½ tsp. ground ginger
½ tsp. nutmeg

Preheat oven to 350°F/180°C/Gas mark 3. Spray a 22cm × 5-cm (13 × 9 × 2-in) pan with non-stick cooking spray. Combine all ingredients in a large bowl and mix until well combined. Pour in pan and bake 40–45 minutes or until a toothpick inserted in the centre of the cake comes out clean.

SERVES 16

Nutrition Facts per Serving

Calories: 220	Sodium: 60mg
Calories from Fat: 70	Total Carbohydrate: 36g
Total Fat: 8g	Dietary Fibre: 3g
Saturated Fat: 1g	Sugar: 23g
Cholesterol: 25mg	Protein: 3g

77. APRICOT OATMEAL BARS

150g (5oz) oatmeal
40g (1½oz) wholemeal flour
1 tsp. baking powder
2 tsp. cinnamon
1 tsp. vanilla extract
240ml (8fl oz) honey
60ml (2fl oz) olive oil
2 eggs
60ml (2oz) skimmed milk or plain soya milk
180g (6oz) dried apricots, chopped

Preheat oven to 350°F/180°C/Gas mark 3. Spray an 28cm × 17-cm (11 × 7-in) pan with oil. Combine all ingredients in a large bowl and mix until well combined. Pat mixture into the pan and bake 20 minutes or until bars feel firm to the touch.

SERVES 12

Nutrition Facts per Serving

Calories: 180	Sodium: 35mg
Calories from Fat: 50	Total Carbohydrate: 29g
Total Fat: 6g	Dietary Fibre: 2g
Saturated Fat: 1g	Sugar: 17g
Cholesterol: 35mg	Protein: 4g

78. PEANUT BUTTER BISCUITS

60ml (2fl oz) light-tasting olive oil
4 level Tbsp. natural unsalted peanut butter
240ml (8fl oz) honey
2 eggs
1 tsp. vanilla extract
200g (6½oz) wholemeal flour
1 tsp. baking powder
25g (¾oz) soya flour
125g (4½oz) seedless raisins
75g (2½oz) unsalted dry roasted peanuts

Preheat oven to 375°F/190°C/Gas mark 4. Line a biscuit tray with baking parchment. Combine all ingredients except raisins and peanuts in a large bowl and mix until well combined. Fold in raisins and peanuts. Roll heaped tablespoons of dough into a ball and flatten with a fork on the biscuit tray. Bake 15 minutes or until biscuits are firm and lightly browned.

YIELD: 24 BISCUITS

Nutrition Facts per Biscuit

Calories: 140
Calories from Fat: 60
Total Fat: 7g
Saturated Fat: 1g
Cholesterol: 20mg

Sodium: 25mg
Total Carbohydrate: 17g
Dietary Fibre: 2g
Sugar: 9g
Protein: 4g

79. CAROB NUT BROWNIES

120ml (4fl oz) light-tasting olive oil
180ml (6fl oz) honey
2 eggs
1 tsp. vanilla extract
75g (2½oz) wholemeal flour
1 tsp. baking powder
100g (3½oz) carob powder (available in health food shops)
50g (1¾oz) walnuts, coarsely chopped

Preheat oven to 350°F/180°C/Gas mark 3. Spray a 22-cm (9-in) square pan with non-stick cooking spray. Combine all ingredients in a large bowl and mix until well combined. Pour in pan and bake 25–30 minutes or until a toothpick inserted in the centre of the cake comes out clean.

SERVES 16

Nutrition Facts per Serving

Calories: 160
Calories from Fat: 90
Total Fat: 10g
Saturated Fat: 1.5g
Cholesterol: 25mg

Sodium: 40mg
Total Carbohydrate: 19g
Dietary Fibre: 2g
Sugar: 11g
Protein: 3g

80. SPICE CAKE

60ml (2fl oz) light-tasting olive oil
120ml (4fl oz) honey
120ml (4fl oz) treacle
2 eggs
1 450g (15oz) can unsalted or low-sodium pinto beans, rinsed and drained and slightly mashed with a fork or your hands
125g (4½oz) seedless raisins
2 tsp. vanilla extract
150g (5oz) wholemeal flour
2 tsp. baking powder
2 tsp. cinnamon
½ tsp. cloves

½ tsp. nutmeg
2 medium apples, peeled and grated

Preheat oven to 350°F/180°C/Gas mark 3. Spray a 34cm × 22cm × 5-cm (13 × 9 × 2-in) pan with non-stick cooking spray. Combine all ingredients in a large bowl and mix until well combined. Pour in pan and bake 50–55 minutes or until a toothpick inserted in the centre of the cake comes out clean.

SERVES 16

Nutrition Facts per Serving

Calories: 180	Sodium: 45mg
Calories from Fat: 40	Total Carbohydrate: 33g
Total Fat: 4.5g	Dietary Fibre: 3g
Saturated Fat: 0.5g	Sugar: 21g
Cholesterol: 25mg	Protein: 3g

81. OATMEAL DATE BISCUITS

20ml (1fl oz) light-tasting olive oil
60ml (2fl oz) honey
2 eggs
¼ tsp. treacle
1 tsp. vanilla extract
150g (5oz) wholemeal flour
1 tsp. baking powder
200g (6½oz) oats
1 tsp. cinnamon
½ tsp. ground ginger
½ tsp. nutmeg
180g (6oz) chopped dates

Preheat oven to 375°F/190°C/Gas mark 4. Line a biscuit tray with baking parchment. Combine all ingredients except dates in a large bowl and mix until well combined. Mix in dates. Drop heaped tablespoons of dough onto the biscuit tray and flatten slightly. Bake 12–14 minutes or until biscuits are firm and lightly browned.

YIELD: 24 BISCUITS

Nutrition Facts per Biscuit

Calories: 120	Sodium: 25mg
Calories from Fat: 35	Total Carbohydrate: 19g
Total Fat: 4g	Dietary Fibre: 2g
Saturated Fat: 0.5g	Sugar: 10g
Cholesterol: 20mg	Protein: 2g

82. LEMON POPPY SEED DIP

160ml (5fl oz) fat-free plain yogurt
4 tsp. honey
1 Tbsp. lemon juice
1 tsp. lemon peel
1 Tbsp. poppy seeds

Combine all ingredients in a small bowl. Store in refrigerator for up to 2 weeks.

YIELD: ABOUT 240ML (8FL OZ)

SERVES 2

Nutrition Facts per Serving

Calories: 100
Calories from Fat: 15
Total Fat: 1.5g
Saturated Fat: 0
Cholesterol: 0

Sodium: 45mg
Total Carbohydrate: 20g
Dietary Fibre: <1g
Sugar: 16g
Protein: 4g

NOTES ON ANGLICIZATION FOR THE UK

Measurements

For ease and accuracy it is recommended that you use standard measuring spoons (1 Tbsp., 1 tsp., ½ tsp., ¼ tsp.) which are available in most supermarkets or kitchenware shops.

Information on low-sodium products

To be in accordance with the low-sodium and salt-free products specified in the ingredients lists it is worth checking sodium content in products. It is not compulsory in the UK to list sodium content, but the majority of products will list this information in the ingredients. Guidelines are given below:

- 'Reduced' – contains 25% less than comparable standard product
- 'Low' – contains less than 40mg (0.04g) per 100g/100ml
- 'Free' – contains less than 5mg (.005g) per 110g/100ml

UK daily guidelines for an average adult of normal weight:

	Men	Women
Energy	2,500kcal	2,000kcal
Sodium	2.5g (7.0g salt)	2g (5.0g salt)

Compared with either the per serving figure for a whole meal, or per 100g (3½oz) for a snack.

	'A lot' is	'A little' is
Sodium	More than 0.5g (1.5g salt)	less than 0.1g (0.3g salt)

Low-sodium and salt-free canned goods such as canned legumes (lentils, kidney etc.) and tomatoes are available at most large supermarkets.

If other low-sodium products are harder to obtain it may be preferable to use fresh produce in these instances, or visit your local health shop, where amongst other products, you can obtain low-sodium stock.

Availability of products

Some of the recipe ingredients are less readily available than others. For general availability of the less common foods try large centres, large supermarkets, health food shops, special health food shops such as Planet Organic and specialist shops such as Chinese or Japanese supermarkets.

Supplements will need to be obtained from health food shops.

If you are having difficulty obtaining foods in your area, *The Inside Story* is a publication worth subscribing to as it has many contacts for less common foods. Contact: Berrydales Publishers, Berrydale House, 5 Lawn Road, London NW3 2XS. Tel: 020 7722 2866 Fax: 020 7722 7685 Email: info@inside-story.com.

The Internet will also give you up-to-date sources of where to order. When doing the search make sure you tick the search only in the UK (or other relevant country) box or you will get mainly US sources.

Amaranth flour – amaranth seeds and flour can be found in speciality shops and health food shops, as well as some Caribbean and Asian shops.

Bran Buds with psyllium – psyllium husks 500mg capsules are available from Holland and Barrett.

Kale – available in large supermarkets.

Nori seaweed – try Chinese and Japanese supermarkets, health food shops or Internet.

Shiitake mushrooms – available dry in health or specialist food shops, and some supermarkets, such as Waitrose.

Soya cheese – available in health food shops.

Soya mayonnaise – available in health food shops including Holland and Barrett

Soya protein powder, soya nuts, soya flakes and Soya grits – try health food shops. They are also available online to order from the US.

Soya yogurts – available in health food shops.

Soya protein – Soya Chunks, Soya Chunks Savoury, Soya Mince, Soya Mince Savoury available from some health shops and to order from Eighth Day, Sidney Street, Manchester M1 7HB. Tel: 0161 273 4878 (shop), Tel: 0161 2731850 (café) Fax: 0161 273 4878 Email: mail@eighth-day.co.uk

OR   49 Old Birley Street, Hulme, Manchester, M15 5RF. Tel: 0161 227 8848 Fax: 0161 273 4878 Email: mail@eighth-day.co.uk

Spelt flour – spelt is closely related to common wheat and has an intense nutty wheaty flavour. The flour is excellent for breadmaking. Spelt flour is available in most health food shops, but pasta and bread are not widely available. Visit www.dovesfarm.co.uk for details of outlets or order from: The Ingredient Company Limited, FREEPOST ANG 3751, Market Deeping, Peterborough, Cambridgeshire PE6 8BR. Tel: 01778 380088 Fax: 01778 380052 *OR* www.dailybread.co.uk

Tempeh – health food or specialist shops such as Holland and Barrett.

Tomato sauces – St Giles Foods Ltd do a range of low-sodium tomato sauces, etc. They are based in Dartford: 5 Church Trading Estate, Slade Green, Kent DA8 2JA. Tel: 01322 337711

Notes on Vitamin A
In the UK the RNI (Reference Nutrient Intake) or recommended daily allowance for Vitamin A is:
700µg retinol equivalents/day for men
600µg retinol equivalents/day for women

The recommended maximum intake for Vitamin A in the UK is:
9,000µg retinol equivalents/day for men
7,500µg retinol equivalents/day for women

Sourced by Kathy Cowbrough

References

CHAPTER 1

1. Albert CM, et al. Fish consumption and risk of sudden cardiac death. *JAMA* 1998;279:23–28.
2. Black HR. Does the evidence from clinical trials justify the treatment of hypertension? *Clin Cornerstone* 1999;2:13–26.
3. Blood Pressure Lowering Treatment Trialists' Collaboration. Effects of ACE inhibitors, calcium antagonists, and other blood pressure-lowering drugs: results of prospectively designed overviews of randomized trials. *Lancet* 2000;356:1955–1964.
4. Burt VL, Whelton P, Roccella EJ, et al. Prevalence of hypertension in the US adult population: results from the Third National Health and Nutrition Examination Survey, 1988–1991. *Hypertension* 1995;25:305–313.
5. Conlin PR, Chow D, Miller ER III, et al. The effect of dietary patterns on blood pressure control in hypertensive patients: results from the Dietary Approaches to Stop Hypertension (DASH) trial. *Am J Hypertens* 2000;13:949–955.
6. Cutler JA, Follmann D, Allender PS. Randomized trials of sodium reduction: an overview. *Am J Clin Nutr* 1997;65:643S–651S.
7. Cutler JA, Follmann D, Elliott P, et al. An overview of randomized trials of sodium reduction and blood pressure. *Hypertension* 1991;17(Suppl 1):127–133.
8. Davis BR, et al. Major cardiovascular events in hypertensive patients randomized to doxazosin vs. chlorthalidone: The Antihypertensive and Lipid-Lowering Treatment to Prevent Heart Attack Trial (ALLHAT). *JAMA* 2000;283:1967–1975.
9. Fleming GA. The FDA, regulations, and the risk of stroke [editorial]. *N Engl J Med* 2000;343:1886–1887.
10. Gress TW, Nieto FJ, Shahar E, et al. Hypertension and antihypertensive therapy as risk factors for type 2 diabetes mellitus. Artherosclerosis Risk in Communities Study. *N Engl J Med* 2000;342:905–912.
11. Hall CL, Higgs CMB, Notarianni L, et al. Home blood pressure recording in mild hypertension: value of distinguishing sustained from clinic hypertension and effect on diagnosis and treatment. *J Hum Hypertens* 1990;4:501–507.
12. Hebert PR, Moser M, Mayer J, et al. Recent evidence on drug therapy of mild to moderate hypertension and decreased risk of coronary heart disease. *Arch Intern Med* 1993;153:578–581.
13. Heidenreich PA, Lee TT, Massie BM. Effect of B-blockade on mortality in patients with heart failure: a meta-analysis of randomized clinical trials. *J Am Coll Cardiol* 1997;30:27–34.
14. Hjalmarson A. Prevention of sudden cardiac death with B-blockers. *Clin Cardiol* 1999;22(suppl 5):V11–V15.

15. Hoegholm A, Kristensen KS, Madsen NH, et al. White coat hypertension diagnosed by 24–h ambulatory monitoring: examination of 159 newly diagnosed hypertensive patients. *Am J Hypertens* 1992;5:64–70.

16. Insua JT, Sacks HS, Lau TS, et al. Drug treatment of hypertension in the elderly: a meta-analysis. *Ann Intern Med* 1994;121:355–362.

17. Joint Health Surveys Unit (1999) Health Survey for England 1998. The Stationery Office: London.

18. Joint National Committee on Detection, Evaluation, and Treatment of High Blood Pressure. *The Fifth Report of the Joint National Committee on Detection, Evaluation, and Treatment of High Blood Pressure*. Bethesda: National Institutes of Health, 1993 (NIH publication no. 93-1088).

19. Kaplan NM. The management of hypertension in patients with type 2 diabetes mellitus: guidelines based on current evidence. *Ann Intern Med* 2001;135:1079–1083.

20. Kernan WN, Viscoli CM, Brass LM, et al. Phenylpropanolamine and the risk of hemorrhagic stroke. *N Engl J Med* 2000;343:1826–1832.

21. Langford HG, Davis BR, Blaufox MD, et al. Effect of drug and diet treatment of mild hypertension on diastolic blood pressure. *Hypertension* 1991;17:210-217.

22. Lazaron J, Pomeranz B, Corey P. Incidence of adverse drug reaction in hospitalized patients. *JAMA* 1998;279:1200-1205.

23. Lusardi P, Zoppi A, Preti P, et al. Effects of insufficient sleep on blood pressure in hypertensive patients: a 24-h study. *Am J Hypertens* 1999;12:63–68.

24. MacMahon S, Neal B. Differences between blood-pressure-lowering drugs. *Lancet* 2000; 356:352–353.

25. Massie BM. Systemic hypertension. In: Tierney LM, et al., eds. *Current Medical Diagnosis and Treatment*. 38th edition. Stamford, CT: Appleton & Lange, 1999:430–452.

26. National Institutes of Health/National Heart, Lung, and Blood Institute. *The Sixth Report of the Joint National Committee on Prevention, Detection, Evaluation and Treatment of High Blood Pressure*. Bethesda, MD: NIH, 1997 (NIH publication no. 98-4080).

27. Neal B, MacMahon S, Chapman N. Effects of ACE inhibitors, calcium antagonists, and other blood-pressure-lowering drugs: results of prospectively designed overviews of randomized trials. *Lancet* 2000;356:1955–1964.

28. Neaton JD, Wentworth D. Serum cholesterol, blood pressure, cigarette smoking, and death from coronary heart disease. Overall findings and differences by age for 316,099 white men. Multiple Risk Factor Intervention Trial Research Group. *Arch Intern Med* 1992;152:56–64.

29. Nygard O, Nordrehaug JE, Refsum H, et al. Plasma homocysteine levels and mortality in patients with coronary artery disease. *N Engl J Med* 1997;337:230-236.

30. Pahor M, Psaty BM, et al. Health outcomes associated with calcium antagonists compared with other first-line anti-hypertensive therapies: a meta-analysis of randomized controlled trials. *Lancet* 2000;356:1949–1954.

31. Pearce KA, Grimm RH Jr., Rao S, et al. Population-derived comparisons of ambulatory and office blood pressures: implications for the determination of usual blood pressure and the concept of white coat hypertension. *Arch Intern Med* 1992;152:750-756.

32. Pickering TG, James GD, Boddie C, et al. How common is white coat hypertension? *JAMA* 1988;259:225–228.

33. Ramsay L, Williams B, Johnston GD, MacGregor G, Poston L, Potter J, Poutten N, Russell G. British Hypertension Society Guidelines for Hypertension Mx 1999: Summary. *BMJ*:319:630–5.

34. Reaven, GM, Chen YDI, Jeppesen J, et al. Insulin resistance and hyperinsulinemia in individuals with small, dense low-density lipoprotein particles. *J Clin Invest* 1993;92:141–146.

35. Ridker, PM, Manson JE, Buring JE, et al. Homocysteine and risk of cardiovascular disease among post-menopausal women. *JAMA* 1999;281(19):1817–1821.

36. Rippe JM, Crossley S, Ringer R. Obesity as a chronic disease: modern medical and lifestyle management. *J Am Diet Assoc* 1998;98:S9–S15.

37. Sacks FM, Svetkey LP, Vollmer WM, et al. Effects on blood pressure of reduced dietary sodium and the dietary approaches to stop hypertension (DASH) diet. *New Engl J Med* 2001;344(1):3–9.

38. Sagie A, Larson MG, Levy D. The natural history of borderline isolated systolic hypertension. *N Engl J Med* 1993;329:1912–1917.

39. Schmidt EB, Skou HA, Christensen JH, Dyerberg J. N-3 fatty acids from fish and coronary artery disease: implications for public health. *Public Health Nutr* 2000;3:91–98.

40. Schotte DE, Stunkard AJ. The effects of weight reduction on blood pressure in 301 obese patients. *Arch Intern Med* 1990;150:1701–1704.

41. SHEP Cooperative Research Group. Prevention of stroke by antihypertensive drug treatment in older persons with isolated systolic hypertension. Final results of the Systolic Hypertension in the Elderly Program (SHEP). *JAMA* 1991;265:3255–3264.

42. Sinatra ST. *Heart Sense for Women.* New York: Plume Publishing, 2001.

43. Stamler J, Stamler R, Neaton JD. Blood pressure, systolic and diastolic, and cardiovascular risks. US population data. *Arch Intern Med.* 1993;153:598–615.

44. Stevens VJ, Obarzanek E, Cook NR, et al. Long-term weight loss and changes in blood pressure: results of the trials of hypertension prevention, phase II. *Annals of Intern Med* 2001;134:1–11.

45. Vollmer WM, Sacks FM, Ard J, et al. Effects of diet and sodium intake on blood pressure: subgroup analysis of the DASH-Sodium Trial. *Ann Intern Med.* 2001;135:1019–1028.

46. Wald DS, Law M, Morris JK. Homocysteine and vascular disease: evidence on causality from a meta-analysis; *BMJ.* 325:1202.

47. Wali RK, Weir MR. Hypertensive cardiovascular disease in African Americans. *Curr Hypertens Rep.* 1999;1:521–528.

48. Web MD on high blood pressure. *Web MD Health.* March 1999, March 2002.

49. Weisser B, Mengden T, Dusing R, et al. Normal values of blood pressure self-measurement in a view of the 1999 World Health Organization–International Society of Hypertension guidelines. *Am J Hypertens* 2000;13:940–943.

50. Wennerblom B, Lurje L, Karlsson T, et al. Circadian variation of heart rate variability and the rate of autonomic change in the morning hours in healthy subjects and angina patients. *Int J Cardiol* 2001;79(1):61–69.

51. Whelton PK, Klag MJ. Epidemiology of high blood pressure. *Clin Geriatr Med* 1989; 5:639–655.

52. World Hypertension League. Physical exercise in the management of hypertension: a consensus statement by the World Hypertension League. *J Hypertens* 1991;9:283–287.

53. Yusuf S, Sleight P, Pogue J, et al. Effects of an angiotensin-converting-enzyme inhibitor, ramipril, on cardiovascular events in high-risk patients. *N Engl J Med* 2000;342:145–153.

CHAPTER 2

1. Alarcon de la Lastra C, Barranco MD, Motilva V, Herrerias JM. Mediterranean diet and health: biological importance of olive oil. *Curr Pharm Des.* 2001;7(10):933–950.
2. Arai Y, Watanabe S, Kimira M, et al. Dietary intakes of flavonols, flavones and isoflavones by Japanese women and the inverse correlation between quercetin intake and plasma LDL cholesterol concentration. *J Nutr* 2000;130(9):2243–2250.
3. Bazzano LA, He J, Ogden LG, et al. Legume consumption and risk of coronary heart disease in US men and women. *Arch Intern Med.* 2001;161:2573–2578.
4. Challem J. *Syndrome X.* New York: John Wiley & Sons, 2000.
5. De Lorgeril M, Salen P. Wine ethanol, platelets, and Mediterranean diet. *Lancet* 1999;353:1067.
6. De Lorgeril M, Salen P, Martin JL, et al. Effects of Mediterranean type of diet on the rate of cardiovascular complications in patients with coronary artery disease. *J Am Coll Cardiol.* 1996;28(5):1103–1108.
7. Despres JP, Lamarche B, Mauriege P, et al. Hyperinsulinism as an independent risk factor for ischemic heart disease. *N Engl J Med.* 1996;334:952–957.
8. Dumesnil JG, Turgeon J, Tremblay A, et al. Effect of a low-glycemic-index–low fat–high protein diet on the atherogenic metabolic risk profile of abdominally obese men. *Br J Nutr.* 2001;86(5):557–568.
9. Edelman SV. Type II diabetes mellitus. *Adv Intern Med.* 1998;43:449–500. Review.
10. Fleming L, Mann JB, Beau J, et al. Parkinson's disease and brain level of organochlorine pesticides. *Ann Neurol.*1994;36(1):100–108.
11. Franklin D. The healthiest women in the world. *Hippocrates.* 1996:51–61.
12. Herzog MC, Feskens EJ, Hollman PC, et al. Dietary antioxidant flavonoids and risk of coronary heart disease: the Zutphen elderly study. *Lancet* 1993;342(8878): 1007–1011.
13. Hoyer AP, Grandiean P, Jorgensen T, Brock JW, Hartrig HG. Organochlorine exposure and risk of breast cancer. *Lancet* 1998;852:1816–1820.
14. Hu FB, Stampfer MJ, Manson JE. Dietary fat intake and the risk of coronary heart disease in women. *N Engl J Med.* 1997;337:1491–1499.
15. Kalus U, Pindur G, Jung F, et al. Influence of the onion as an essential ingredient of the Mediterranean diet on arterial blood pressure and blood fluidity. *Arzneimittelforschung.* 2000;50(9):795–801.
16. Knekt P, Jarvinen R, Reunanen A, Maatela J. Flavonoid intake and coronary mortality in Finland: a cohort study. *BMJ* 1996;312(7029):478–481.
17. Kouris-Blazos A, Wahlqvist ML. The traditional Greek food pattern and overall survival in elderly people. *Australian J Nutr and Dietetics* 1998;55(4):S20–S23.
18. Kushi LH, Lenart EB, Willett WC. Health implications of Mediterranean diets in light of contemporary knowledge. Meat, wine, fats, and oils. *Am J Clin Nutr.* 1995;61(suppl): 1416S–1427S.
19. Marques-Lopes I, Ansorena D, Astiasaran I, et al. Postprandial de novo lipogenesis and metabolic changes induced by a high-carbohydrate, low-fat meal in lean and overweight men. *Am J Clin Nutr.* 2001;73:253–261.

20. Massaro M, Carluccio MA, De Caterina R. Direct vascular antiatherogenic effects of oleic acid: a clue to the cardioprotective effects of the Mediterranean diet. *Cardiologia* 1999;44(6):507–513.

21. Maxwell S, Cruickshank A, Thorpe D. Red wine and antioxidants activity in serum. *Lancet* 1994;344:193–194.

22. Oster KR, Ross DJ, Richmond-Dawkins HH. The XO Factor: Homogenized Milk May Cause Your Heart Attack. New York: Park City Press, 1983.

23. Renaud S, deLorgeril M. Wine, alcohol, platelets and the French paradox for coronary heart disease. *Lancet* 1992;339:1523–1526.

24. Siscovick DS, Raghunathan TE, King I, et al. Dietary intake and cell membrane levels of long-chain n-3 polyunsaturated fatty acids and the risk of primary cardiac arrest. *JAMA* 1995;274(17):1363–1367.

25. Stone NJ. The Gruppo Italiano per lo Studio della Sopravvivenza nell'Infarto Miocardio (GISSI) Prevenzione. Trial on fish oil and vitamin E supplementation in myocardial infarction survivors. *Curr Cardiol Rep.* 2000;2(5):445–451.

26. Visioli F, Galli C. Oleuropein protects low density lipoprotein from oxidation. *Life Sciences* 1994;55(24):1965–1971.

27. Visioli F, Galli C. The effect of minor constituents of olive oil on cardiovascular disease: New findings. *Nutr Rev.* 1998;56(5):142–147.

28. Weisburger JH. Evaluation of the evidence on the role of tomato products in disease prevention. *Proc Soc Exp Biol Med.* 1998;218(2):140–143.

29. Willett WC, Sacks F, Trichopoulo A, et al. Mediterranean diet pyramid: A cultural model for health eating. *Am J Clin Nutr.* 1995;61(suppl):1402S–1406S.

30. Wilson PW, Kannel WB. Clustering of risk factors, obesity, and Syndrome X. *Nutr Clin Care.* 1998;1:44–50.

31. Wolk A, Manson JE, Stampfer MJ, et al. Long-term intake of dietary fibre and decreased risk of coronary heart disease among women. *JAMA* 1999;28(21): 1998–2004.

CHAPTER 3

1. Allander PS, Culter JA, Follmann D, et al. Dietary calcium and blood pressure: a meta-analysis of randomized clinical trials. *Am J Intern Med* 1996;124:825.

2. Anderson JW, Johnstone BM, Cook-Newell M. Meta-analysis of the effects of soya protein intake on serum lipids. *N Engl J Med* 1995;333:276–282.

3. Anderson JW, Smith BM, Washnock CS. Cardiovascular and renal benefits of dry bean and soyabean intake. *Am J Clin Nutr* 1999;70:464S–474S.

4. Ascherio A, Rimm EB, Herman MA, et al. Intake of potassium, magnesium, calcium, and fibre and risk of stroke among US men. *Circulation* 1998;98(12): 1198–1204.

5. Benjafield AV, Morris BJ. Association analysis of endothelial nitric oxide synthase gene polymorphisms is essential in hypertension. *Am J Hypertens* 2000;13:994–998.

6. Boaz M, Smetana S, Weistein T, et al. Secondary prevention with antioxidants of cardiovascular disease in endstage renal disease (SPACE): randomized placebo-controlled trial. *Lancet* 2000;356(9237):1213–1218.

7. Burke BE, Neuenschwander R, Olson RD. Randomized, double-blind, placebo-controlled trial of coenzyme Q$_{10}$ in isolated systolic hypertension. *Southern Med J* 2001;94(11):1112–1117.

8.   Burke V, Hodgson JM, Beilin LJ, et al. Dietary protein and soluble fibre reduce ambulatory blood pressure in treated hypertensives. *Hypertension*. 2001;38(4): 821–826.

9.   Cheitlin MD, Hutter AM Jr, Brindis RG, et al, for the Technology and Practice Executive Committee. Use of sildenafil (Viagra) in patients with cardiovascular disease. *Circ* 1999;99:168–177.

10. Chopra RK, Goldman R, Sinatra ST, Bhagavan HN. Relative bioavailability of coenzyme Q_{10} formulations in human subjects. *Int J Vitamin Nutr Res* 1998;68: 109–113.

11. Cooke JP. Nutriceuticals for cardiovascular health. *Am J Cardiol* 1998;82(10A): 43S–46S.

12. Denke MA. Dietary retinol—a double-edged sword. *JAMA* 2002;287(1):102–104.

13. Digiesi V, Cantini F, Oradei A, et al. Coenzyme Q_{10} in essential hypertension. *Mol Aspects Med* 1994;15:S257–S263.

14. Duffy SJ, Gokce N, Holbrook M, et al. Treatment of hypertension with ascorbic acid. *Lancet* 1999;354:2048–2049.

15. Ewy GA. Antioxidant therapy for coronary artery disease. *Arch Inter Med* 1999;159: 1279–1280.

16. Feskanich D, Singh V, Willett WC, Colditz GA. Vitamin A intake and hip fractures among postmenopausal women. *JAMA* 2002;287(1):47–54.

17. Freedman JE, Cheney K, Eaney JR. Vitamin E inhibition of platelet aggregation is independent of antioxidant activity. *J Nutr* 2000;131:374S–377S.

18. Fukai T, Siegfried MR, Ushio-Fukai M, et al. Regulation of the vascular extracellular superoxide dismutase by nitric oxide and exercise training. *J Clin Invest* 2000;105: 1631–1639.

19. Greenberg ER, Baron JA, Karagas MR, et al. Mortality associated with low plasma concentration of beta carotene and the effect of oral supplementation. *JAMA* 1996;275:699–703.

20. Herbert V. Does mega-C do more good than harm, or more harm than good? *J Am Diet Assoc* 1992;92:1502–1509.

21. Huang PL, Huang ZH, Mashimo H, et al. Hypertension in mice lacking the gene for endothelial nitric oxide synthase. *Nature* 1995;377:239–242.

22. Jialal I, Traber M, Deveraj S. Is there a vitamin E paradox? *Curr Opinion Lipidol* 2001;12:49–53.

23. Kardinaal AF, Kok FJ, Ringstad J, et al. Antioxidants in adipose tissue and risk of myocardial infarction: the EURAMIC Study. *Lancet* 1993;342:1379–1384.

24. Kh R, Khullar M, Kashyap M, et al. Effect of oral magnesium supplementation on blood pressure, platelet aggregation and calcium handling in deoxycorticosterone acetate induced hypertension in rats. *J Hypertens* 2000;18:919–926.

25. Khaw KT, Bingham S, Welch A, et al. Relation between plasma ascorbic acid and mortality in men and women in EPIC-Norfolk Prospective Study: a prospective population study. *Lancet* 2001;357:657–663.

26. Khaw KT, Barrett-Connor E. Dietary potassium and stroke-associated mortality. A 12–year prospective population study. *N Engl J Med* 1987;316(5):235–240.

27. Koneth I, Suter PM, Vetter W. Potassium and arterial hypertension—are potassium supplements helpful? *Schweiz Rundsch Med Prax* 2000;89(38):1499–1505.

28. Langsjoen PH, Langsjoen AM. Overview of the use of CoQ_{10} in cardiovascular disease. *BioFactors* 1999;9:273–284.

29. Langsjoen H, Langsjoen P, Langsjoen P, et al. Usefulness of coenzyme Q$_{10}$ in clinical cardiology: a long-term study. *Mol Aspects Med* 1994;15:S165–S175.

30. Langsjoen P, Langsjoen P, Willis R, Folkers K. Treatment of essential hypertension with coenzyme Q$_{10}$. *Mol Aspects Med* 1994;15:S65–S72.

31. Laufs U, Lafata V, Plutzky J, Liao JK. Upregulation of endothelial nitric oxide synthase by HMG CoA reductase inhibitors. *Circulation* 1998;97:1129–1135.

32. Lin KF, Chao L, Chao J. Prolonged reduction of high blood pressure with human nitric oxide synthase gene delivery. *Hypertension* 1997;30:307–313.

33. McLean RM. Magnesium and its therapeutic uses: a review. *Am J Med* 1994;96:63–76.

34. Meagher EA, Barry OP, Lawson JA, et al. Effects of vitamin E on lipid peroxidation in healthy persons. *JAMA* 2001;285(9):1178–1182.

35. Mehta J, Yang B, Nichols W. Free radicals, antioxidants and coronary heart disease. *J Myocardial Ischemia* 1993;5:31–41.

36. Messina MJ. Legumes and soybeans: overview of their nutritional profiles and health effects. *Am J Clin Nutr* 1999;70:439S–450S.

37. Moncada S, Higgs A. The L-arginine–nitric oxide pathway. *N Engl J Med* 1993;329:2002–2012.

38. Ness AR, Chee D, Elliott P. Vitamin C and blood pressure—an overview. *J Hum Hypertens* 1997;11:343–350.

39. Noguchi T, Ikeda K, Sasaki Y, et al. Effects of vitamin E and sesamin on hypertension and cerebral thrombogenesis in stroke-prone spontaneously hypertensive rats. *Hypertens Res* 2001;24(6):735–742.

40. Nuttall SL, Kendall MJ, Martin U. Antioxidant therapy for the prevention of cardiovascular disease. *QJ Med* 1999;92:239–244.

41. Ohashi Y, Kawashima S, Hirata K, et al. Hypotension and reduced nitric oxide–elicited vasorelaxation in transgenic mice overexpressing endothelial nitric oxide synthase. *J Clin Invest* 1998;102:2061–2071.

42. Omenn GS, Goodman GE, Thornquist MD, et al. Effects of a combination of beta carotene and vitamin A on lung cancer and cardiovascular disease. *N Engl J Med* 1996;334(18):1150-1155.

43. Ortiz MC, Manriquez MC, Romero JC, Juncos LA. Antioxidants block angiotensin II-induced increases in blood pressure and endothelin. *Hypertension* 2001;38(3 pt 2):655–659.

44. Ozer NK, Azzi A. Effect of vitamin E on the development of atherosclerosis. *Toxicology* 2000;148(2–3):179–185.

45. Rapola JM, Virtamo J, Ripatti S, et al. Randomized trial of alpha-tocopherol and beta-carotene supplements on incidence of major coronary events in men with previous myocardial infarction. *Lancet* 1997;349:1715–1720.

46. Retter AS. Carnitine and its role in cardiovascular disease. *Heart Disease* 1999;1:108–113.

47. Sander M, Chavoshan B, Victor RG. A large blood-pressure-raising effect of nitric oxide synthase inhibition in humans. *Hypertension* 1999;33:937–942.

48. Shechter M. Oral magnesium in coronary artery disease: Fresh insight on thrombus inhibition. *The Magnesium Report* 1999:1–4.

49. Shechter M, Merz CN, Paul-Labrador M, et al. Oral magnesium supplementation inhibits platelet-dependent thrombosis in patients with coronary artery disease. *Am J Cardiol* 1999;84(2):152–156.

50. Siani A, Strazzullo P, Russo L, et al. Controlled trial of long-term oral potassium supplements in patients with mild hypertension. *Br Med J (Clin Res Ed)* 1987; 294(6604):961.

51. Sinatra ST. Coenzyme Q_{10} and the heart. *Keats Good Health Guide*. New Canaan, CT: Keats Publishing, 1998.

52. Sinatra ST, DeMarco J. Free radicals, oxidative stress, oxidized low density lipoprotein (LDL), and the heart: antioxidants and other strategies to limit cardiovascular damage. *Conn Med* 1995;59:579–588.

53. Singh RB, Niaz MA, Rastogi SS, et al. Effect of hydrosoluble coenzyme Q_{10} on blood pressures and insulin resistance in hypertensive patients with coronary artery disease. *J Hum Hypertens* 1999;13:203–208.

54. Singh RB, Wander GS, Rastogi A, et al. Randomized, double-blind, placebo-controlled trial of coenzyme Q_{10} in patients with acute myocardial infarction. *Cardiov Drugs Ther* 1998;12:347–353.

55. Stephens NG, Parsons A, Schofield PM, et al. Randomized controlled trial of vitamin E in patients with coronary disease: Cambridge Heart Antioxidant Study. *Lancet* 1996; 347:781–786.

56. Teede HJ, Dalais FS, Kotsopoulos D, et al. Dietary soya has both beneficial and potentially adverse cardiovascular effects: a placebo-controlled study in men and post-menopausal women. *J Clin Endocrinol Metab* 2001;86(7):3053–3060.

57. The Alpha-tocopherol, Beta-carotene Therapy Cancer Prevention Study Group: The effect of vitamin E and beta-carotene on the incidence of lung cancer and other cancers in male smokers. *N Engl J Med* 1994;330:1029–1035.

58. Thomas GD, Zhang W, Victor RG. Nitric oxide deficiency as a cause of clinical hypertension. *JAMA* 2001;285(16):2055–2057.

59. Ting HH, Creager MA, Ganz P, et al. Vitamin C improves endothelium-dependent vasodilation in forearm resistance vessels of humans with hypercholesterolemia. *Circ* 1997:2617–2622.

60. Watson PS, Scalia GM, Galbraith A, et al. Lack of effect of coenzyme Q_{10} on left ventricular function in patients with congestive heart failure. *J Am Coll Cardiol* 1999; 33:1549–1552.

61. Weiner CP, Lizasoain I, Baylis SA, et al. Induction of calcium-dependent nitric oxide synthases by sex hormones. *Proc Natl Acad Sci USA* 1994;91:5212–5216.

62. Whelton PK, He J. Potassium in preventing and treating high blood pressure. *Semin Nephrol* 1999;19:494–499.

63. Whelton PK, He J, Cutler JA, et al. Effects of oral potassium on blood pressure. Meta-analysis of randomized controlled clinical trials. *JAMA* 1997;277(20): 1624–1632.

64. White LR, et al. Brain aging and midlife tofu consumption. *J Amer Coll Nutr* 2000;19:242–255.

65. Williams AW, Boileau TW, Zhou JR, et al. Beta-carotene modulates human prostate cancer cell growth and may undergo intracellular metabolism to retinol. *J Nutr* 2000; 130:728–732.

66. Wolf G. Gamma-tocopherol: an efficient protector of lipids against nitric oxide—initiated peroxidative damage. *Nutr Rev* 1997;55(10):376–378.

67. Yamagami T, Shibata N, Folkers K. Bioenergetics in clinical medicine. VIII. Administration of coenzyme Q_{10} to patients with essential hypertension. *Res Commun Chem Pathol Pharmacol* 1976;14:721–727.

68. Yamagami T, Shibata N, Folkers K. Study of coenzyme Q₁₀ in essential hypertension. In: Folkers K, Yamamura Y. (eds.) *Biomedical and Clinical Aspects of Coenzyme Q₁₀*. Vol. 1. Amsterdam: Elsevier, 1977:231–242.

CHAPTER 4

1. Albert CM, Hennekens CH, O'Donnell CJ, et al. Fish consumption and risk of sudden cardiac death. *JAMA* 1998;279:23–28.
2. Anderson RA. Nutritional factors influencing the glucose/insulin system: chromium. *J Am Coll Nutr* 1997;16:404–410.
3. Bensiek D, Kyle D. Socioeconomic differences in the consumption of polyunsaturated fatty acids in the United States. *J Am Coll Nutr* 1999;18(5):543–544.
4. Burke V, Hodgson JM, Beilin LJ, et al. Dietary protein and soluble fibre reduce ambulatory blood pressure in treated hypertensives. *Hypertension* 2001;38(4):821–826.
5. Cunnane SC, et al. High a-linoleic flax seed (*Linum usitatissimum*): Some nutritional properties. *Br J Nutr* 1993;69:443–453.
6. Department of Health Dietary Reference Values for Food Energy and Nutrients for the United Kingdom. 1991. Report of the Panel on Dietary Reference. Values of the Committee on Medical Aspects of Food Policy.
7. Despres JP, Larmarche B, Mauriege P, et al. Hyperinsulinism as an independent risk factor for ischemic heart disease. *N Engl J Med* 1996;334:952–957.
8. GISSI-Prevenzione Investigators. Dietary supplementation with n-3 polyunsaturated fatty acids and vitamin E after myocardial infarction: results of the GISSI-Prevenzione trial. *Lancet* 1999;354:447–455.
9. Golomb LM, Solidum AA, Warren MP, et al. Primary dysmenorrhea and physical activity. *Med Sci Sports Exerc* 198;30(6):906–909.
10. Horrocks LA, Yeo YK. Health benefits of docosahexaenoic acid (DHA). *Pharmacol Res* 1999;40(3):211–225.
11. Horton ES. Exercise and decreased risk of NIDDM (editorial). *N Engl J Med* 1991;325: 196–197.
12. Hu FB, Stampfer MJ, Colditz GA, et al. Physical activity and risk of stroke in women. *JAMA* 2000;283(22):2961–2967.
13. Hutchins AM, Lampe J, et al. Vegetables, fruits, and legumes: effect on urinary phytoestrogen and lignan excretion. *J Am Diet Assoc* 1995;95:769–774.
14. Kasch FW, et al. Ageing of the cardiovascular system during 33 years of aerobic exercise. *Age Ageing* 1999;28:531–536.
15. Kushi LH, Fee RM, Folsom AR, et al. Physical activity and mortality in postmenopausal women. *JAMA* 1997;277(16):1287–1292.
16. Lee IM, Rexrode KM, Cook NR, et al. Physical activity and coronary heart disease in women: Is "no pain, no gain" passé? *JAMA* 2001;285(11):1447–1454.
17. Manson JE, Hu FB, Rich-Edwards JW, et al. A prospective study of walking as compared with vigorous exercise in the prevention of coronary heart disease in women. *N Engl J Med* 1999;341(9):650–658.
18. McCartney N, McKelvie R, Haslam D, Jones N. Usefulness of weight lifting training in improving strength and maximal power output in coronary artery disease. *Am J Cardiol* 1991;67:939–945.
19. Mitchell S. Omega-3 fatty acids may have beneficial effects on blood pressure, platelets. *Reuters Health* June 2000.

20. Mori TA, Bao DQ, Burke V, et al. Docosahexaenoic acid, but not eico-sapentaenoic acid, lowers ambulatory blood pressure and heart rate in humans. *Hypertension* 1999;34(2): 253–260.

21. Mori TA, Beilin LJ. Long-chain omega-3 fatty acids, blood lipids and cardiovascular risk reduction. *Curr Opin Lipidol* 2001;12:11–17.

22. Murray MT. *The Healing Power of Herbs*. Rocklin, CA: Prima Publishing, 1995.

23. O'Keefe J, Harris W. Omega-3 fatty acids: Time for clinical implementation? *Am J Cardiol* 2000;85.

24. Pramik MJ. Exercise may improve insulin sensitivity. *Med Tribune Diabetes* 1996:7.

25. Simon JA, Fong J, Bernert JT Jr., et al. Dietary alpha-linolenic acid lowers the risk of stroke. *Modern Medicine* 1995;63:45.

26. Simopoulos AP, Leaf A, Salem N Jr., et al. Workshop on the essentiality of and recommended dietary intakes for omega-6 and omega-3 fatty acids. *J Am Coll Nutr* 1999;18(5):487–489.

27. Sinatra ST, et al. Effects of continuous passive motion, walking and a placebo intervention on physical and psychological well-being. *J Cardiopulmonary Rehab* 1990;10:279–286.

28. Terry P, Lichtenstein P, Feychting M, et al. Fatty fish consumption and risk of prostate cancer. *Lancet* 2001;357:1764–1766.

29. Tham D, Gardner CD, Haskel WL. Potential health benefits of dietary phytoestrogens: A review of the clinical, epidemiological, and mechanistic evidence. *J Endocrinol Metab* 1997;83(7):2223–2235.

30. Westerterp KR. Pattern and intensity of physical activity. *Nature* 2001; 410(6828):539.

31. Whelton SP, Ashley C, Xin X, Jiang H. Effect of aerobic exercise on blood pressure: A meta-analysis of randomized, controlled trials. *Ann Inter Med* 2002;136(7): 493–503.

32. Yosefy C, et al. The effect of fish oil on hypertension, plasma lipids and hemostasis in hypertensive, obese, dyslipidemic patients with and without diabetes mellitus. *Prostaglandins Leukot Essent Fatty Acids* 1999;61(2):83–87.

CHAPTER 5

1. Achterberg J, Dossey L, et al. *Rituals of Healing: Using Imagery for Health and Wellness*. New York: Bantam, 1994.

2. Benson H, Alexander S, Feldman CL. Decreased premature ventricular contractions through use of the relaxation response in patients with stable ischemic heart disease. *Lancet* 1975;2:380–382.

3. Chan L. *101 Miracles of Natural Healing*. West Chester, Ohio: Benefactor Press, 1999.

4. Jahnke R. *The Healer Within: Using Traditional Chinese Techniques to Release Your Body's Own Medicine*. San Francisco: Harper, 1999.

5. Kuang A, Wang C, Xu D, Qian Y. Research on the anti-aging effect of qigong. *J Tradit Chin Med* 1991;11(2):153–158.

6. Kelly BS, Alexander JW, Dreyer D, et al. Oral arginine improves blood pressure in renal transplant and hemodialysis patients. *J Parenter Enteral Nutr* 2001;25(4): 194–202.

7. Mayer M. Qigong and hypertension: a critique of research. *J Altern Complement Med* 1999;5(4):371–382.

8. Sancier KM. Medical applications of qigong. *Alt Ther* 1996;2(1):40–46.
9. Siani A, Pagano E, Iacone R, et al. Blood pressure and metabolic changes during dietary L-arginine supplementation in humans. *Am J Hypertens* 2000;13(5 pt 1): 547–551.
10. Sinatra ST, Chawla S. Aortic dissection associated with anger, suppressed rage, and acute emotional stress. *J Cardiopulmonary Rehabil* 1986;6:197–199.
11. Wang C, Xu D, Qian Y, Shi W. Effects of qigong on preventing stroke and alleviating the multiple cerebrocardiovascular risk factors: a follow-up report on hypertensive cases over 30 years. *Proceedings* from the Second World Conference for Academic Exchange of Medical Qigong: Beijing, China; 1993:125.

CHAPTER 6

1. Eliot, RS, Breo DL. *Is It Worth Dying For?* New York: Bantam, 1986.
2. Fitzpatrick DF, Fleming RC, Bing B, et al. Isolation and characterization of endothelium-dependent vasorelaxing compounds from grape seeds. *J Agric Food Chem* 2000;48(12): 6384–6390.
3. Lerman-Garber I, Ichazo-Cerro S, Zamora-Gonzalez J, et al. Effect of a high-monounsaturated fat diet enriched with avocado in NIDDM patients. *Diabetes Care* 1994; 17(4):311–315.
4. Maffetone P. *In Fitness and in Health.* Stamford, NY: David Barmore Productions, 1997.
5. Meunier MT, et al. Inhibition of angiotensin-I converting enzyme by flavonolic compounds: in vitro and in vivo studies. *Planta Medica* 1987;54:112–115.
6. Preuss HG, Wallerstedt D, Talpur N, et al. Effects of niacin-bound chromium and grape seed proanthocyanidin extract on the lipid profile of hypercholesterolemic subjects: a pilot study. *J Med* 2000;31(5–6):227–246.
7. Sinatra ST. *Heartbreak and Heart Disease.* New Canaan, CT: Keats Publishing, 1996.
8. Smith EA. Purple power: drug topics. *Gale Encylopedia of Alternative Medicine,* June 1, 1998, www.gale.com.
9. Spencer JW, Jacobs JJ. *Complementary Alternative Medicine.* St. Louis, MO: Mosby, 1999.

CHAPTER 7

1. Ackermann RT, Mulrow CD, Ramirez G, et al. Garlic shows promise for improving some cardiovascular risk factors. *Arch Intern Med* 2001;161:813–824.
2. Bazzano LA, He J, Ogden LG, et al. Legume consumption and risk of coronary heart disease in US men and women. *Arch Intern Med* 2001;161:2573–2578.
3. Bernardi L, Sleight P, Bandinelli G, et al. Effect of rosary prayer and yoga mantras on autonomic cardiovascular rhythms: comparative study. *BMJ* 2001;323(7327): 1446–1449.
4. Fraser GE, et al. A possible protective effect of nut consumption on risk of coronary heart disease. *Arch Intern Med* 1992;152:1416–1424.
5. Kidd PM. Use of mushrooms, glucans and proteoglycans in cancer treatment. *Alt Med Rev* 2000;5(1):4–27.
6. Konno S. Maitake D-fraction: apoptosis inducer and immune enhancer. *Alternative and Complementary Ther* 2001:102–107.

7.   McMahon FG, Vargas R. Can garlic lower blood pressure? A pilot study. *Pharma-cotherapy* 1993;13:406–407.
8.   Mohamadi A, Jarrell ST, Shi SJ, et al. Effects of wild versus cultivated garlic on blood pressure and other parameters in hypertensive rats. *Heart Disease* 2000;2:3–9.
9.   Murugesan R, Govindarajulu N, Bera TK. Effect of selected yogic practices on the management of hypertension. *Indian J Physiol Pharmacol* 2000;44(2):207–210.
10.   Nanba H. Maitake D-fraction: Healing and preventive potential for cancer. *J Ortho-molecular Med* 1997;12:43–49.
11.   Rose KD, Croissant PD, Parliament CF, et al. Spontaneous spinal epidural hematoma with associated platelet dysfunction from excessive garlic ingestion: A case report. *Neurosurgery* 1990;26:880–882.
12.   Sabate J, Fraser GI. The probable role of nuts in preventing coronary heart disease. *Primary Cardiology* 1993;19(11):65–76.
13.   Silagy C, Neil A. Garlic as a lipid lowering agent—a meta-analysis. *J R Coll Physi-cians Lond* 1994;28:39–45.
14.   Silagy CA, Neil HA. A meta-analysis of the effect of garlic on blood pressure. *J Hypertens* 1994;12:463–468.
15.   Sinatra ST. Alternative medicine for the conventional cardiologist. *Heart Disease* 2000;2:16–30.
16.   Sinatra ST. *Optimum Health*. New York: Bantam Books, 1997.
17.   Spencer JW, Jacobs JJ. *Complementary Alternative Medicine*. St. Louis, MO Mosby, Inc., 1999.

CHAPTER 8

1.   Bahorun T, Trotin F, Pommery J, et al. Antioxidant activities of *Crataegus monogyna* extracts. *Planta Med* 1994;60:323–328.
2.   Busse W. Standardized crataegus extract clinical monograph. *Quar Rev Natl Med* 1996;189–197.
3.   Dulloo AG, Duret C, Rohrer D, et al. Efficacy of a green tea extract rich in catechin polyphenols and caffeine in increasing 24-h energy expenditure and fat oxidation in humans. *Am J Clin Nutr* 1999;70(6):1040–1045.
4.   Dulloo AG, Seydoux J, Girardier L, et al. Green tea and thermogenesis: interactions between catechin-polyphenols, caffeine and sympathetic activity. *Int J Obes Relat Metab Disord* 2000;24(2):252–258.
5.   Ishikawa T, Suzukawa M, Ito T, et al. Effect of tea flavonoid supplementation on the susceptibility of low-density lipoprotein to oxidative modification. *Am J Clin Nutr* 1997; 66(2):261–266.
6.   Kim SH, Kang KW, Kim KW, Kim ND. Procyanidins in crataegus extract evoke endothelium-dependent vasorelaxation in rat aorta. *Life Sci.* 2000;67:121–131.
7.   Landers KA, Hunter GR, Wetzstein CJ, et al. The interrelationship among muscle mass, strength, and the ability to perform physical tasks of daily living in younger and older women. *J Gerontol A Biol Sci Med Sci* 2001;56(10):443–448.
8.   Lane JD, et al. Caffeine raises blood pressure at work. *Psychosom Med* 1998;60: 327–330.
9.   Minami J, Yoshii M, Todoroki M, et al. Effects of alcohol restriction on ambulatory blood pressure, heart rate, and heart rate variability in Japanese men. *Am J Hyper-tens* 2002;15(2 pt 1):125–129.

10. Maruta TC, Colligan RC, Malinschoc M, Offord KP. Optimists vs. pessimists: Survival rate among medical patients over a 30-year period. *Mayo Clinic Proceedings* 2000;75:140–143.
11. Schussler M, Holzl J, Fricke U. Myocardial effects of flavonoids from *Crataegus* species. *Arzneim Forsch* 1995;45(8):842–845.
12. Sinatra ST. *Heartbreak and Heart Disease*. New Canaan, CT: Keats Publishing, 1998.
13. Valcic S, Timmermann BN, Alberts DS, et al. Inhibitory effect of six green tea catechins and caffeine on the growth of four selected human tumor cell lines. *Anticancer Drugs* 1996;7(4):461–468.
14. Yucha CB, Clark L, Smith M, et al. The effect of biofeedback in hypertension. *Appl Nurs Res* 2001;14(1):29–35.

CHAPTER 9

1. Allen K, Golden LH, Izzo JL Jr, et al. Normalization of hypertensive responses during ambulatory surgical stress by perioperative music. *Psychosom Med* 2001;63(3):487–492.
2. Ebeling P, Koivisto VA. Physiological importance of dehydroepiandrosterone. *Lancet* 1994;343:1479–1482.
3. Eisenberg DM, Davis RB, Ettner SL, et al. Trends in alternative medicine use in the United States, 1990–1997: the results of a follow-up national survey. *JAMA* 1998; 280:1569–1575.
4. Feldman HA, Johannes CB, Araujo AB, et al. Low dehydroepiandrosterone and ischemic heart disease in middle-aged men: prospective results from the Massachusetts Male Aging Study. *Am J Epidemiol* 2001;153(1):79–89.
5. Knight WE, Rickard NS. Relaxing music prevents stress-induced increases in subjective anxiety, systolic blood pressure, and heart rate in healthy males and females. *Music Ther* 2001; 38(4):254–272.
6. Mitchell LE, et al. Evidence for an association between dehydroepiandrosterone sulfate and nonfatal, premature myocardial infarction in male. *Circulation* 1994;89(1):89–93.
7. Morales AJ, Nolan JJ, Nelson JC, Yen SSC. Effects of replacement dose of dehydroepiandrosterone in men and women of advancing age. *J Clin Endocrinol Metab* 1994;78(6):1360–1367.
8. Newcomer LM, Manson JE, Barbieri RL, et al. Dehydroepiandrosterone sulfate and the risk of myocardial infarction in US male physicians: a prospective study. *Amer J Epidem* 1994;140(10):870–875.
9. Peabody F. The care of the patient. *JAMA* 1927;88:877–882.
10. Reiter WJ, Schatzl G, Mark I, et al. Dehydroepiandrosterone in the treatment of erectile dysfunction in patients with different organic etiologies. *Urol Res* 2001;29(4):278–281.
11. Sinatra ST. Alternative medicine for the conventional cardiologist. *Heart Disease* 2000; 2:16–30.

Glossary

Alpha Lipoic Acid (ALA): ALA is a fat- and water-soluble molecule that functions as an antioxidant, while also helping to recycle vitamins C and E (as well as glutathione), which enhances all of their antioxidant properties. ALA has also been shown to help prevent cataracts, improve the immune system, and enhance the liver's ability to detoxify metals. It has also shown promising results in treating diabetic nerve damage and improving blood flow to the peripheral nerves.

Antioxidants: Substances that prevent or reverse the damage of free-radical stress. For example, antioxidants such as beta-carotene and vitamins C and E can neutralize oxygen and free radicals to help prevent fats from becoming oxidized or rancid. Antioxidants can help prevent many of the degenerative diseases of the twentieth century.

Arachidonic Acid: An unsaturated, 20-carbon long, omega-6 fatty acid, which is a principle precursor to "unfavorable" eicosanoids. It is synthesized via the omega-6 pathway. Arachidonic acid is a highly inflammatory compound produced by cells in the presence of free radicals that sets the stage for inflammatory events.

Arteriosclerosis: Damage in blood vessels characterized by thickening and loss of the elasticity of arterial walls. Much of this damage is thought to be due to free-radical stress and inflammation.

Atherosclerosis: A common form of arteriosclerosis in which deposits of yellowish plaque (atheromas) containing cholesterol, clotted blood, and other lipids form within the walls of arteries causing compromised circulation.

Beta-Carotene: A form of provitamin A (vitamin A precursor) found mainly in yellow and/or orange fruits and vegetables. When vitamin A levels are insufficient, ingested beta-carotene will be converted to vitamin A as needed by the body.

Calcium: The most abundant mineral in the body. Its major function is building and maintaining bones and teeth, but it is also an important part of most of the body's enzyme activity. The contraction of muscles, release of neurotransmitters, regulation of heartbeat, and the clotting ability of the blood all depend on calcium.

Carcinogens: Cancer-producing substances such as chemicals, heavy metals, free radicals, radiation, viruses, and insecticides and pesticides.

Coenzyme Q10: CoQ10 is a powerful antioxidant that enhances energy at the cellular level. It supports cardiac function by stabilizing cardiac cellular membranes, and enhances stamina and energy by providing ATP support. When taken in higher dosages, it can help the heart to pump blood more efficiently, promote healthy blood pressure levels, and help maintain healthy Lp(a) and cholesterol levels. It's vitally important to take coenzyme Q10 when taking statin drugs as statins reduce the synthesis of CoQ10 in the body. It is also essential for antioxidant defense.

C-reactive Protein (CRP): A phase-reacting protein substance that reflects the presence of a previous infectious agent in the blood stream. High C-reactive protein levels are a major prognostic indicator of coronary heart disease, as it tends to be the main inflammatory risk factor for the heart.

Docosahexaenoic Acid (DHA): An unsaturated, 22-carbon long, omega-3 fatty acid found mainly in fish, algae, and marine plants. One of the best ways of obtaining DHA is in purified fish oil preparations. DHA is vitally important for brain and eye development, prevention of cancer, and especially in the prevention of sudden death and cardiovascular disease.

Eicosanoids: Hormone-like substances resulting from an overabundance of omega-3 fatty acids and arachidonic acid. Eicosanoids are classified into prostaglandins and leukotrienes. Eicosanoids can be either "bad" or "good," and they can help influence blood pressure, blood clotting, and allergic responses, as well as the body's response to infection.

Eicosapentaenoic Acid (EPA): An unsaturated, 20-carbon long, omega-3 fatty acid found in fish, algae, and marine plants. EPA is particularly useful for arthritis by helping to produce "good" eicosanoids acting as anti-inflammatories.

Essential Fatty Acids: These are fatty acids that the body cannot synthesize but are required for normal metabolism and hemostasis. Essential fatty acids include linoleic and linolenic acids. Linolenic acid is broken down in the body into small amounts of other essential fatty acids, i.e., DHA/EPA. Deficiency of essential fatty acids can cause skin and hair problems. Plaque rupture and coronary thrombosis or heart attack have also been associated with essential fatty acid deficiency.

Fibrinogen: An inflammatory clot-promoting substance in the blood. Higher fibrinogen levels are associated with coronary heart disease.

Flavonoids: Phytochemicals (plant-based chemicals) found in nature with strong antioxidant properties. There are over 4,000 flavonoids in nature possessing potent anti-inflammatory capabilities.

Flaxseed Oil: Flaxseed oil is the primary source of alpha-linolenic acid (an omega-3 essential fatty acid), which helps to regulate many metabolic functions in the body, especially inflammatory responses.

Free Radicals: Unstable molecules that are highly activated and highly charged, which interact with body tissues causing inflammation and ageing. Free radicals are also produced by the body in response to inflammation as well as in the mitochondrial respiratory chain.

Garlic: Garlic has antibiotic, antifungal, antiparasitic, antitoxin, antiviral, expectorant, and blood thinner properties. It also lowers blood pressure.

Homocysteine: A dangerous amino acid that promotes free-radical oxidation and premature vascular disease. Higher homocysteine levels are associated with cardiovascular disease and Alzheimer's.

Hypertension: High blood pressure.

Inflammation: A localized protective response attempting to destroy or neutralize an injurious agent. Chronic inflammation can also cause injury to the surrounding tissue. Coronary heart disease is now thought to be a response to inflammation.

Leukotrienes: Compounds produced by the arachidonic acid pathway that produce inflammatory changes throughout the body.

Lipoprotein A, Lp(a): A small cholesterol particle that causes inflammation and clogging of blood vessels.

Lycopene: An antioxidant compound found in tomatoes, which helps to prevent prostate cancer and coronary artery disease.

Magnesium: This mineral is needed for bone growth and maintenance, as well as carbohydrate and protein utilization. It aids the function of the nerves and muscles, including regulation of heart rhythm, blood pressure, and body temperature.

N-Acetyl-Cysteine: This nutrient helps repair oxidative damage in cells, and also helps prevent dysfunction of endothelial cells. It has also been shown to support red blood cell function, eliminate heavy metals, and increase levels of the antioxidant enzyme glutathione peroxidase.

Omega-3 Essential Fatty Acid: Refers to the third carbon in the fatty molecule, which is unsaturated in the carbon terminal end. These anti-inflammatory essential fatty acids found in fish, nuts, and soya were shown to reduce the risk of heart disease and cancer, as well as to reduce high blood pressure and sudden cardiac death.

Omega-6: Refers to the sixth carbon in the fatty acid molecule, which is unsaturated. Omega-6 compounds are found mainly in vegetable oils. There is a high concentration of omega-6 essential fatty acids in processed foods, as well as margarines and multiple oils, resulting in an overabundance.

Oxidative Stress: A highly deleterious environment within cells where there is an excess of free radicals and a lack of antioxidants, resulting in injury to the tissue. When there is a paucity of antioxidants to neutralize free radicals, oxidative stress and accelerated ageing of tissues occur.

Oxidized LDL: An ominous form of cholesterol that enhances inflammation resulting in plaque formation.

Polyphenols: Antioxidant bioflavonoids found in tea, onions, and red wine.

Polyunsaturated: Fatty acids with more than one unsaturated carbon. Polyunsaturated oils freeze at lower temperatures than monounsaturated and saturated oils.

Proanthocyanidins: Potent antioxidants found in grape seeds, blueberries, pine bark, and hawthorn. They have high bioavailability and are able to cross the blood-brain barrier.

Quercetin: A potent polyphenol found in onions, apples, tea, and red wine. Quercetin is often referred to as the nutriceutical responsible for the "French paradox", which suggests a lower incidence of coronary heart disease due to the polyphenol/red wine effect.

Serum Ferritin: Can also reflect inflammation, but most often reflects high levels of iron in the body. When serum ferritin levels are high, an evaluation of an iron overload state needs to be done.

Thromboxane: A type of eicosanoid that causes stickiness of platelets and clotting of blood.

Triglycerides: The common fat that is in our abdominal area, often referred to as the "love handles". Triglycerides are made up of three molecules of fatty acids and one molecule of glycerol. High triglycerides are part of the insulin resistance syndrome and are an important cardiovascular risk factor.

Vitamin A: A fat-soluble vitamin that helps form and maintain healthy skin, hair, and mucous membranes. It promotes bone growth, tooth development, and reproductive function, and enhances the body's immune system. Also, it aids in treatment of eye disorders such as night blindness.

Vitamin B6: This vitamin acts as a coenzyme in many reactions involved in the metabolism of amino acids and essential fatty acids. Therefore it is needed for proper growth and maintenance of almost all of our body functions. It also helps maintain chemical balance among body fluids. Additionally, it has been shown to help normalize function of the brain, promote normal red blood cell formation, and regulate the excretion of water.

Vitamin B12: This vitamin acts as a coenzyme for fat and carbohydrate metabolism, and therefore promotes normal growth and development. It is also involved in the production of myelin, which is the sheath of "insulation" that covers nerves. This vitamin is present only in animal products, so those following a vegan diet need to supplement it.

Vitamin C: A water-soluble vitamin that promotes healthy capillaries, gums, and teeth, and helps heal wounds and broken bones. It promotes iron absorption (thereby enhancing red blood cell formation), and helps form collagen in connective tissues.

Vitamin D: A fat-soluble vitamin that regulates growth, as well as hardening and repair of bone by controlling absorption of calcium and phosphorus. In a healthy person, vitamin D is synthesized in the skin when the skin is exposed to sunlight.

Vitamin E: A fat-soluble vitamin that functions mainly as an antioxidant in protecting cell membranes from free-radical damage. It promotes normal growth and development, as well as red blood cell formation, and also acts as an anti-blood clotting agent.

Zinc: This mineral functions as an essential component of hormones, insulin, and enzymes. It helps maintain normal growth and development by promoting cell division, cell repair, and cell growth. Also, it aids in wound healing and the maintenance of normal taste and smell.

Resources

The British Longevity Society
PO Box 71
Hemel Hempstead HP3 9DN

National Heart Forum
Tavistock House South
Tavistock Square
London WC1H 9LG
Tel: 020 7383 7638
E-mail: www.heartforum.org.uk

British Naturopathic Association
Goswell House
2 Goswell Road
Street
Somerset BA16 0JG
Tel: 08707 456 984
Fax: 08707 456 985
E-mail: admin@naturopaths.org.uk
www.naturopaths.org.uk

British Cardiac Society
9 Fitzroy Square
London W1T 5HW
Tel: 020 7383 3887
Fax: 020 7388 0903
E-mail: enquiries@bcs.com
www.bcs.com

British Heart Foundation
14 Fitzhardinge Street
London W1H 4DH
Tel: 020 7935 0185
www.bhf.org.uk

NUTRITIONAL SUPPLEMENTS

UK

Higher Nature
Burwash Common
East Sussex TN19 7LX
Tel: 01435 882880
www.highernature.co.uk

Solgar Vitamins Ltd
Aldbury
Tring
Hertfordshire HP23 5PT
Tel: 01442 890355
www.solgar.com

US

Optimum Health International, L.L.C.
257 East Center Street
Manchester, CT 06040
Tel: 001 800-228-1507
Tel: 001 860-647-9729
Fax: 001 860-643-2531
www.optimumhealthintl.com
Complete line of pharmaceutical-grade nutriceutical supplements, including hydrosoluble coenzyme Q_{10}.

Clinical Creations, L.L.C.
377 Research Parkway
Meriden, CT 06450
Tel: 001 888-823-7837
www.clinicalcreations.com
Topical coenzyme Q_{10} cream and nutritional supplements

Vita-Net
6540 Riverside Drive
Dublin, OH 43017
Tel: 001 800-807-8080
http://store.yahoo.com/vitanet/index.html
Maitake Products.

NEWSLETTERS

Sinatra Health Report
Phillips Publishing, L.L.C.
7811 Montrose Road
Potomac, MD 20859-1350
Tel: 001 800-861-5970
Tel: 001 800-211-7643
www.drsinatra.com

Health Wisdom for Women by Christiane Northrup, M.D.
Phillips Publishing, L.L.C.
7811 Montrose Road
Potomac, MD 20859
Tel: 001 800-804-0935
www.drnorthrup.com

Index

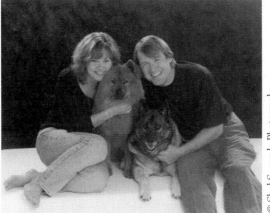

About the Authors

STEPHEN T. SINATRA is a board-certified cardiologist and certified psycho-therapist with more than twenty-five years' clinical experience. At his New England Heart and Longevity Center he integrates conventional and complementary therapies for treating heart disease. He is a fellow of the American College of Cardiology and former chief of cardiology at Manchester Memorial Hospital where he is currently director of education. He is also assistant clinical professor of medicine at the University of Connecticut School of Medicine and the author of eight previous books.

JAN SINATRA is an advanced practice nurse in psychiatric nursing, with a master's degree in psychiatric liaison nursing, a specialty that explores the link between medical illness and psychological factors. She practised for fifteen years as a registered nurse in a coronary care unit, a cardiac rehabilitation CCU, an exercise testing laboratory, and a pain clinic. She has been coordinator of a hospital-based weight management programme and has edited and coauthored various peer review publications and books.

Also By Stephen T. Sinatra

OPTIMUM HEALTH: A NATURAL LIFESAVING PRESCRIPTION FOR YOUR BODY AND MIND

THE COENZYME Q10 PHENOMENON

COENZYME Q10 AND THE HEART

HEART SENSE FOR WOMEN: YOUR PLAN FOR NATURAL PREVENTION AND TREATMENT

L-CARNITINE AND THE HEART

LOSE TO WIN: A CARDIOLOGIST'S GUIDE TO WEIGHT LOSS AND NUTRITIONAL HEALING

HEARTBREAK AND HEART DISEASE: A MIND/BODY PRESCRIPTION FOR HEALING THE HEART

Visit the Piatkus website!

Piatkus publishes a wide range of best-selling fiction and non-fiction, including books on health, mind, body & spirit, sex, self-help, cookery, biography and the paranormal.

If you want to:
- read descriptions of our popular titles
- buy our books over the Internet
- take advantage of our special offers
- enter our monthly competition
- learn more about your favourite Piatkus authors

VISIT OUR WEBSITE AT: www.piatkus.co.uk